Bronchopulmonary Dysplasia: An Update

Editors

SUHAS G. KALLAPUR
GLORIA S. PRYHUBER

CLINICS IN PERINATOLOGY

www.perinatology.theclinics.com

Consulting Editor
LUCKY JAIN

December 2015 • Volume 42 • Number 4

ELSEVIER

1600 John F. Kennedy Boulevard • Suite 1800 • Philadelphia, Pennsylvania, 19103-2899

http://www.theclinics.com

CLINICS IN PERINATOLOGY Volume 42, Number 4
December 2015 ISSN 0095-5108, ISBN-13: 978-0-323-39577-9

Editor: Kerry Holland
Developmental Editor: Casey Jackson

Clinics in Perinatology (ISSN 0095-5108) is published quarterly by Elsevier Inc., 360 Park Avenue South, New York, NY 10010-1710. Months of issue are March, June, September, and December. Business and Editorial Offices: 1600 John F. Kennedy Blvd., Ste. 1800, Philadelphia, PA 19103-2899. Customer Service Office: 3251 Riverport Lane, Maryland Heights, MO 63043. Periodicals postage paid at New York, NY and additional mailing offices. Subscription prices are $285.00 per year (US individuals), $445.00 per year (US institutions), $340.00 per year (Canadian individuals), $545.00 per year (Canadian institutions), $420.00 per year (international individuals), $545.00 per year (international institutions), $135.00 per year (US students), and $195.00 per year (Canadian and international students). International air speed delivery is included in all Clinics subscription prices. All prices are subject to change without notice. **POSTMASTER:** Send address changes to *Clinics in Perinatology*, Elsevier Health Sciences Division, Subscription Customer Service, 3251 Riverport Lane, Maryland Heights, MO 63043. **Customer Service: Telephone: 1-800-654-2452** (U.S. and Canada); **1-314-447-8871** (outside U.S. and Canada). **Fax: 1-314-447-8029. E-mail: journalscustomerservice-usa@elsevier.com** (for print support); **journalsonlinesupport-usa@elsevier.com** (for online support).

Reprints. For copies of 100 or more, of articles in this publication, please contact the Commercial Reprints Department, Elsevier Inc., 360 Park Avenue South, New York, NY 10010-1710. Tel. 212-633-3874; Fax: 212-633-3820; E-mail: reprints@elsevier.com.

Clinics in Perinatology is also pubilshed in Spanish by McGraw-Hill Interamericana Editores S.A., P.O. Box 5-237, 06500 Mexico D.F., Mexico.

Clinics in Perinatology is covered in *MEDLINE/PubMed (Index Medicus) Current Contents, Excepta Medica, BIOSIS and ISI/BIOMED.*

Printed in the United States of America.

Contributors

CONSULTING EDITOR

LUCKY JAIN, MD, MBA
Richard W. Blumberg Professor and Interim Chairman, Emory University School of Medicine, Department of Pediatrics, Executive Medical Director & Interim Chief Academic Officer, Children's Healthcare of Atlanta, Atlanta, Georgia

EDITORS

SUHAS G. KALLAPUR, MD
Professor of Pediatrics, Division of Neonatology and Pulmonary Biology, Cincinnati Children's Hospital Medical Center, University of Cincinnati, Cincinnati, Ohio

GLORIA S. PRYHUBER, MD
Professor of Pediatrics and Environmental Medicine, Division of Neonatology, University of Rochester Medical Center, Rochester, New York

AUTHORS

STEVEN H. ABMAN, MD
Professor of Pediatrics, Section of Pulmonary Medicine, Pediatric Heart Lung Center, Department of Pediatrics, University of Colorado, School of Medicine, Aurora, Colorado

NAMASIVAYAM AMBALAVANAN, MD
Professor, Division of Neonatology, Department of Pediatrics, Women and Infants Center, University of Alabama at Birmingham, Birmingham, Alabama

RAOUF S. AMIN, MD
Director, Division of Pulmonary Medicine, Cincinnati Children's Hospital Medical Center; Professor of Pediatrics, University of Cincinnati College of Medicine, Cincinnati, Ohio

JUDY L. ASCHNER, MD
Departments of Pediatrics and Obstetrics and Gynecology and Women's Health, Children's Hospital at Montefiore, Albert Einstein College of Medicine of Yeshiva University, Bronx, New York

ELENA CIARMOLI, MD
Neonatal Intensive Care Unit, MBBM Foundation, San Gerardo Hospital, Monza, Italy

BRIAN A. DARLOW, MD, FRCP, FRACP, FRCPCH
Professor, Cure Kids Professor of Paediatric Research, Department of Paediatrics, University of Otago at Christchurch, Christchurch, New Zealand

JULIANN M. DI FIORE, BSEE
Biomedical Engineer, Case Western Reserve University; Division of Neonatology, Department of Pediatrics, Rainbow Babies & Children's Hospital, Cleveland, Ohio

ELIZABETH E. FOGLIA, MD
Division of Neonatology, Department of Pediatrics, The Children's Hospital of Philadelphia, The University of Pennsylvania, Philadelphia, Pennsylvania

ERIK A. JENSEN, MD
Division of Neonatology, Department of Pediatrics, The Children's Hospital of Philadelphia, The University of Pennsylvania, Philadelphia, Pennsylvania

SUHAS G. KALLAPUR, MD
Professor of Pediatrics, Division of Neonatology and Pulmonary Biology, Cincinnati Children's Hospital Medical Center, University of Cincinnati, Cincinnati, Ohio

MARTIN KESZLER, MD, FAAP
Department of Pediatrics, Women and Infants Hospital of Rhode Island, Alpert Medical School of Brown University, Providence, Rhode Island

CHARITHARTH VIVEK LAL, MD
Assistant Professor, Division of Neonatology, Department of Pediatrics, Women and Infants Center, University of Alabama at Birmingham, Birmingham, Alabama

THOMAS J. MARIANI, PhD
Associate Professor of Pediatrics, Division of Neonatology and Pediatric Molecular and Personalized Medicine Program, University of Rochester Medical Center, Rochester, New York

CAMILIA R. MARTIN, MD, MS
Assistant Professor of Pediatrics, Beth Israel Deaconess Medical Center, Harvard Medical School, Boston, Massachusetts

RICHARD J. MARTIN, MD
Professor, Pediatrics, Reproductive Biology & Physiology & Biophysics, Case Western Reserve University School of Medicine; Drusinsky/Fanaroff Professor, Division of Neonatology, Department of Pediatrics, Rainbow Babies & Children's Hospital, Cleveland, Ohio

CINDY T. McEVOY, MD, MCR
Department of Pediatrics, Oregon Health and Science University, Portland, Oregon

COLIN J. MORLEY, MD, FRCPCH
Honorary Lecturer, Department of Obstetrics and Gynaecology, University of Cambridge, Cambridge, United Kingdom

PETER M. MOURANI, MD
Associate Professor of Pediatrics, Section of Pediatric Critical Care, Pediatric Heart Lung Center, Department of Pediatrics, University of Colorado, School of Medicine, Aurora, Colorado

MARIA PIERRO, MD
Department of Clinical Sciences and Community Health, Fondazione IRCCS Cà Granda Ospedale Maggiore Policlinico, University of Milan, Milan, Italy; Neonatal Intensive Care Unit, IRCCS Istituto Giannina Gaslini, Genova, Italy

BRENDA B. POINDEXTER, MD, MS
Professor of Pediatrics, Director of Clinical and Translational Research, Perinatal Institute, Cincinnati Children's Hospital Medical Center, Cincinnati, Ohio

GLORIA S. PRYHUBER, MD
Professor of Pediatrics and Environmental Medicine, Division of Neonatology, University of Rochester Medical Center, Rochester, New York

MICHAEL J. RUTTER, MBChB, FRACS
Division of Pediatric Otolaryngology–Head and Neck Surgery, Cincinnati Children's Hospital Medical Center; Professor of Otolaryngology-Head and Neck Surgery, University of Cincinnati College of Medicine, Cincinnati, Ohio

GUILHERME SANT'ANNA, MD, PhD, FRCPC
Department of Pediatrics, Neonatal Division, Montreal Children's Hospital, McGill University, Montreal, Quebec, Canada

BARBARA SCHMIDT, MD, MSc
Division of Neonatology, Department of Pediatrics, The Children's Hospital of Philadelphia, The University of Pennsylvania, Philadelphia, Pennsylvania

BERNARD THÉBAUD, MD, PhD
Division of Neonatology, Department of Pediatrics, Children's Hospital of Eastern Ontario; Regenerative Medicine Program, Sprott Center for Stem Cell Research, Ottawa Hospital Research Institute, The Ottawa Hospital; Department of Cellular and Molecular Medicine, University of Ottawa, Ottawa, Ontario, Canada

ROSE MARIE VISCARDI, MD
Professor of Pediatrics, University of Maryland School of Medicine, Baltimore, Maryland

LAURA L. WALKUP, PhD
Division of Pulmonary Medicine, Department of Radiology, Center for Pulmonary Imaging Research, Cincinnati Children's Hospital Medical Center, Cincinnati, Ohio

MICHELE C. WALSH, MD, MSEpi
Professor, Pediatrics, Case Western Reserve University School of Medicine; Chief, Division of Neonatology; William and Lois Briggs Professor; Interim Chair, Department of Pediatrics, Rainbow Babies and Children's Hospital, Cleveland, Ohio

JASON C. WOODS, PhD
Division of Pulmonary Medicine, Department of Radiology, Center for Pulmonary Imaging Research, Cincinnati Children's Hospital Medical Center, Cincinnati, Ohio

Contents

Update on Molecular Biology of Lung Development—Transcriptomics   685

Thomas J. Mariani

This article highlights some of the significant advances in our understanding of lung developmental biology made over the last few years, which challenge existing paradigms and are relevant to a fundamental understanding of this process. Additional comments address how these new insights may be informative for chronic lung diseases that occur, or initiate, in the neonatal period. This is not meant to be an exhaustive review of the molecular biology of lung development. For a more comprehensive, contemporary review of the cellular and molecular aspects of lung development, readers can refer to recent reviews by others.

Postnatal Infections and Immunology Affecting Chronic Lung Disease of Prematurity   697

Gloria S. Pryhuber

Premature infants suffer significant respiratory morbidity during infancy with long-term negative consequences on health, quality of life, and health care costs. Enhanced susceptibility to a variety of infections and inflammation play a large role in early and prolonged lung disease following premature birth, although the mechanisms of susceptibility and immune dysregulation are active areas of research. This article reviews aspects of host-pathogen interactions and immune responses that are altered by preterm birth and that impact chronic respiratory morbidity in these children.

Role of *Ureaplasma* Respiratory Tract Colonization in Bronchopulmonary Dysplasia Pathogenesis: Current Concepts and Update   719

Rose Marie Viscardi and Suhas G. Kallapur

Respiratory tract colonization with the genital mycoplasma species *Ureaplasma parvum* and *Ureaplasma urealyticum* in preterm infants is a significant risk factor for bronchopulmonary dysplasia (BPD). Recent studies of the ureaplasmal genome, animal infection models, and human infants have provided a better understanding of specific virulence factors, pathogen-host interactions, and variability in genetic susceptibility that contribute to chronic infection, inflammation, and altered lung development. This review provides an update on the current evidence supporting a causal role of ureaplasma infection in BPD pathogenesis. The current status of antibiotic trials to prevent BPD in *Ureaplasma*-infected preterm infants is also reviewed.

The pathogenesis of bronchopulmonary dysplasia (BPD) is multifactorial, and the clinical phenotype of BPD is extremely variable. Several clinical and laboratory biomarkers have been proposed for the early identification of infants at higher risk of BPD and for determination of prognosis of infants with a diagnosis of BPD. The authors review available literature on prediction tools and biomarkers of BPD, using clinical variables and biomarkers based on imaging, lung function measures, and measurements of various analytes in different body fluids that have been determined to be associated with BPD either in a targeted manner or by unbiased omic profiling.

Bronchopulmonary dysplasia (BPD) is the most common chronic complication of extreme preterm birth. The authors applied the Grading of Recommendations Assessment, Development, and Evaluation (GRADE) methodology to pharmacologic therapies found to prevent BPD. Caffeine and vitamin A are the only medications shown in high-quality studies to prevent BPD without the risk of clinically important adverse effects. Dexamethasone is effective for the prevention of BPD; but for many infants, the increased risks of hypertrophic cardiomyopathy, gastrointestinal perforation, and cerebral palsy outweigh this benefit. Several medications are currently under investigation for the prevention of BPD, but few are novel agents.

Mechanical ventilation is an important potentially modifiable risk factor for the development of bronchopulmonary dysplasia. Effective use of noninvasive respiratory support reduces the risk of lung injury. Lung volume recruitment and avoidance of excessive tidal volume are key elements of lung-protective ventilation strategies. Avoidance of oxidative stress, less invasive methods of surfactant administration, and high-frequency ventilation are also important factors in lung injury prevention.

Bronchopulmonary dysplasia (BPD) remains a common morbidity of prematurity. Although the pathogenesis of BPD is recognized to be both multifactorial and complex, the role of nutrition in the pathophysiology of BPD is typically limited to management after a diagnosis has been made. Infants born small for gestational age and those who experience postnatal growth failure are more likely to have BPD. Therapies for lung disease, such as fluid restriction, diuretics, and corticosteroids, can negatively impact post-natal growth. Future research is needed to optimize nutritional strategies in the neonatal intensive care unit and following hospital discharge.

Oxygen saturation targeting is widely used in neonatal intensive care, but the optimal target range in very preterm infants has been uncertain and is the subject of recent debate and research. This review briefly discusses the technology of oxygen monitoring and the role of oxygen toxicity in pre-term infants. The background to the recent trials of oxygen saturation tar-geting in acute and continuing care of very preterm infants is reviewed, and the findings and implications of the recent trials, particularly with respect to bronchopulmonary dysplasia, are discussed.

Hypoxic episodes are troublesome components of bronchopulmonary dysplasia (BPD) in preterm infants. Immature respiratory control seems to be the major contributor, superimposed on abnormal respiratory func-tion. Relatively short respiratory pauses may precipitate desaturation and bradycardia. This population is predisposed to pulmonary hyperten-sion; it is likely that pulmonary vasoconstriction also plays a role. The nat-ural history has been well-characterized in the preterm population at risk for BPD; however, the consequences are less clear. Proposed associa-tions of intermittent hypoxia include retinopathy of prematurity, sleep disordered breathing, and neurodevelopmental delay. Future study should address whether these associations are causal relationships.

Despite advances in the care of preterm infants, these infants remain at risk bronchopulmonary dysplasia (BPD), which results in prolonged need for supplemental oxygen, recurrent respiratory exacerbations, and exer-cise intolerance. Recent investigations have highlighted the important contribution of the developing pulmonary circulation to lung development, showing that these infants are also at risk for pulmonary vascular disease (PVD), including pulmonary hypertension (PH) and pulmonary vascular ab-normalities. Several epidemiologic studies have delineated the incidence of PH in preterm infants and the impact on outcomes. These studies have also highlighted gaps in the understanding of PVD in BPD.

This article presents an overview of the diagnosis and management of airway problems encountered in infants with severe bronchopulmonary

PROGRAM OBJECTIVE
The goal of *Clinics in Perinatology* is to keep practicing perinatologists, neonatologists, obstetricians, practicing physicians and residents up to date with current clinical practice in perinatology by providing timely articles reviewing the state of the art in patient care.

TARGET AUDIENCE
Perinatologists, neonatologists, obstetricians, practicing physicians, residents and healthcare professionals who provide patient care utilizing findings from *Clinics in Perinatology*.

LEARNING OBJECTIVES
Upon completion of this activity, participants will be able to:
1. Review early diagnosis and biomarkers of bronchopulmonary dysplasia.
2. Discuss stem cell therapies, mechanical ventilation, and pharmacological therapies for bronchopulmonary dysplasia.
3. Recognize issues associated with bronchopulmonary dysplasia, such as hypoxic episodes and pulmonary hypertension.

ACCREDITATION
The Elsevier Office of Continuing Medical Education (EOCME) is accredited by the Accreditation Council for Continuing Medical Education (ACCME) to provide continuing medical education for physicians.

The EOCME designates this enduring material for a maximum of 15 *AMA PRA Category 1 Credit*(s)™. Physicians should claim only the credit commensurate with the extent of their participation in the activity.

All other health care professionals requesting continuing education credit for this enduring material will be issued a certificate of participation.

DISCLOSURE OF CONFLICTS OF INTEREST
The EOCME assesses conflict of interest with its instructors, faculty, planners, and other individuals who are in a position to control the content of CME activities. All relevant conflicts of interest that are identified are thoroughly vetted by EOCME for fair balance, scientific objectivity, and patient care recommendations. EOCME is committed to providing its learners with CME activities that promote improvements or quality in healthcare and not a specific proprietary business or a commercial interest.

The planning committee, staff, authors and editors listed below have identified no financial relationships or relationships to products or devices they or their spouse/life partner have with commercial interest related to the content of this CME activity:
Steven H. Abman, MD; Raouf S. Amin, MD; Judy L. Aschner, MD; Elena Ciarmoli, MD; Brian A. Darlow, MD, FRCP, FRACP, FRCPCH; Juliann M. Di Fiore, BSEE; Elizabeth E. Foglia, MD; Anjali Fortna; Kerry Holland; Lucky Jain, MD, MBA; Erik A. Jensen, MD; Suhas G. Kallapur, MD; Charitharth Vivek Lal, MD; Thomas J. Mariani, PhD; Camilia R. Martin, MD, MS; Cindy T. McEvoy, MD, MCR; Colin J. Morley, MD, FRCPCH; Peter M. Mourani, MD; Palani Murugesan; Maria Pierro, MD; Brenda B. Poindexter, MD, MS; Gloria S. Pryhuber, MD; Guilherme Sant'Anna, MD, PhD, FRCPC; Barbara Schmidt, MD, MSc; Megan Suermann; Bernard Thébaud, MD, PhD; Rose M. Viscardi, MD; Laura L. Walkup, PhD; Michele C. Walsh, MD, MSEpi.

The planning committee, staff, authors and editors listed below have identified financial relationships or relationships to products or devices they or their spouse/life partner have with commercial interest related to the content of this CME activity:
Namasivayam Ambalavanan, MD is a consultant/advisor for Mallinckrodt, with research support from Pfizer Inc.
Martin Keszler, MD, FAAP is a consultant/advisor for Draegerwerk AG & Co; Discovery Laboratories, Inc; and Medipost America, with research support from Draegerwerk AG & Co.
Richard J. Martin, MD is a consultant/advisor for Sancilio & Company, Inc. and Alcresta, and has research support from Abbott Nutrition; Gilead; Sancilio & Company, Inc.; and Alcresta.
Michael J. Rutter, MBChB, FRACS is a consultant/advisor for, with royalties/patents from, Bryan Medical Inc.
Jason C. Woods, PhD is a consultant/advisor for, with stock ownership in, Vertex Pharmaceuticals Incorporated.

UNAPPROVED/OFF-LABEL USE DISCLOSURE
The EOCME requires CME faculty to disclose to the participants:
1. When products or procedures being discussed are off-label, unlabelled, experimental, and/or investigational (not US Food and Drug Administration [FDA] approved); and

2. Any limitations on the information presented, such as data that are preliminary or that represent ongoing research, interim analyses, and/or unsupported opinions. Faculty may discuss information about pharmaceutical agents that is outside of FDA-approved labelling. This information is intended solely for CME and is not intended to promote off-label use of these medications. If you have any questions, contact the medical affairs department of the manufacturer for the most recent prescribing information.

TO ENROLL
To enroll in the *Clinics in Perinatology* Continuing Medical Education program, call customer service at 1-800-654-2452 or sign up online at http://www.theclinics.com/home/cme. The CME program is available to subscribers for an additional annual fee of $235 USD.

METHOD OF PARTICIPATION
In order to claim credit, participants must complete the following:
1. Complete enrolment as indicated above.
2. Read the activity.
3. Complete the CME Test and Evaluation. Participants must achieve a score of 70% on the test. All CME Tests and Evaluations must be completed online.

CME INQUIRIES/SPECIAL NEEDS
For all CME inquiries or special needs, please contact elsevierCME@elsevier.com.

CLINICS IN PERINATOLOGY

Foreword

Why the Bronchopulmonary Dysplasia Improvement Curve Lags Behind

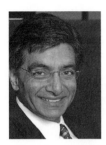

Lucky Jain, MD, MBA
Consulting Editor

In a recent publication from the Neonatal Network of the National Institute of Child Health and Human Development, Stoll and colleagues[1] report trends in morbidity and mortality of extremely preterm neonates from 1993 to 2012. This twenty-year epoch represents a critical period in our journey as a subspecialty, one marked by widespread adoption of antenatal steroids (**Fig. 1**),[1] broader application of surfactant, new modes of ventilation, and novel therapies such as inhaled nitric oxide. These advances have led to gains, albeit modest for some gestations, in the overall survival as well as survival without morbidity.[2,3] Yet, one morbidity (**Fig. 2**)[1] stands out as a recalcitrant rebel, seemingly oblivious of the singular attention it has received from the entire subspecialty: bronchopulmonary dysplasia (BPD)!

So why doesn't BPD toe the line? Or is it possible that our measures are faulty and that gains have been made, but our definitions mask them? A review of the published literature would suggest that it is some of both. The initial report of BPD by Northway and colleagues[4] described a disease very different from the one we see today. Over the years, it is rare to see the extensive cystic BPD seen in those early reports; instead, oxygen requirement at 36 weeks corrected age or at 28 days after birth (for bigger babies) is what is most commonly used. With the widespread use of oxygen supplementation and oxygen saturation monitoring, many babies who are discharged home on small amounts of oxygen are often still receiving supplemental oxygen weeks later, qualifying them to be in the BPD cohort whether or not a radiograph with corroborating evidence is available. This, coupled with the improved survival of extremely low birth weight infants who carry the highest risk of BPD, has contributed to the rise in BPD.

This does not mean that opportunities don't exist to reduce the burden of BPD. Nearly thirty years ago, Avery and colleagues[5] showed that significant differences

Clin Perinatol 42 (2015) xv–xvii
http://dx.doi.org/10.1016/j.clp.2015.09.002
0095-5108/15/$ – see front matter © 2015 Published by Elsevier Inc.

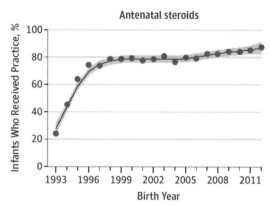

Fig. 1. Antenatal steroid use in infants born at gestational ages 22 through 28 weeks from 1991 to 2011 at the NICHD Neonatal Research Network Centers. (*Adapted from* Stoll BJ, Hansen NI, Bell EF, et al. Trends in care practices, morbidity, and mortality of extremely preterm neonates, 1993-2012. JAMA 2015;314:1043.)

existed in the incidence of BPD between premier institutions even when birth weight, race, and sex were controlled for. Similar differences persist even today,[6] challenging us to evaluate carefully how we care for these babies. A recent workshop[7] organized by the National Heart, Lung, and Blood Institute concluded that, despite decades of promising research, primary prevention of BPD has remained elusive. It called for a shift in research priorities and targeted bench-to-bedside research into primary prevention of BPD.

In this issue of *Clinics in Perinatology*, Drs Kallapur and Pryhuber have put together a state-of-the-art compilation of articles related to this complex disease covering the entire spectrum of the disease from molecular biology of lung development to an integrated approach to primary prevention.

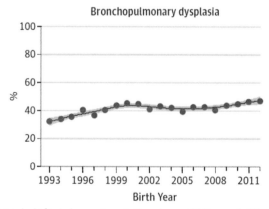

Fig. 2. BPD incidence in infants born at gestational ages 22 through 28 weeks from 1991 to 2011 at the NICHD Neonatal Research Network Centers. (*Adapted from* Stoll BJ, Hansen NI, Bell EF, et al. Trends in care practices, morbidity, and mortality of extremely preterm neonates, 1993-2012. JAMA 2015;314:1044.)

I want to thank the editors, authors, and the publishing team at Elsevier (Kerry Holland and Casey Jackson) for bringing together another superb issue of the *Clinics in Perinatology* for you.

Lucky Jain, MD, MBA
Emory University School of Medicine
Department of Pediatrics
Children's Healthcare of Atlanta
2015 Uppergate Drive
Atlanta, GA 30322, USA

E-mail address:
ljain@emory.edu

REFERENCES

1. Stoll BJ, Hansen NI, Bell EF, et al. Trends in care practices, morbidity, and mortality of extremely preterm neonates, 1993-2012. JAMA 2015;314:1039–51.
2. Fanaroff AA, Wright LL, Stevenson DK, et al. Very-low-birth weight outcomes of the National Institutes of Child Health and Human Development Research Network, May 1991 through December 1992. Am J Obstet Gynecol 1995;173: 1423–31.
3. Patel RM, Kandefer S, Walsh MC, et al. Causes and timing of death in extremely premature infants from 2000-2011. N Engl J Med 2015;372:331–40.
4. Northway WH Jr, Rosan RC, Porter DY. Pulmonary disease following respirator therapy of hyaline-membrane disease. Bronchopulmonary dysplasia. N Engl J Med 1967;276:357–68.
5. Avery ME, Tooley WH, Keller JB, et al. Is chronic lung disease in low birth weight infants preventable? A survey of eight centers. Pediatrics 1987;79:26–30.
6. Rysavy MA, Li L, Bell EF, et al. Between-hospital variation in treatment and outcomes in extremely preterm infants. N Engl J Med 2015;372:1801–11.
7. McEvoy CT, Jain L, Schmidt B, et al. Bronchopulmonary dysplasia: NHLBI Workshop on the Primary Prevention of Chronic Lung Diseases. Ann Am Thorac Soc 2014;11:S146–53.

Preface

Bronchopulmonary Dysplasia— The Search for Answers Continues

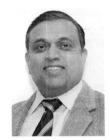 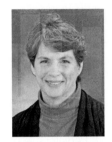

Suhas G. Kallapur, MD   Gloria S. Pryhuber, MD
Editors

Bronchopulmonary dysplasia (BPD) has been recognized as a chronic lung disease affecting preterm infants for more than 45 years. However, little progress has been made in the prevention and treatment of the disease resulting from injury and abnormal repair occurring in structurally immature lung. BPD continues to be a source of major morbidity affecting preterm infants both in the Neonatal Intensive Care Unit and as young children. Studies in preadolescent children demonstrate that abnormal lung function originating in BPD persists well into childhood. The severity of the lung disease in infants with BPD also correlates with risk for adverse neurodevelopmental outcome. Potential lasting effects of the disease into adulthood are also suspected but not yet well-documented. Thus, BPD imposes a significant burden of adverse health outcomes in infants born prematurely.

Despite the lack of overall progress in BPD, there have been recent developments in the understanding, diagnosis, and management of this disease. In this issue of the *Clinics in Perinatology*, we present an update on different aspects of BPD written by experts in the field. The major risk factors for BPD are prematurity, mechanical ventilation (article by Drs Keszler and Sant'Anna), exposure to noxious insults such as oxygen (article by Drs Darlow and Morley), and prenatal as well as postnatal infections (articles by Dr Pryhuber and Drs Viscardi and Kallapur). New basic science and clinical research studies are revealing novel details of pathogenesis (article by Mariani), biomarkers (article by Drs Lal and Ambalavanan), newer imaging modalities (article by Drs Walkup and Woods), and possible new treatment strategies for the future, including stem cell therapy (article by Drs Pierro, Thébaud, and Ciarmoli). Management continues to evolve with significant changes in the application of ventilation (article by Drs Keszler and Sant'Anna), oxygenation (article by Drs Darlow and Morley), nutrition (article by Drs Poindexter and Martin), and evidence-based therapies (article by Drs

Clin Perinatol 42 (2015) xix–xx
http://dx.doi.org/10.1016/j.clp.2015.09.001
0095-5108/15/$ – see front matter © 2015 Published by Elsevier Inc.

perinatology.theclinics.com

Jensen, Foglia, and Schmidt) in just recent years. Major sources of frustration for the bedside clinician caring for a sick infant with BPD are the hypoxic spells (article by Drs Martin, Di Forte, and Walsh), pulmonary hypertension (article by Drs Mourani and Abman), and the dilemmas in caring for chronic ventilator-dependent infants (article by Drs Amin and Rutter). Finally, we present the natural history of BPD and of lung function of infants as they grow older and make the case for primary prevention of the disease (article by Drs McEvoy and Aschner). Our approach in this issue has been to balance new information with an adequate review of classic topics. We anticipate that the issue will be of interest to a broad array of readership, including clinical neonatologists, pulmonologists, and investigators.

Suhas G. Kallapur, MD
Division of Neonatology and Pulmonary Biology
Cincinnati Children's Hospital Medical Center
3333 Burnet Avenue
Cincinnati, OH 45229, USA

Gloria S. Pryhuber, MD
Pediatrics and Environmental Medicine
Division of Neonatology
University of Rochester Medical Center
Box 651, 601 Elmwood Avenue
Rochester, NY 14642, USA

E-mail addresses:
suhas.kallapur@cchmc.org (S.G. Kallapur)
Gloria_Pryhuber@URMC.Rochester.edu (G.S. Pryhuber)

Update on Molecular Biology of Lung Development—Transcriptomics

Thomas J. Mariani, PhD

KEYWORDS

- Epithelium • Mesenchyme • Airway • Alveoli • Progenitor cells

KEY POINTS

- The past 2 decades have witnessed tremendous growth in our understanding of fundamental regulatory processes and networks responsible for coordinating the development of the mammalian lung; high-throughput, genome-wide analyses have facilitated this growth.
- Recent seminal observations regarding cellular heterogeneity and lineage relationships demonstrate we have much yet to learn.
- Recent developments in single-cell transcriptome analysis are likely to transform our appreciation of cellular heterogeneity with the respiratory system and help to determine whether this heterogeneity is programmed, stochastic, or a combination.
- The precise role of environmental cues, both normal (eg, oxygen) and foreign (eg, microbes), in the coordinated regulation of lung development remains poorly defined.
- Multi-scale integration of molecular information, such as that defined by comprehensive profiling of miRNA and mRNA expression, will ultimately be necessary for a complete explanation of lung development.

INTRODUCTION

This article highlights some of the significant advances in our understanding of lung developmental biology made over the last few years, which challenge existing paradigms and are relevant to a fundamental understanding of this process. Additional comments address how these new insights may be informative for chronic lung diseases that occur, or initiate, in the neonatal period. This is not meant to be an exhaustive review of the molecular biology of lung development. For a more comprehensive, contemporary review of the cellular and molecular aspects of lung development, readers can refer to recent reviews by others.[1–7]

Disclosure: Dr T.J. Mariani is supported by HL101813 (NHLBI), HL101794 (NHLBI), HL122700 (NHLBI) and HHSN272201200005C (NIAID) grants.
Division of Neonatology and Pediatric Molecular and Personalized Medicine Program, University of Rochester Medical Center, 601 Elmwood Avenue, Box 850, Rochester, NY 14642, USA
E-mail address: Tom_Mariani@urmc.rochester.edu

Clin Perinatol 42 (2015) 685–695
http://dx.doi.org/10.1016/j.clp.2015.08.001
0095-5108/15/$ – see front matter © 2015 Elsevier Inc. All rights reserved.

DISCUSSION
Introduction to Lung Development

Historically, the process of lung development has been conceptualized as a linear set of stages, typically including 4 or 5 discrete parts, aligned with the age of the organism. These stages were defined largely on histologic and morphologic changes in lung structure that occur during fetal development. The embryonic stage of lung development is recognized as encompassing the initiation of lung formation and, as a reference, occurs from 4 to 6 weeks postmenstrual age (PMA) in humans and embryonic day 9.5 (E9.5) to E10.5 in mice. This stage involves budding of a patch of ventral foregut endoderm, located between the thymus and liver, to form a distinct organ primordium. A central role for retinoic acid (RA) in this process has been appreciated, and recent studies uncovered a Wnt/Tgfbeta/Fgf10 regulatory network controlled by RA to drive the formation of the lung bud.[8]

The pseudoglandular stage of lung development largely involves establishment of the airway structure of the mature rodent and occurs from 6 to 16 weeks' PMA in the human and E10.5 to E16.5 in the mouse. Formation of the airways results from recursive branching morphogenesis, similar to that which occurs in other glandular organs with a branched tubular structure (eg, salivary, mammary). Branching morphogenesis in the lung seems to be regulated locally by FGF10/FGFR2 and BMP4/Shh signaling, to promote tube elongation or branch-point formation, respectively. Some investigators have suggested conversely that FGF10 controls epithelial differentiation.[9] Although it was largely presumed that this local regulation occurred stochastically, seminal studies by Metzger and colleagues[10,11] demonstrated that these events are programmed in both time and space.

Once the major airway architecture of the lung has been established during the pseudoglandular stage, the canalicular stage of lung development involves initiation of the formation of the functional (acinar) portion of the lung and initiation of the differentiation of distinct respiratory cell types. This stage occurs from 16 to 26 weeks' PMA in the human; but for some reason, it is much more condensed in mice, occurring from E16.5 to E17.5. The establishment of a proximal-distal differentiation pattern of lung epithelium has been described[12,13] and seems to be regulated by a complex set of regulatory molecules and transcription factors driven by the activation of Wnt/b-catenin signaling. The emergence of morphologically distinguishable alveolar epithelial cell types, which are essential for facilitating gas exchange, also begins at this stage. As discussed later, although it is now clear that mesenchyme undergoes analogous processes to specify various cell types,[14] and can play a direct role in developmentally associated lung diseases,[15,16] an understanding of how this process is regulated for mesenchymal cells is less clear.

The saccular stage of lung development involves the formation of frank, functional airspace capable of gas exchange. This stage is associated with the emergence of the expression of numerous cell type–specific markers and expansion of the density of the alveolar capillary bed. In the human, the saccular stage takes place entirely in utero, initiating at approximately 26 weeks' PMA and continuing through 36 weeks' PMA. In the mouse, for reasons that are not entirely clear, this stage spans birth, initiating at E17.5 and continuing through approximately the first 4 to 7 postnatal days (P4-7). The initiation of functional pulmonary surfactant production and surfactant secretion is a key physiologic event that occurs during this stage. Functional surfactant is essential to maintain airspace patency, and its absence is a major cause of morbidity and mortality in babies born before this time.[17]

The alveolar stage is the ultimate stage of lung development, and it initiates at 36 weeks' PMA in humans and at approximately P4-7 in mice. The major events of the alveolar stage include a dramatic expansion of surface area, through secondary crest formation and elongation, and reorganization of the alveolar capillary bed to ensure close apposition of the blood supply to alveolar surfaces. Although acinar units are sometimes referred to as alveoli, this term is appropriately applied only to fully mature airspaces derived from secondary crest elongation. The complexity of alveolar formation, essentially the processes that guide secondary crest formation and elongation, is widely appreciated, but is poorly understood relative to the preceding stages, and has been a focus of recent investigation. Among the complexity of this process, the organized deposition of elastin fibers at alveolar entrance rings, at a location consistent with elongating secondary crests, seems to be among the most critical. Processes that block events leading up to the formation of these fibers, either through disruption of signaling events[18] or emergence of cell types,[19,20] or that interfere with proper elastin fiber organization[19] or function[21] block or attenuate proper alveolar size and number. Therefore, this stage is arguably most important to human health because abnormalities in this process are compatible with life (whereas abnormalities in earlier stages are much more likely to lead to defects that are not survivable) but can have sustained impacts on long-term health and susceptibility to disease.

There is some debate as to the timing at which the alveolar stage ends and when the formation of new alveoli ceases. In the mouse, it is widely appreciated that alveolar formation peaks in the first week of life and is complete by the end of the first month of life, at the time of animal maturity. The precise timing for the end of the mouse alveolar stage has apparently not been rigorously evaluated. In humans, it was long held that development occurred in utero and that all or most of alveoli were formed at or shortly after the time of birth. However, this dogma has been reprised over the past decade by careful morphometric analyses in humans and other primates, which suggest that alveoli are formed after birth.[22] It is now appreciated that alveolar formation continues in humans through the first decade of life. As in the case of the mouse, these data support a termination of the alveolar stage at about the time of maturity.

Molecular Stages of Development

Numerous recent studies have codified an appreciation of the overly simplistic nature of this linear stage model of development and underscored the heterogeneity of both the processes and cell types involved. As an example, a physiologic model of lung development would focus on the binary nature of the organ before and after its necessity for functional gas exchange at birth. Similarly, ontological models of lung development, focusing on biological processes that occur during and across overlapping stages, have been proposed for decades. More recently, genome-wide molecular expression analysis of lung development has helped to understand how the complexity of lung development can be explained from an alternate, molecular perspective. Consistent with a functional, physiologic model of development, early transcriptomic studies suggested that the regulation of processes associated with preparing for time of birth exhibited the greatest molecular impact on lung development.[23] Furthermore, although gene expression differences between species could be readily identified, this signature of time to birth was conserved.

These observations should not be interpreted to suggest that histologic stage-specific genome-wide expression patterns were not recognizable, or of significant importance. Before the recognition of this molecular signature of time to birth, analysis demonstrated a substantial impact of the initiation of the alveolar stage on the developing mouse lung transcriptome.[24] Indeed, secondary to birth, alveolar formation seems to have the greatest influence on gene expression patterns across development in the mouse.[23] These data provide for an alternate means to identify process- and stage-specific gene expression patterns and regulatory networks that may contribute to these processes.

Analogous studies in the human thus far have been restricted to the earlier epochs of development, before the end of the canalicular stage, and do not provide an equivalent degree of clarity.[25] However, these studies do clearly demonstrate that global genome-wide expression during human lung development follows patterns that are not entirely correlated with classic histologic stages. In early human lung development, there seem to be 2 temporal demarcations in the transcriptome. Interestingly, one of these demarcations occurs exactly at the time of transition from the pseudoglandular to the canalicular stages of development. However, another occurs in the middle of the pseudoglandular stage and seems to demarcate an early from a late phase of pseudoglandular lung development. Unlike the case whereby demarcations in the mouse lung transcriptome have identifiable biological correlates, the biological processes that these demarcations in human lung development represent are currently not entirely clear. Regardless, cumulatively, these data support the appreciation of molecular phases of lung development, which integrate stages and processes, and can be considered analogous to classic histologic stages.

Ontogeny of Lung Epithelial Cells

The hierarchical nature of cell ontogeny during lung development has not been completely defined. Although tremendous diversity in pulmonary cell types has been appreciated for more than half a century,[26] the last decade has seen a tremendous growth in the characterization of cellular heterogeneity. For a large part, this progress has focused on epithelial cells, whereas progress on the mesenchyme has lagged, as is the case for most of our understanding of the pulmonary system. Arguably, a new appreciation of this diversity among the major epithelial cell types was stimulated by observations regarding the differential sensitivities of airway epithelial cells to toxins and their differing capacity for regenerating the airway following injury, the identification and characterization of so-called variant club cells that contribute to repopulation of the airway.[27] Another watershed discovery was the identification of bronchioalveolar stem cells (BASCs) that reside at the entrance to alveolar ducts and have the capacity to produce progeny of an alveolar (Alveolar Type II cell (AT2)/ Alveolar Type I cell [AT1]) or airway (club cells) fate. There is little evidence that these BASCs actually give rise to alveolar lineages during development. However, the paradigm that airway epithelial progenitor cells can contribute to alveoli following injury or during lung regeneration has been further supported by recent work from the laboratories of McKeon and Chapman. Chapman and colleagues[28] have reported that epithelial cells located in the proximity of the bronchioalveolar duct junction (BADJ) (and/or within the alveolus) that express Itgb4, but not Sftpc, can differentiate to alveolar epithelial cell types in a fibrotic model. Furthermore, distal airway stem cells coexpressing p63 and Krt5 are essential for alveolar repair in models of severe viral-derived or cytotoxin-mediated respiratory destruction.[29–31]

Classically, alveolar epithelial cells were thought to exist in 2 forms: the squamous type I epithelial cell (AT1) that allows apposition of airspace and vasculature and the cuboidal type II cell (AT2) that is responsible for production and secretion of pulmonary surfactant. Markers of AT2 can be observed at the earliest time points of lung formation,[32] and for decades these cells have been described as the progenitors for AT1 during development and in response to injury. A seminal study from Desai and colleagues[33] used lineage tracing and molecular analysis to demonstrate that AT1 and AT2 arise from a common bipotential progenitor during lung development. A follow-up study by Treutlein and colleagues[34] described using single-cell transcriptional profiling of epithelial cells isolated from the developing lung to construct hierarchical relationships between AT1 and AT2 and their progenitors, as well as their genomic profiles. Also included in this analysis were airway ciliated and secretory cell types. These studies expanded, by an order of magnitude or more, the number of cell type-specific markers associated with individual lung epithelial cell types. These studies also support a model whereby frank bipotential progenitors, defined by the coexpression of Sftpc and Pdpn, emerge around E18.5 and are responsible for the formation of both mature alveolar epithelial cell types. The work by Desai and colleagues[33] also clearly showed, as had long been held, that fully differentiated AT2 give rise to AT1 in mature lungs following injury. However, this capacity was apparently restricted to a subset of long-lived AT2 that was also capable of self-renewal. It remains unclear whether these mature AT2 progenitor cells are programmed or stochastically determined. Regardless, the data clearly indicate a distinction in the origin of alveolar epithelial cells during development and during homeostasis following injury/repair.

With regard to epithelial cell diversity in the pseudostratified airway of the lung, basal cells are thought to be progenitors for differentiated secretory and ciliated cells, both during lung development and during repair responses to injury. Two recent reports have further clarified how these airway progenitors are specified during development, restricted from the distal lung, and function in homeostatic maintenance.[35,36] The Hippo/Yap pathway seems to be central to controlling the specification of the airway and the progenitor capacity of basal cells, at least in part by driving the expression of the cardinal airway epithelial cell transcriptional regulator Sox2. Intriguingly, the ability of Hippo signaling to specify the airway is associated with subcellular redistribution of Yap from a nuclear to a cytoplasmic pool.[36] Furthermore, Yap is necessary and sufficient to maintain the pseudostratified airway epithelium and form the appropriate distribution of ciliated and secretory cells.[35] This ability of Yap to promote/maintain basal progenitors occurs through the coordinated regulation of a p63-dependent transcriptional program.

Regulation of Diversity of Lung Mesenchyme

The field has been slow to appreciate that similar diversity exists for epithelial and mesenchymal cells in the lung; the mesenchyme is sometimes referred to as relatively homogeneous, which is clearly not accurate. A preponderance of data in the literature over the last few decades quite clearly demonstrates significant diversity among frank smooth muscle cells, be it airway or vascular smooth muscle, muscularized and nonmuscular, lipid-laden parenchymal fibroblasts and various vascular support cells, including pericytes. Kumar and colleagues[14] have provided perhaps the most complete assessment of mesenchymal specification and airway smooth muscle (ASM) cell diversity during lung development. Using a strategy to target individual airway-associated mesenchymal cells during lung development, they characterized the location and dynamics of ASM progenitor niches. Unlike the case for epithelial progenitors, it seems that mesenchymal progenitor niches are not fixed in space or time. Conversely, an ASM niche originates along with each airway branch and migrates along with the developing airways, and cells from each niche are restricted to that specific airway structure. Interestingly, the ASM progenitor niche seems to be localized around the tips of growing airway branches. Transcriptomic analysis revealed mesenchyme from these growing tips display a signature of Wnt activation, suggesting this ligand family may be a key factor in defining the ASM progenitor niche. Genome-wide profiling of ASM progenitors obtained from outside of the niche, treated with Wnt ligand in vitro, demonstrated regulatory effects ontologically associated with motility and migration, consistent with Wnt controlling the migration and differentiation of these cells. Wnt treatment of these cells also resulted in them assuming a phenotype more reminiscent of mesenchymal progenitors within the niche. It is unclear whether Wnt5a may be a key family member contributing to this process and whether this partially explains the distal mesenchyme phenotype observed in the Wnt5a-deficient mouse.[37]

A Molecular Basis for Dysanapsis?

Dysanapsis, or the disproportionate growth of airways and lung parenchyma, has been put forth as an explanation for respiratory physiology deficiencies in certain disease states, most notably in the argument for a developmental origin for asthma.[38–40] However, little evidence exits for the theory of variability in airway growth or length. A paradigm-establishing study recently published by Chen and colleagues[41] indicates that the length of airways, and the point at which the respiratory portion of the lung begins as demarcated by the BADJ, is genetically programmed. This study describes 2 waves of regulatory control during lung development; the first associated with establishing Sox9 expression and generally defining lung patterning through branching morphogenesis and the second associated with establishing Sox2 expression and specifying the end of the conducting airway and the location of the BADJ. Importantly, genetic manipulation could alter the location of the BADJ and, thus, airway length, independent of differentiation of the full complement of proximal and distal cell types.

Establishment of the location for BADJ formation was shown to be associated with changes in endogenous glucocorticoid signaling in vivo and affected by exogenous glucocorticoids, but not retinoids, in an ex vivo model of lung development. Furthermore, excess glucocorticoids promoted precocious alveolar formation proximal to the default location of the BADJ. Transcriptomics analysis demonstrated this was associated with widespread increases in alveolar cell markers. It seems there exists a population of Sox2-negative cells in the developing terminal airway, capable of responding to hormonal cues and differentiating toward an alveolar fate, that will otherwise go on to form conducting airway. Given the importance of endogenous glucocorticoids to biochemical (eg, surfactant) and structural (eg, elastin) aspects of lung maturation, and the use of exogenous glucocorticoids to promote lung maturation in late fetal development, these novel observations have potential relevance to lung disease occurring in the perinatal period. Furthermore, by analogy with dysanapsis, these data indicate that airway length may be a clinically relevant structural parameter with implications for lung function and disease susceptibility.

Integrated Genomics Analysis of Development

Although many comprehensive characterizations of lung development using high-throughput methods have been published, relatively few have successfully integrated data sets to formulate a thorough understanding of regulatory processes. A notable success would be the studies of Bar-Joseph, Kaminski, and Ambalavanan and colleagues,[42] who used a computational systems biology approach to integrate genome-wide miRNA and mRNA expression patterns to identify dynamic regulatory networks. This approach involved the development of a computational tool, which they named the MIRna Dynamic Regulatory Events Miner. Leveraging this probabilistic modeling approach, they were able to identify known and novel miRNA/transcription factor–regulated networks that are associated with specific stages and processes during lung development.

More recently, the same group used genome-wide transcriptomics and DNA methylation analyses to study relationships between chromatin modifications and gene expression in the perinatal period in both mice and humans.[43] In the mouse, a subset of genes with known roles in the regulation of lung development displayed an inverse correlation between DNA methylation and gene expression, including those associated with Wnt signaling, proximal-distal epithelial cell specification, capillary vascular formation, and extracellular matrix formation. In the human lung, integration of DNA methylation patterns in normal development and expression profiles in chronic lung disease following preterm birth (bronchopulmonary dysplasia) identified genes/pathways suspected to play a role in defining susceptibility to disease. These data are consistent with the hypothesis that chromatin remodeling influences the regulatory processes controlling lung development in the perinatal period and that failure of this coordination may be involved in associated disease states.

A Molecular Atlas for Lung Development

An ongoing National Heart, Lung, and Blood Institute–supported multi-institutional, collaborative program (termed the developing LUNG Molecular Atlas Program [Lung-MAP]) is developing a map of human (and mouse) lung development at the structural, cellular, and molecular levels, with a focus on the perinatal period including the saccular and alveolar stages. This active program involves developing and leveraging high-throughput and multi-scale anatomic imaging, cellular and molecular methods to provide the research community benchmark data regarding normal developmental processes, which will aid in our understanding of abnormalities associated with diseased states. One product of the LungMAP is an interactive, Web-based portal (www.lungmap.net), including the BREATH data repository (www.lungmap.net/breath/), to be used for frequent prepublication data distribution. These resources were made available for public access in May 2015 in conjunction with the American Thoracic Society International Conference. Other products of the LungMAP will include high-resolution, detailed ontologies to formalize terminology for describing the developing lung anatomy,[44] including dynamic cell populations, and molecular functions important for the respiratory system.

Transcriptomics of Bronchopulmonary Dysplasia

For at least the last decade, microarray analysis has been used to characterize animal models of chronic lung disease initiated in the newborn period by exposure to excessive concentrations of oxygen.[45,46] These data have provided critical insights into disease-associated mechanisms. Early studies in the mouse confirmed responses involved aberrant expression of chemokines and proteases, changes in reactive oxygen species, and reductions in fibroblast growth factor - and vascular endothelial growth factor–related signaling.[46] Other studies dissected the involvement of specific pathways and, for instance, uncovered Nrf2-dependent and independent responses.[45] A more recent study suggested that neonatal hyperoxic lung injury in mice, which is associated with BPD-related phenotypes, centrally involves p21/Cdkn1 and Aryl-hydrocarbon receptor–related pathways.[47]

Over the past 5 years, genome-wide transcriptional assays have been applied to gain a better understanding of expression changes associated with bronchopulmonary dysplasia (BPD) in samples derived from human subjects. A focused but multifactorial analysis of angiogenesis-related gene expression in the lungs of preterm infants born at less than 27 weeks of gestation and receiving short-term ventilatory support identified a switch from proangiogenic factors to antisprouting regulators, consistent with deficiencies in alveolar vascularization.[48] In a study of samples collected at autopsy from preterm subjects with severe BPD leading to mortality and preterm controls with no lung disease or no BPD, microarray analysis was used to identify genes and pathways dysregulated in diseased lung tissue.[49] In what seems to have been the first study to perform such a comprehensive assessment of the BPD transcriptome, some obvious disease-related pathways were identified, including those involved in the regulation of cell proliferation, oxidative stress, control of vascular development, and inflammation. The most remarkable finding was a predominant and consistent signature of mast cell accumulation in the lungs of these preterm infants dying of severe BPD. Importantly, this signature was not of the typical mucosal mast cells normally found within the respiratory system. The signature was clearly of connective tissue-type mast cells (CTMC), which are rarely observed in the lung. Validation studies demonstrated a robust, albeit with variable magnitude, accumulation of CTMC in the airspaces in BPD lung tissue. In a preterm baboon model of hyperoxia-induced lung injury leading to BPD-like phenotypes, microarray analysis of lung tissue identified increased expression of genes related to chromosomal maintenance, proliferation, and differentiation.[50] Additionally, and of note, in this model there seemed to be an increase in genes associated with the inhibition of inflammation.

A more recent study characterized mRNA expression in peripheral blood mononuclear cells (PBMC) from preterm infants at risk for BPD.[51] In this study, peripheral blood was collected from 111 infants born at less than 32 weeks of gestational age, within the first week after birth, 2 weeks after birth, or at 1 month of life; PBMC RNA was interrogated by microarray analysis. When comparing those infants receiving a diagnosis of BPD (n = 68) with those who did not develop BPD (n = 43), approximately 10% of the genome was differentially expressed. These expression patterns were associated with a significant inhibition of the T-cell receptor signaling pathway as well as changes in cell proliferation. Equally of note, these data establish that disease-related responses are detectable in peripheral samples that can be obtained with minimally invasive procedures, as can be seen in many other diseases.

Similar transcriptomic studies have attempted to understand miRNA responses in human BPD and in animal models of disease. In another study of the neonatal mouse hyperoxia model, 14 miRNAs displaying increased expression and 7 miRNAs displaying decreased expression were identified, some of which seem to target cell proliferation genes.[52] Another comparison of miRNA expression in PBMC cells from 15 subjects with BPD and 15 controls identified 4 miRNAs (miR-152, miR-30a-3p, miR-133b, and miR-7) with aberrant expression levels. These observations included reduced expression of miR-152 and miR-30a-3p and increased expression of miR-133b and miR-7.[53] Results of a meta-analysis of BPD-related miRNA profiling identified 4 consistently upregulated miRNAs (miRNA-21, miRNA-34a, miRNA-431, and Let-7f) and one consistently downregulated miRNA (miRNA-335) in BPD lung tissues.[54] Additional miRNAs (miRNA-146b, miRNA-29a, miRNA-503, miRNA-411, miRNA-214, miRNA-130b, miRNA-382, and miRNA-181a-1*) seemed to be regulated in lung development and affected in BPD. Putative targets for these miRNAs included transcripts for genes previously demonstrated to show aberrant expression, such as HPGD and NTRK. Finally, at least one study has attempted to integrated comprehensive miRNA and mRNA expression profiles, using the neonatal mouse hyperoxia exposure model.[55] This study identified treatment-related effects on cell proliferation, adhesion/migration, inflammation, and angiogenesis and also implicated a significant role of miR-29.

REFERENCES

1. Whitsett JA, Weaver TE. Alveolar development and disease. Am J Respir Cell Mol Biol 2015;53(1):1–7.

2. Herriges M, Morrisey EE. Lung development: orchestrating the generation and regeneration of a complex organ. Development 2014;141(3):502–13.
3. Hagood JS, Ambalavanan N. Systems biology of lung development and regeneration: current knowledge and recommendations for future research. Wiley Interdiscip Rev Syst Biol Med 2013;5(2):125–33.
4. Ornitz DM, Yin Y. Signaling networks regulating development of the lower respiratory tract. Cold Spring Harb Perspect Biol 2012;4(5):a008318.
5. Rock JR, Hogan BL. Epithelial progenitor cells in lung development, maintenance, repair, and disease. Annu Rev Cell Dev Biol 2011;27:493–512.
6. Morrisey EE, Hogan BL. Preparing for the first breath: genetic and cellular mechanisms in lung development. Dev Cell 2010;18(1):8–23.
7. Warburton D, El-Hashash A, Carraro G, et al. Lung organogenesis. Curr Top Dev Biol 2010;90:73–158.
8. Chen F, Cao Y, Qian J, et al. A retinoic acid-dependent network in the foregut controls formation of the mouse lung primordium. J Clin Invest 2010;120(6):2040–8.
9. Volckaert T, Campbell A, Dill E, et al. Localized Fgf10 expression is not required for lung branching morphogenesis but prevents differentiation of epithelial progenitors. Development 2013;140(18):3731–42.
10. Metzger RJ, Klein OD, Martin GR, et al. The branching programme of mouse lung development. Nature 2008;453(7196):745–50.
11. Metzger RJ, Krasnow MA. Genetic control of branching morphogenesis. Science 1999;284(5420):1635–9.
12. Shu W, Guttentag S, Wang Z, et al. Wnt/beta-catenin signaling acts upstream of N-myc, BMP4, and FGF signaling to regulate proximal-distal patterning in the lung. Dev Biol 2005;283(1):226–39.
13. Mucenski ML, Wert SE, Nation JM, et al. beta-Catenin is required for specification of proximal/distal cell fate during lung morphogenesis. J Biol Chem 2003;278(41):40231–8.
14. Kumar ME, Bogard PE, Espinoza FH, et al. Mesenchymal cells. Defining a mesenchymal progenitor niche at single-cell resolution. Science 2014;346(6211):1258810.
15. Chao CM, El Agha E, Tiozzo C, et al. A breath of fresh air on the mesenchyme: impact of impaired mesenchymal development on the pathogenesis of bronchopulmonary dysplasia. Front Med (Lausanne) 2015;2:27.
16. Ahlfeld SK, Conway SJ. Aberrant signaling pathways of the lung mesenchyme and their contributions to the pathogenesis of bronchopulmonary dysplasia. Birth Defects Res A Clin Mol Teratol 2012;94(1):3–15.
17. Avery ME, Mead J. Surface properties in relation to atelectasis and hyaline membrane disease. AMA J Dis Child 1959;97(5 Pt 1):517–23.
18. McGowan S, Jackson SK, Jenkins-Moore M, et al. Mice bearing deletions of retinoic acid receptors demonstrate reduced lung elastin and alveolar numbers. Am J Respir Cell Mol Biol 2000;23(2):162–7.
19. Srisuma S, Bhattacharya S, Simon DM, et al. Fibroblast growth factor receptors control epithelial-mesenchymal interactions necessary for alveolar elastogenesis. Am J Respir Crit Care Med 2010;181(8):838–50.
20. Bostrom H, Willetts K, Pekny M, et al. PDGF-A signaling is a critical event in lung alveolar myofibroblast development and alveogenesis. Cell 1996;85(6):863–73.
21. Kumarasamy A, Schmitt I, Nave AH, et al. Lysyl oxidase activity is dysregulated during impaired alveolarization of mouse and human lungs. Am J Respir Crit Care Med 2009;180(12):1239–52.

22. Herring MJ, Bhattacharya S, Mecham BH, et al. Growth of alveoli during postnatal development in humans based on stereological estimation. Am J Physiol Lung Cell Mol Physiol 2014;307(4):L338–44.

23. Kho AT, Bhattacharya S, Mecham BH, et al. Expression profiles of the mouse lung identify a molecular signature of time-to-birth. Am J Respir Cell Mol Biol 2009; 40(1):47–57.

24. Mariani TJ, Reed JJ, Shapiro SD. Expression profiling of the developing mouse lung: insights into the establishment of the extracellular matrix. Am J Respir Cell Mol Biol 2002;26(5):541–8.

25. Kho AT, Bhattacharya S, Mecham BH, et al. Transcriptomic analysis of human lung development. Am J Respir Crit Care Med 2010;181(1):54–63.

26. Dunsmore SE, Rannels DE. Extracellular matrix biology in the lung. Am J Physiol 1996;270(1 Pt 1):L3–27.

27. Reynolds SD, Giangreco A, Power JH, et al. Neuroepithelial bodies of pulmonary airways serve as a reservoir of progenitor cells capable of epithelial regeneration. Am J Pathol 2000;156(1):269–78.

28. Chapman HA, Li X, Alexander JP, et al. Integrin alpha6beta4 identifies an adult distal lung epithelial population with regenerative potential in mice. J Clin Invest 2011;121(7):2855–62.

29. Vaughan AE, Brumwell AN, Xi Y, et al. Lineage-negative progenitors mobilize to regenerate lung epithelium after major injury. Nature 2015;517(7536):621–5.

30. Zuo W, Zhang T, Wu DZ, et al. p63(+)Krt5(+) distal airway stem cells are essential for lung regeneration. Nature 2015;517(7536):616–20.

31. Kumar PA, Hu Y, Yamamoto Y, et al. Distal airway stem cells yield alveoli in vitro and during lung regeneration following H1N1 influenza infection. Cell 2011; 147(3):525–38.

32. Perl AK, Wert SE, Nagy A, et al. Early restriction of peripheral and proximal cell lineages during formation of the lung. Proc Natl Acad Sci U S A 2002;99(16): 10482–7.

33. Desai TJ, Brownfield DG, Krasnow MA. Alveolar progenitor and stem cells in lung development, renewal and cancer. Nature 2014;507(7491):190–4.

34. Treutlein B, Brownfield DG, Wu AR, et al. Reconstructing lineage hierarchies of the distal lung epithelium using single-cell rna-seq. Nature 2014;509(7500):371–5.

35. Zhao R, Fallon TR, Saladi SV, et al. Yap tunes airway epithelial size and architecture by regulating the identity, maintenance, and self-renewal of stem cells. Dev Cell 2014;30(2):151–65.

36. Mahoney JE, Mori M, Szymaniak AD, et al. The hippo pathway effector Yap controls patterning and differentiation of airway epithelial progenitors. Dev Cell 2014; 30(2):137–50.

37. Li C, Xiao J, Hormi K, et al. Wnt5a participates in distal lung morphogenesis. Dev Biol 2002;248(1):68–81.

38. Munakata M, Ohe M, Homma Y, et al. Pulmonary dysanapsis, methacholine airway responsiveness and sensitization to airborne antigen. Respirology 1997; 2(2):113–8.

39. Kauffmann F. Sex-specific dysanapsis and the effect of passive smoking among asthmatics. Pediatrics 1990;86(4):646–7.

40. Mead J. Dysanapsis in normal lungs assessed by the relationship between maximal flow, static recoil, and vital capacity. Am Rev Respir Dis 1980;121(2): 339–42.

41. Alanis DM, Chang DR, Akiyama H, et al. Two nested developmental waves demarcate a compartment boundary in the mouse lung. Nat Commun 2014;5:3923.

42. Schulz MH, Pandit KV, Lino Cardenas CL, et al. Reconstructing dynamic microRNA-regulated interaction networks. Proc Natl Acad Sci U S A 2013; 110(39):15686–91.

43. Cuna A, Halloran B, Faye-Petersen O, et al. Alterations in gene expression and DNA methylation during murine and human lung alveolar septation. Am J Respir Cell Mol Biol 2015;53(1):60–73.

44. Wert SE, Deutsch GH, Pan H. A comprehensive anatomical ontology for the developing lung, in American Thoracic Society international conference. Denver May 15-20, 2015.

45. McGrath-Morrow SA, Lauer T, Collaco JM, et al. Transcriptional responses of neonatal mouse lung to hyperoxia by Nrf2 status. Cytokine 2014;65(1):4–9.

46. Wagenaar GT, ter Horst SA, van Gastelen MA, et al. Gene expression profile and histopathology of experimental bronchopulmonary dysplasia induced by prolonged oxidative stress. Free Radic Biol Med 2004;36(6):782–801.

47. Bhattacharya S, Zhou Z, Yee M, et al. The genome-wide transcriptional response to neonatal hyperoxia identifies Ahr as a key regulator. Am J Physiol Lung Cell Mol Physiol 2014;307(7):L516–23.

48. De Paepe ME, Greco D, Mao Q. Angiogenesis-related gene expression profiling in ventilated preterm human lungs. Exp Lung Res 2010;36(7):399–410.

49. Bhattacharya S, Go D, Krenitsky DL, et al. Genome-wide transcriptional profiling reveals connective tissue mast cell accumulation in bronchopulmonary dysplasia. Am J Respir Crit Care Med 2012;186(4):349–58.

50. Das KC, Wasnick JD. Biphasic response of checkpoint control proteins in hyperoxia: exposure to lower levels of oxygen induces genome maintenance genes in experimental baboon BPD. Mol Cell Biochem 2014;395(1–2):187–98.

51. Pietrzyk JJ, Kwinta P, Wollen EJ, et al. Gene expression profiling in preterm infants: new aspects of bronchopulmonary dysplasia development. PLoS One 2013;8(10):e78585.

52. Zhang X, Peng W, Zhang S, et al. MicroRNA expression profile in hyperoxia-exposed newborn mice during the development of bronchopulmonary dysplasia. Respir Care 2011;56(7):1009–15.

53. Wu YT, Chen WJ, Hsieh WS, et al. MicroRNA expression aberration associated with bronchopulmonary dysplasia in preterm infants: a preliminary study. Respir Care 2013;58(9):1527–35.

54. Yang Y, Qiu J, Kan Q, et al. MicroRNA expression profiling studies on bronchopulmonary dysplasia: a systematic review and meta-analysis. Genet Mol Res 2013;12(4):5195–206.

55. Dong J, Carey WA, Abel S, et al. MicroRNA-mRNA interactions in a murine model of hyperoxia-induced bronchopulmonary dysplasia. BMC Genomics 2012;13: 204.

Postnatal Infections and Immunology Affecting Chronic Lung Disease of Prematurity

Gloria S. Pryhuber, MD[a,b,*]

KEYWORDS

- Prematurity • Neonatal immunology • Neonatal infection • Virus • Lymphocytes
- Bronchopulmonary dysplasia • Chronic lung disease of prematurity • Preterm

KEY POINTS

- In the first year of life, preterm infants are rehospitalized twofold to fivefold times more frequently than infants born at term, primarily for respiratory symptoms.
- Mediators of inflammation tend to enhance lung maturation but impair alveolar septation and developmental vascular remodeling.
- The developmental age of the immune system at birth, and at early-age infections, may significantly alter the acute response, and the sequelae, to inflammatory stimuli.
- Prenatal and postnatal infection and immune responses contribute to the severity of chronic lung disease of prematurity.

INTRODUCTION

Each year, approximately 1 in 9 infants in the United States, more than 440,000 infants yearly, are born prematurely (<37 weeks gestation).[1] These infants suffer from complications of exposure to a diverse environment at a time in development when the respiratory tract and immune system are intended to be protected and maintained in a relatively naïve intrauterine state. During infancy and early childhood, premature infants suffer significant inflammatory and infectious respiratory morbidities with extended negative consequences for health, quality of life, and health care costs.

Funding Source: Department of Pediatrics, University of Rochester Medical Center, NIH/NHLBI/-NICHD 1U01 HL101813, NIH/NHLBI 1U01 HL122628, NIH/NIAID HHSN272201200005C.
Disclosures: The authors have no conflicts of interest or relevant financial interests to disclose.
[a] Division of Neonatology, Department of Pediatrics, University of Rochester Medical Center, 601 Elmwood Avenue, Box 651, Rochester, NY 14642, USA; [b] Department of Environmental Medicine, University of Rochester Medical Center, 601 Elmwood Avenue, Rochester, NY 14642, USA
* Division of Neonatology, Department of Pediatrics, University of Rochester Medical Center, 601 Elmwood Avenue, Box 651, Rochester, NY 14642.
E-mail address: gloria_pryhuber@urmc.rochester.edu

Clin Perinatol 42 (2015) 697–718
http://dx.doi.org/10.1016/j.clp.2015.08.002
0095-5108/15/$ – see front matter © 2015 Elsevier Inc. All rights reserved.
perinatology.theclinics.com

As compared with approximately 8% of full-term newborns, 17% of late-preterm (LPT, born at 34 0/7–36 6/7 weeks) and 30% to 40% of early preterm infants (EPT, born at <32 weeks) are rehospitalized within the first year of life, most commonly for viral respiratory infections.[2–4] Respiratory infections that are less severe, not requiring hospitalization, are even more common, recurrent and, in total, costly in the very young.[5] The incidence and severity of respiratory tract infections in infants younger than 1 year is attributed at least in part to immune immaturity, a problem magnified by preterm birth and influenced by genetic traits and environmental exposures. Differences in gastrointestinal tract colonization patterns and the development and balance of the intestinal microbiome have been shown to influence immunologic development in full-term infants, and have begun to be evaluated in the premature.[6–8] Viral infections, either subclinical or severe, may also alter immunologic development both directly and by altering the bacterial microflora. Preterm infants are exposed to maternal and hospital-based flora, frequently with additional pressures of antibiotics, indwelling catheters, and tubes, that alter the establishment of diverse, health-promoting microbiota on the skin and respiratory mucosa, as well as in the gastrointestinal tract, and increase the risk of invasive disease with predominant organisms.

Recurrence of respiratory symptoms in the first year of life correlates inversely with gestational age at birth, directly with in utero exposure to inflammation (chorioamnionitis), and with non-white race. The pathogenesis of chronic lung disease of prematurity, bronchopulmonary dysplasia (BPD), has been recently reviewed and is closely correlated with in utero inflammation, oxygen toxicity, ventilator-induced trauma, and prealveolar lung development at birth (**Fig. 1**).[9–11] Premature birth induces a slowing or arrest of lung development that underlies BPD and likely occurs in a spectrum of severity in all prematurely born infants. Perinatal therapeutic and environmental exposures, most notably oxygen exposure and environmental tobacco smoke, have been reproducibly related to chronic respiratory morbidity, independent of mechanical ventilation and

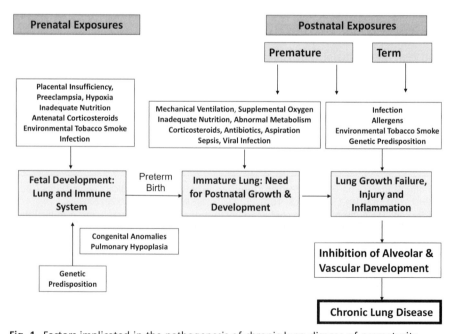

Fig. 1. Factors implicated in the pathogenesis of chronic lung disease of prematurity.

the diagnosis of BPD. A recent study of very low birth weight (VLBW) infants without BPD demonstrated significant relationships between an integrated estimate of oxygen exposure in the first 3 to 14 days of life and symptomatic respiratory disease (SRD) over the first year of life.[12] Lower gestational age, non-white race, greater oxygen exposure, and chorioamnionitis significantly increased the odds ratio of infants having SRD. A recent murine model demonstrated that early neonatal exposure to hyperoxia dramatically increases, in a dose-responsive manner, the severity of influenza infection when induced in adulthood, with markedly enhanced inflammation and fibrotic repair.[9,10] These observations, and an increasing understanding of the preterm infant immune system, as well as their exposures, colonization, and infections with microorganisms, suggest that interventions to modify the immunologic response may significantly improve respiratory and general outcome for these children. This article reviews prenatal and postnatal exposures that induce lung inflammation in preterm infants in the context of unique susceptibility factors that occur because of premature delivery.

INFLAMMATION AS A MECHANISM FOR RESPIRATORY MORBIDITY

Several lines of evidence suggest that the inflammatory response of the fetal or premature lung to injury or infection, if not causative of disease, exacerbates the severity of chronic lung disease in infants at risk.[11,13] Recent reviews highlight the current understanding of the role of inflammatory mediators and the immunobiology of BPD.[14–16] Increased levels of proinflammatory mediators in amniotic fluid,[17,18] early tracheal effluents,[19–24] lung tissue,[23] and serum[25,26] of at-risk premature infants support a role for both intrauterine and extrauterine inflammation in the development and severity of BPD. Airway and bronchoalveolar lavage samples demonstrate increased inflammatory cells and multiple proinflammatory mediators in ventilated, oxygen-exposed infants progressing toward BPD.[19–23] Genome-wide expression profiling of BPD lungs, as compared with gestational age–matched controls, identified 159 differentially expressed genes.[27] Pathway analysis identified cell cycle, immunodeficiency signaling, and B-cell development pathways associated with BPD. In addition, of the top 25 differentially expressed gene sets, 9 were related to chymase-expressing mast cells, the presence of which was confirmed by polymerase chain reaction (PCR) and immunohistochemistry. Consistent with active inflammation, the transcription factor, NF-κB, a prototypical regulator of inflammation and cell survival, was elevated in neutrophils and macrophages in preterm infant airways, correlating with the presence of *Ureaplasma urealyticum* and need for prolonged mechanical ventilation.[28] Interestingly, NF-κB activation in fetal lung and fetal lung macrophages has been shown to inhibit airway morphogenesis and activity of fibroblast growth factor 10, a critical factor in lung development, linking inflammation to the growth arrest of the preterm lung.[29,30] Several animal models demonstrate that mediators of inflammation, including endotoxins, tumor necrosis factor α (TNF-α), and transforming growth factor α, enhance lung maturation but also impair alveolar septation and vascular remodeling, and thus contribute to the development of BPD even without frank tissue destruction.[31–33]

Proinflammatory stimuli come from multiple sources in the premature infant both prenatally and after birth. The most common causes are considered next.

PRENATAL INDUCTION OF INFLAMMATION AND RESPIRATORY MORBIDITY
Chorioamnionitis

Once thought to be sterile, modern molecular techniques independent of culture demonstrated that amniotic fluid and placental tissues frequently contain microbes.[34–40] Maternal-fetal inflammation is clinically identified as chorioamnionitis by maternal fever with one or more of maternal/fetal tachycardia, maternal leukocytosis, uterine tenderness, and/or foul amniotic fluid. A recent study, using amniocentesis to sample amniotic fluid of 46 mothers with signs and symptoms of clinical chorioamnionitis, detected microorganisms by culture and/or PCR/mass spectrometry, frequently more than one microbe, in 61%.[41] Fifteen percent had neither inflammation nor infection and 24% had amniotic fluid evidence of inflammation without detectable microorganisms, suggesting other noninfectious causes of clinical symptoms. Of those with clinical chorioamnionitis, 51% to 62% also have histologic evidence of placental inflammation.[41,42] Severity of acute histologic chorioamnionitis has been correlated with amniotic fluid matrix-metalloproteinase-8 and interleukin (IL)-6 levels supporting the presence of active inflammation.[43,44] It is not uncommon, however, to have evidence of acute histologic chorioamnionitis without detectable microorganisms, ranging from 30% to more than 50%. The cause of "sterile inflammation" of the fetal-placental tissues may be noninfectious disease or lack of sensitivity for microbial detection. Inflammatory placental lesions of a more chronic form, characterized by lymphocytes, plasma cells, and macrophages, sometimes eosinophils, also occur in association with preterm birth and recurrent placental failure. Most frequently, these lesions are of unknown etiology.[45]

Chorioamnionitis has been associated with chronic lung disease of prematurity in multiple small series[46] and in focused studies of specific organisms, such as *Ureaplasma*.[47] In experimental models, chorioamnionitis caused by intra-amniotic injections of endotoxin or *Ureaplasma* initially cause fetal lung inflammation followed by persistent low-grade inflammation and evidence of enhanced lung maturation.[48–50] A more aggressive inflammatory response to oxygen or mechanical ventilation in newborns with a history of chorioamnionitis has been suggested in animal models[51] and some clinical reports.[52] The severity of the fetal inflammatory response to infection, as indicated by amniotic fluid IL-6, is inversely related to gestational age, suggesting that more premature infants are at greater risk of inflammatory injury.[44]

The most common organisms isolated from infected amniotic fluid and placentas are *Ureaplasma parvum* and *U urealyticum*. Likewise, it is relatively common to identify these organisms in the bodily fluids of preterm infants. Compelling evidence for an association between pulmonary *Ureaplasma* colonization and BPD in preterm infants has been recently reviewed.[53,54] Further details and discussion of clinical trials for treatment of *Ureaplasma* found in respiratory secretions of preterm infants are reviewed by Viscardi and Kallapur.[55]

However, the role of chorioamnionitis as a risk factor for BPD remains controversial and recently debated.[56,57] Several large studies question the relationship of in utero infection to chronic lung disease. As part of the Extremely Low Gestational Age Newborns (ELGAN) Study, exhaustive placental bacterial cultures were done from deliveries at 23 to 27 weeks of gestation.[58] There was no correlation between placental culture results and the phenotypes of the infants assessed by oxygen need at day of life 14 or the development of BPD. The Canadian Neonatal Network also reported that 3094 infants born at less than 33 weeks' gestation exposed to clinical chorioamnionitis had no increase in the incidence of BPD.[59] Further, Lahra and colleagues[60] reported, using a 13-year experience from Sydney, that a fetal inflammatory response was protective for BPD.

These and other similar studies demonstrate that clinical or culture-proven chorioamnionitis are not good predictors of BPD. Chorioamnionitis/infection has a major association with preterm premature rupture of membranes and preterm labor at early gestations.[61,62] Also, chorioamnionitis is associated with inflammation in lungs of preterm infants soon after birth[63] and causes lung inflammation and altered immune modulation in animal models where the type and duration of fetal exposures can be controlled.[64] Clinically, variation in detection and virulence of causative organisms, as well as in the duration of infection and the maternal-fetal inflammatory response, complicates the determination of effect on outcomes. The assessment of influence on preterm infant chronic lung disease is further confounded by the imprecise diagnosis of BPD.[65]

Other Prenatal Proinflammatory Exposures

As outlined in **Fig. 1**, there are a number of other maternal-fetal-placental abnormalities that alter lung growth and/or induce fetal inflammation. The association of maternal preeclampsia, placental insufficiency, and associated intrauterine growth restriction with BPD, however, remains controversial, with some studies suggesting increased and others decreased or no effect.[66–72] Antenatal corticosteroids enhance fetal lung maturation and likely reduce inflammation but, although one study suggested that corticosteroids reduced BPD in those with histologic chorioamnionitis, overall they have had little effect on rates of BPD.[73]

POSTNATAL INDUCTION OF INFLAMMATION AND RESPIRATORY MORBIDITY

Many exposures in the postnatal period promote inflammation.[52]

Oxygen and Mechanical Ventilation

Both oxygen and mechanical ventilation, together and independently, induce inflammation via direct cellular injury, induction of cytokines and chemokines, recruitment of neutrophils and macrophages, and oxidation of DNA, lipids, and proteins. Oxygen toxicity and barotrauma or volutrauma are important hazards of mechanical ventilation that are associated with the release of inflammatory cytokines and chemokines that cause pulmonary injury.[74] Higher levels of cytokines correlate with more prolonged duration of ventilation.[74] Supplemental oxygen also contributes to inflammation through biochemical pathways of oxidant stress.[75–77]

Bacterial Infection and Sepsis

Sepsis beyond the first days of life is frequent in extremely low birthweight (ELBW) infants at risk of BPD and often presents with respiratory instability.[60] Both early and late microbial presence in neonatal lung fluid samples was significantly associated with the development of chronic lung disease, suggesting that both antenatal and postnatal infection play a role in the development of disease.[24] Numerous studies associate postnatal sepsis, both early-onset and late-onset and typically with common infectious agents, such as coagulase-negative *Staphylococcus* and gram-negative bacteria, with BPD, suggesting that sepsis-induced inflammation compromises lung development and healing.[52,78–82] Administration of intravenous immunoglobulin, however, although associated with a small reduction in sepsis, was not shown by meta-analysis of randomized controlled trials to reduce the incidence of BPD.[83]

Viral Infections

Broad respiratory virus surveillance in the neonatal intensive care unit (NICU) is a relatively new approach augmented by more readily available culture-independent methods of detection. Previous NICU viral studies targeted patients with threshold symptoms. With this approach, small pandemics of viral infection, such as with adenovirus or respiratory syncytial virus (RSV) were detected, but the overall infection rate in

NICUs appeared relatively low.[84] As example, using a symptom-based testing strategy, viral infection was confirmed in 51 (1%) of 5396 infants admitted to the NICU; of these, 20 (39%) had an enterovirus/*Parechovirus* infection, 15 (29%) RSV, 5 (10%) rotavirus, 3 (6%) cytomegalovirus (CMV), 2 (4%) adenovirus, 2 (4%) parainfluenza virus, 2 (4%) herpes simplex virus, 1 (2%) rhinovirus, and 1 (2%) rubella virus.[85]

Recent data, including that from our collection of expedited autopsy human neonatal distal lung tissue, suggest a relatively high prevalence of lung viral infections in those who succumb to respiratory failure in the NICU; 21 of 63 samples tested were virus positive (Ref.[86] and data not shown). Coronavirus, rhinovirus, parainfluenza, and CMV were detected by reverse-transcriptase PCR (RT-PCR). Interestingly, in this small postmortem sample, RSV, influenza A and B, parainfluenza type 1, and metapneumovirus were not detected.

Surveillance studies using PCR and genomic sequencing for detection have begun to report a closer to true incidence of nosocomial viral respiratory infections (NVRI) in neonates and children hospitalized in pediatric intensive care units and NICUs. In a NICU surveillance study, nasal brush samples were taken weekly from all neonates (age ≤28 days) and children (age >28 days) hospitalized through a winter viral season. Of a total of 120 patients enrolled (64 neonates and 56 children), 20 patients were virus positive by PCR (incidence 16.7%). Seven positive samples for human coronaviruses were detected (incidence 11%). Risk factors for NVRI in the neonates were duration of hospitalization, antibiotic treatment, and duration of parenteral nutrition ($P<.01$).[87]

A 1-year NICU surveillance study of infants born at less than 33 weeks' gestation, using PCR detection of 17 viral subtypes, identified at least one positive respiratory virus during the hospitalization in 26 of 50 subjects, most asymptomatic. Testing positive was associated with longer length of stay and length of mechanical ventilation, as well as diagnosis of BPD. Similar ongoing studies should determine if viral infection is such a common occurrence in the NICU as to warrant more frequent surveillance and development of interventions to reduce exposure and illness.

Neonatal Cytomegalovirus

Human CMV, a Betaherpesvirinae virus, latent in leukocytes, is highly prevalent in the human population; approximately 50% of adults are CMV seropositive and 60% of mothers of preterm infants. Congenital, in utero, infection of the fetus occurs in 0.1% to 2.0% of all pregnancies and may arise through primary infection of the mother, reactivation during pregnancy of a latent infection or reinfection with a different strain of CMV. Postnatal, the virus is spread even more efficiently from mother to the newborn via breastmilk. Because it reactivates in 95% or more of CMV-seropositive women in the postpartum period and can be detected in breastmilk as early as 3.5 days after delivery, CMV is a relatively common viral infection of the newborn period.[88] Transmission to full-term newborns is reported in approximately 40%, whereas in preterm infants it varies from 6% to 55%, potentially due to differing strains, use of fresh/frozen milk, and maternal factors affecting viral shedding.[88] A surveillance study of 175 NICU neonates, testing serum CMV-titers and CMV-DNA, demonstrated an overall prevalence of CMV of 12.6%. Ten (5.71%) of the infants had congenital infection, whereas 12 cases (6.86%) had perinatal infection.[89] Postnatal infection in the newborn can be detected by molecular diagnostics as early as 12 days of life. Infection remains clinically silent in most, but 9% to 12% of postnatally infected low birth weight preterm infants have been reported to demonstrate severe, sepsislike infection.[90] Although infants at lower gestational age are at increased risk of developing symptoms with postnatal infection and are also at greatest risk of BPD, there remains relatively little evidence of cause and effect. Prosch and colleagues[91] found approximately 29% of VLBW infants with BPD to be CMV positive, but 12% of those without BPD. This study and others have found postnatal infection symptoms in preterms to be transient and to have no effect on neonatal outcome including BPD or necrotizing enterocolitis.[92,93] A review of PubMed articles describing CMV pneumonitis, however, concludes that CMV infection can be protracted with diffuse interstitial pneumonitis associated with fibrosis and BPD.[94] It would appear that more surveillance and outcome studies are needed to determine if a causative relationship exists and if anti-CMV therapy or methods to reduce transmission of CMV to the fetus and neonates could effectively reduce disease.

Interestingly, CMV has a notable influence on the human immune system inducing a substantial cytolytic CD8+ T-cell population.[95] CMV infection in infants induces the differentiation of not only phenotypically mature cells, but also functionally active cells that produce interferon gamma (IFN-γ) on restimulation.[96] Serum cytokine concentrations measured in CMV congenitally infected infants show evidence of a strong Th1 bias with a predominance of IFN-γ, IL-2, IL-12, and IL-8 production and diminished IL-4.[97] Because the generation of IFN-γ secreting T cells and CD8+ effector cells is associated with successful recovery from viral infections in general and RSV in particular, such data suggest that CMV infection in infancy could be beneficial. There is, however, concern that CMV-induced immuno-ageing of lymphocytes may ultimately result in immunosuppression suggested by poor vaccine response in the elderly.[98]

Respiratory Syncytial Virus and Other Common Viruses

Recurrent wheezing in later childhood has been associated with infections with RSV, metapneumovirus (hMPV), parainfluenza (PIV), rhinovirus, and human coronavirus NL63.[99–103] RSV infections have best demonstrated that effects of viral respiratory tract infections in infancy may be long-lived. In premature infants born at less than 32 weeks' gestation, with and without BPD, those with a history of RSV lower respiratory tract infection (LRTI) were found to have more days of cough and wheeze at 1 year of age than those without RSV LRTI.[104] Additionally, those with RSV LRTI and hMPV LRTI were found to have increased airway resistance at 1 year of age on pulmonary function testing.[102] In some infants, airway function has been shown to deteriorate during the first years of life.[105] When the group with BPD was followed up at school entry, those who had been hospitalized with RSV LRTI or another respiratory illness within the first 2 years of life had a greater cumulative number of outpatient visits and costs of care compared with former premature infants with BPD without a respiratory hospitalization.[106] A subset of these children with pulmonary function testing at 8 to 10 years of age demonstrated significantly reduced lung function (lower forced expiratory volume in 0.75 s [FEV0.75], FEV0.75/forced vital capacity, and flows at 50% and 75% of vital capacity) in those with an RSV LRTI compared with children without. Whether viral LRTIs cause subsequent airway disease or are merely markers for preexisting abnormal lung function has not been definitively determined.[101] The role of atopy, predisposition to asthma, and postinfection airway remodeling in relationship to LRTI and subsequent wheezing in childhood is also not clear.[101,107] A combination of viral factors and innate and adaptive immune responses, in the setting of a susceptible genetic background and a young or elderly host appear to drive clinical outcome.[108,109] An ongoing study of premature infants and viral LRTIs, including baseline pulmonary function testing, seeks to determine if the viral respiratory infection is causal of the increased long-term morbidity or merely a marker for children with more severe preexisting lung disease, as has been suggested for term infants (ClinicalTrials.gov NCT01789268). This question is important when evaluating selective vaccine strategies to prevent severe LRTI and chronic disease.

SUSCEPTIBILITY FACTORS FOR ENHANCED INFLAMMATION

The immune system is a double-edged sword: too little response and microbes invade and injure, too robust a host response may result in bystander injury and disease. In addition to exposure to infectious agents, there appear to be certain intrinsic factors that result in enhanced inflammatory responses in some individuals as adult, child, or preterm infant, when compared with others. There is evidence to suggest that preterm infants may be affected by both relative immunosuppression and more robust immune responses than full-term infants. We conclude this article with a review of susceptibility factors identified or suggested to enhance inflammation in the prematurely born.

Genetics

Genetics that predispose to shortened pregnancy, especially if related to increased inflammation, naturally increase the risk of inflammatory lung disease of prematurity. For example, elevated mid-trimester vaginal IL-1β is associated with increased risk for spontaneous preterm birth. Homozygous carriers of IL1RN*1, a single nucleotide polymorphism (SNP) in the IL-1 receptor antagonist (IL-1ra) gene, a genotype associated with elevated IL-1β, are at increased risk for preterm birth and an example of genetic polymorphisms that affect the innate immune system and risks of prematurity.[110] In women who had a preterm birth, the combination of clinical chorioamnionitis and IL-10 (-1082)*G allele was associated with an increased risk for delivery before 29 weeks' gestation, suggesting a gene-environment interaction.[111]

In infants, twin studies suggest significant genetic susceptibility to BPD.[112] Relative to inflammation, genotype analysis, after multiple comparisons correction, revealed 2 significant SNPs, rs3771150 (IL-18RAP) and rs3771171 (IL-18R1), in African American individuals with BPD (vs African American individuals without BPD; q <0.05). No associations with Caucasian BPD, African American or Caucasian respiratory distress syndrome (RDS), or prematurity in either African American or Caucasian individuals were identified with these SNPs.[113] Functional polymorphisms in the promoter of NFKBIA that encodes IκBα, a negative regulator of NF-κB, is associated with differential susceptibility to severe bronchopulmonary dysplasia, as well as other common inflammatory diseases of infant lung.[114] A number of additional studies, evaluating exome sequencing in extremes of disease, epigenomic regulation, transcriptome responses to exposures such as hyperoxia, and pathway analyses are ongoing to identify gene and gene regulatory susceptibility factors involved in pathogenesis of BPD.[115–125]

Alterations in Immune Responses Due to Developmental Window of Preterm Delivery

Recent developments in miniaturization of technologies, including assays based on polychromatic flow cytometry, multiplexed protein assays, and low-input transcriptional analyses, have begun to advance the field of neonatal immunology. Dowling and Levy[126] provide a recent review of both in vivo and in vitro approaches to studying early-life immuno-development, as well as a summary of unique characteristics of the preterm and term innate and adaptive immune systems.

The innate immune responses of full-term infants, including the function and recruitment of granulocytes, natural killer (NK) cells, and antigen-presenting cells are characterized as immature and functionally suppressed.[126] Innate immune responses in human preterm infants have been less well characterized.[127,128] Fetal cells, including NK cells, have enhanced sensitivity to the immuno-suppressive effects of transforming growth factor beta.[129] Early-life antigen-presenting cells tend to produce more IL-6, IL-10, and IL-27, predominantly immunosuppressive cytokines. Intriguingly, a recent study has in addition suggested that CD71+ nucleated red blood cells (erythroid precursor cells) that are typically increased in fetal blood, especially in pregnancies complicated by placental insufficiency, appear to suppress phagocyte and antigen-presenting cell stimulus-induced TNF-α production suggesting an immunosuppressive function.[127]

Lymphocytes and the adaptive immune system provide a critical defense against intracellular, including viral, infections. Reduced CD4+ T cells result in impaired immune response to pathogens. CD8+ T cells and NK cells provide protection from viral infection but also contribute to immunopathology by contact-dependent effector functions (eg, perforin and FasL). IFN-γ and, particularly, TNF-α are thought to be primary perpetrators of T-cell–mediated lung injury, yet are also important for antimicrobial defense.[130]

The fetal and neonatal periods are unique immune developmental stages in which adaptive responses are highly plastic and dependent on gestational age.[131,132] Although relatively little literature refers to detailed phenotyping of lymphocytic maturation in the prematurely born infant, investigators have numerically evaluated classes of lymphocytes in the human fetus and young child. The total circulating white cell counts increase through the latter half of gestation until term delivery and then decrease slightly to adult levels. The percentage of lymphocytes decreases from approximately 80% at 18 to 36 weeks (median 26 weeks) to 40% at term delivery to 21% in the adult human, based on cord blood sampling at delivery or cordocentesis.[133,134] The proportion of CD3+ cells, however, increases with gestational age and in the presence of an infection. In normal pregnancies, circulating CD4+ T-cell numbers are inversely related to gestational age and the fetal percentage of CD8+ T cells was reduced, increasing before term (9.5%–15.7%) such that CD4+/CD8+ ratios also vary inversely with gestational age, higher in VLBW infants than full-term.[135,136] Maternal disease may alter fetal lymphocytes. Preeclampsia had a significant effect on T-cell distribution associating with fewer CD4+ cells and CD4+CD8+ double-positive cells, decreased CD4+/CD8+ ratios, reduced Th2 and regulatory T-cell subsets in cord blood, whereas maternal betamethasone therapy also associates with higher CD3+ cell proportion and a lower proportion of NK cells.[137,138]

Evidence for Lymphocytic Abnormalities in Premature Infants with Lung Disease

Several lines of investigation suggest a role for dysregulation of CD4+ responses in BPD. In animal models, T cells accumulate in the lungs of preterm lambs exposed to lipopolysaccharide in utero[139] and preterm baboons that develop BPD were found to have abundant CD4+ T cells in the lung parenchyma.[140] Significant infiltrates of T cells were noted in distal lung of infants who died with BPD as compared with gestational age–matched infants without lung disease.[141] In serial blood samples from premature infants with RDS born 1200 g and less than 30 weeks' gestation, Ballabh and colleagues[142] demonstrated a reduction in absolute lymphocyte count, as well as the percentage and the absolute number of CD4+ T cells, in those who progressed to BPD (*P*<.03), significant even on day 1 of life. More activated T cells in those who go on to develop BPD may reflect sequestration and activation of cells within the lung.[142,143] CD4+ T-cell percentage continued to decrease with postnatal age. Berrington and colleagues[144] measured lymphocyte subclasses in premature infants just before first immunizations. At 7 to 8 weeks of age, prematurely born infants had lower absolute lymphocyte, T-cell, B-cell, and T-helper cell counts, and lower CD4+/CD8+ T-cell ratio, than term infants, as well as increased proportion of T-regulatory (Treg) (CD4+CD25+) cells and decreased CD45RA + naïve cells. By 6 months, the B-cell population had numerically normalized but T-cell abnormalities persisted.

Recent studies have challenged the concept that CD3+ T-cell responses are uniformly impaired in neonates, especially in preterm infants. Although most of the newborn CD4+ T cells are naïve, activation markers like CD25, CD69, and CD45RO+ are enhanced on CD4+ cells of prematurely born infants.[145] Likewise, the proportion of cord blood CD8+ T cells that are CD45RO+, suggesting activation, is also higher at lower gestational age.[146] Several reports now demonstrate a correlation between T-cell activation, as measured by CD45RO expression, and premature infants' adverse outcomes, such as BPD, necrotizing enterocolitis, and periventricular leukomalacia.[25,142,147] CD4+ and CD8+ T cells at lower gestational age are also shown to have enhanced cytokine production with in vitro stimulation, suggesting that enhanced CD45RO expression in preterms is accompanied by inducible effector functions that may contribute to the severity of lung disease.[146,148] A report that regulatory CD4+ T cells (CD4+CD25^{hi}FoxP3+CD127Dim) were significantly reduced in cord blood of preterm infants who developed BPD further raises the potential for enhanced inflammation due to reduced inhibitory control.[148] It has been suggested that the relatively activated CD4+ and CD8+ T-cell phenotype at early gestational ages is reminiscent of recovery from bone marrow ablation in adults and represents rapid homeostatic expansion in a lymphopenic host.[147] Further, intra-amniotic administration of IL-1beta to rhesus monkeys at 80% gestation resulted in reduction in frequency of Treg cells in lymphoid organs, whereas Th17, IL-17A-producing, cells were increased, potentially linking in utero innate immune activity to inflammatory lymphocyte-mediated injury.[149]

Some insight into potential T-cell immunopathology in BPD may be gained from animal and adult models of inflammatory lung disease. In a baboon model of BPD, thymic involution, increased peripheral T cells carrying markers of maturation, robust nonspecific cytokine secretion, and increased autoreactive CD4+ T cells in the lung interstitium, were associated with an increase in bombesin-like peptides (BLP).[140,150] Treatment with a neutralizing antibody to BLP corrected the thymic and lung pathology seen in preterm baboons treated with 100% oxygen.[140] BLP is also elevated in preterm human infants with BPD,[151] suggesting a mechanism linking lymphocyte dysregulation and BPD.

Age at First Infection

The degree of lung and immune system maturation at the time of infection influences cytopathogenic responses to virus and perhaps bacteria but also appears to set a trajectory of immune response to subsequent challenge. Newborn mice infected with RSV have, compared with mice infected at a slightly later age, increased bronchoalveolar lavage fluid numbers of Th2 type CD4+IL-4+ cells and fewer CD4+IFN-γ+ cells when reinfected in adulthood.[152] Likewise, mice infected with influenza A within 1 week of birth showed enhanced airway hyperreactivity, chronic pulmonary inflammation, and diffuse emphysematous-type lesions as adults. An adaptive immune insufficiency was most apparent in the neonatal CD8+ T cells. Newborn infection was associated with reduced and delayed IFN-γ responses as compared with infection in older animals. RSV-infected neonatal mice recruited CD8+ T cells defective in IFN-γ production in association with mild symptoms. Reinfection as adults, however, resulted in limited viral replication but enhanced inflammation and T-cell recruitment, including Th2 cells and eosinophils.[153,154] Depletion of CD8+ T cells (but not CD4) cells during the primary neonatal infection was protective against the adult challenge. Recall responses from neonatal-primed and adult-primed mice were associated with IFN-γ secretion, indicative of a Th1 response. However, IL-4 and IL-5 secretion were enhanced only in neonatal-primed mice. Rechallenge of these mice, primed as newborns, was also associated with increased concentrations of monocyte chemoattractant protein-1 (MCP-1), macrophage inflammatory protein-1α (MIP-1α), and RANTES in the lung. It is suggested then that neonatal T cells, in particular IFN-γ–deficient CD8+ T cells, play a crucial role in regulation of immune responses after neonatal infection. In these neonatal animal models, adoptive transfer of naive CD8+ cells, from wild-type but not from IFN-γ–deficient donors, significantly lowered pulmonary viral titers and greatly improved pulmonary function as adults, supporting the importance of IFN-γ secreting CD8+ T cells in determining disease outcome.[155]

A strong argument has now been advanced that childhood wheezing and atopy are related to reduced cord blood IFN-γ. In a study of infants predisposed to asthma and atopy, less robust mitogen-induced or specific antigen-induced IFN-γ and IL-13 responses from cord blood cells were associated with more wheezing episodes in the first year of life in children infected with RSV and rhinovirus.[156] In the Childhood Origins of Asthma (COAST) Project, cytokine-response profiles of cord blood and 1-year mononuclear cells stimulated in vitro identified that cord blood IFN-γ responses were inversely related to the frequency of viral respiratory infections and wheezing in infancy while enhanced IFN-γ responses at 1 year correlated positively with the frequency of preceding viral infections.[157] Severity of asthma has been associated with excessive IFN-γ production, particularly by CD8+ T cells, potentially reflecting the cytotoxic effect of the cytokine. These data suggest that neonatal IFN-γ responses influence subsequent antiviral activity. Conversely, the frequency of viral infections in infancy can influence IFN-γ responses.

Neutralizing antibodies provide important antiviral protection in infants. Higher RSV neutralizing antibody titers in both premature and term infants are associated with protection from infection and LRTI, an effect also supported by the success of palivizumab in preventing severe RSV disease in premature infants.[158] Transplacental transfer of maternal antibodies is inversely related to length of gestation such that the more preterm infants have relatively less humoral protection contributing to disease risk. Because viral loads of RSV, hMPV, PIV, and rhinovirus correlate with the severity of clinical disease,[159–162] it is suggested that infants with a greater ability to control viral replication on first infection, via the presence of neutralizing antibody and a more robust IFN-γ response, are successful in limiting excessive antigen presentation, generating protective immune responses associated with viral clearance, and avoiding immuno-pathogenesis. To date, no study has evaluated antibody and cellular immune phenotype together with viral load measurements in infants with respiratory infections. Additionally, the association between these factors and disease severity has not been explored in premature infants.

Overall, alterations in lymphocyte-related immunity occur and are dependent on gestational age, maternal influences, postnatal oxidant stress, and viral diseases. There are burgeoning data in this area in premature infants, although as yet minimal knowledge of specific mechanisms by which lymphocytes participate in respiratory outcomes in premature infants.

Altered Establishment of Colonizing Microbiota

A developing body of research suggests that both the acquisition and maintenance of bacterial populations in the gut soon after birth are important drivers of the development of both systemic and mucosal immunity.[7] Recent advances in high-throughput sequencing technology have provided insight into the gut microbiome and are beginning to describe the diversity and dynamics of the microbial populations in both health and disease. Although the exact factors that control the interactions between the gut epithelial cells, the gut-associated lymphoid tissue, and the gut microbiome are not yet clear, all 3 components appear to play a significant role in the induction of immune tolerance to luminal bacterial antigens and the maintenance of homeostasis. Proposed mechanisms identified in animal models include the blocking of innate signaling via Toll-like receptor-4, the development or expansion of Fox P3+ Treg cells, and enhanced IL-10 production in the gut induced by commensal bacteria.[163,164] The presence of specific species of bacteria also may be crucial to the development of gut tolerance as suggested by the relatively decreased amounts of *Bacteroides*, *Bifidobacterium*, and *Lactobacillus* species in patients with inflammatory bowel disease.[7] Additionally, the timing of acquisition of gut bacteria may be critical for the positive effects on health. Neonatal IL-10–deficient mice exposed to bacterial antigens had delayed development of colitis at 18 weeks of age compared with those not exposed. Decreased IFN-γ and IL-17 production in explanted intestinal tissue and spleen cells following stimulation with gut bacteria also suggests that exposure of the neonatal immune system to antigens of the microbiome is associated with both mucosal and systemic immune tolerance.[8] These findings may be especially relevant to the preterm infant in view of recent data showing an inverse relationship between antibiotic therapy and parenteral nutrition with fecal diversity in the infants born at less than 29 weeks' gestation.[165] A recent study in elderly adults also suggests improved protection from influenza infection with oral provision of a *Bifidobacterium longum* species.[166]

Attention has recently turned to determining the microbiome of the respiratory tract in premature infants. The conventional theory that the lower airways are sterile has been challenged by identification of organisms in the deep lung of adults and now infants and children, initially, not surprisingly associated with diseases such as cystic fibrosis, chronic obstructive pulmonary disease, and asthma, but also now as a "normal microbiome" in healthy patients.[167–169] In preterm infants, Lohmann and colleagues[170] described nonsterile tracheal aspirates with a predominance of *Acinetobacter* in samples taken at intubation in the delivery room, and a persistent decrease in diversity of organisms over the first month of life in those who went on to develop BPD. Early sustained airway bacterial colonization in infants less than 1250 g at birth and intubated for at least 3 weeks was detected within 7 days of life, dominated by *Staphylococcus* and *Ureaplasma*.[171] Ongoing studies promise further longitudinal intestinal and respiratory microbiome and viral infection data and correlations to respiratory outcomes in preterm and full-term infants (Clinicaltrials.gov: NCT01607216 and NCT01789268, funding U01HL101813 and HHSN272201200005C, respectively).

That the microbes, the bacteria, viruses, fungi, and others, that flourish on human skin and mucosa affect the metabolism, immune system, health, and disease of their host is becoming more clear. Just what those effects are in the premature infant and how they affect susceptibility to infections and alter respiratory outcomes is an important area of current research.

REFERENCES

1. Martin JA, Hamilton BE, Osterman MJ, et al. Births: final data for 2013. Natl Vital Stat Rep 2015;64(1):1–65.
2. McLaurin KK, Hall CB, Jackson EA, et al. Persistence of morbidity and cost differences between late-preterm and term infants during the first year of life. Pediatrics 2009;123(2):653–9.
3. Gunville CF, Sontag MK, Stratton KA, et al. Scope and impact of early and late preterm infants admitted to the PICU with respiratory illness. J Pediatr 2010; 157(2):209–14.e1.
4. Underwood MA, Danielsen B, Gilbert WM. Cost, causes and rates of rehospitalization of preterm infants. J Perinatol 2007;27(10):614–9.
5. Wade KC, Lorch SA, Bakewell-Sachs S, et al. Pediatric care for preterm infants after NICU discharge: high number of office visits and prescription medications. J Perinatol 2008;28(10):696–701.
6. Dimmitt RA, Staley EM, Chuang G, et al. Role of postnatal acquisition of the intestinal microbiome in the early development of immune function. J Pediatr Gastroenterol Nutr 2010;51(3):262–73.
7. Conroy ME, Shi HN, Walker WA. The long-term health effects of neonatal microbial flora. Curr Opin Allergy Clin Immunol 2009;9(3):197–201.
8. Sydora BC, McFarlane SM, Doyle JS, et al. Neonatal exposure to fecal antigens reduces intestinal inflammation. Inflamm Bowel Dis 2011;17(4): 899–906.
9. O'Reilly MA, Marr SH, Yee M, et al. Neonatal hyperoxia enhances the inflammatory response in adult mice infected with influenza A virus. Am J Respir Crit Care Med 2008;177(10):1103–10.
10. Maduekwe ET, Buczynski BW, Yee M, et al. Cumulative neonatal oxygen exposure predicts response of adult mice infected with influenza A virus. Pediatr Pulmonol 2014. [Epub ahead of print].
11. Speer CP. New insights into the pathogenesis of pulmonary inflammation in preterm infants. Biol Neonate 2001;79(3–4):205–9.
12. Stevens TP, Dylag A, Panthagani I, et al. Effect of cumulative oxygen exposure on respiratory symptoms during infancy among VLBW infants without bronchopulmonary dysplasia. Pediatr Pulmonol 2010;45(4):371–9.
13. Jobe AH, Ikegami M. Mechanisms initiating lung injury in the preterm. Early Hum Dev 1998;53(1):81–94.
14. Viscardi RM. Perinatal inflammation and lung injury. Semin Fetal Neonatal Med 2012;17(1):30–5.
15. Bhandari V. Postnatal inflammation in the pathogenesis of bronchopulmonary dysplasia. Birth Defects Res A Clin Mol Teratol 2014;100(3):189–201.
16. Ryan RM, Ahmed Q, Lakshminrusimha S. Inflammatory mediators in the immunobiology of bronchopulmonary dysplasia. Clin Rev Allergy Immunol 2008; 34(2):174–90.
17. Baud O, Emilie D, Pelletier E, et al. Amniotic fluid concentrations of interleukin-1beta, interleukin-6 and TNF-alpha in chorioamnionitis before 32 weeks of gestation: histological associations and neonatal outcome. Br J Obstet Gynaecol 1999;106(1):72–7.
18. Viscardi RM, Muhumuza CK, Rodriguez A, et al. Inflammatory markers in intrauterine and fetal blood and cerebrospinal fluid compartments are associated with adverse pulmonary and neurologic outcomes in preterm infants. Pediatr Res 2004;55(6):1009–17.

19. Kotecha S, Wilson L, Wangoo A, et al. Increase in interleukin (IL)-1 beta and IL-6 in bronchoalveolar lavage fluid obtained from infants with chronic lung disease of prematurity. Pediatr Res 1996;40(2):250–6.
20. Kotecha S, Mildner RJ, Prince LR, et al. The role of neutrophil apoptosis in the resolution of acute lung injury in newborn infants. Thorax 2003;58(11):961–7.
21. Baier RJ, Majid A, Parupia H, et al. CC chemokine concentrations increase in respiratory distress syndrome and correlate with development of bronchopulmonary dysplasia. Pediatr Pulmonol 2004;37(2):137–48.
22. Munshi UK, Niu JO, Siddiq MM, et al. Elevation of interleukin-8 and interleukin-6 precedes the influx of neutrophils in tracheal aspirates from preterm infants who develop bronchopulmonary dysplasia. Pediatr Pulmonol 1997;24(5):331–6.
23. Bose CL, Dammann CE, Laughon MM. Bronchopulmonary dysplasia and inflammatory biomarkers in the premature neonate. Arch Dis Child Fetal Neonatal Ed 2008;93(6):F455–61.
24. Beeton ML, Maxwell NC, Davies PL, et al. Role of pulmonary infection in the development of chronic lung disease of prematurity. Eur Respir J 2011;37(6): 1424–30.
25. Ambalavanan N, Carlo WA, D'Angio CT, et al, Eunice Kennedy Shriver National Institute of Child Health and Human Development Neonatal Research Network. Cytokines associated with bronchopulmonary dysplasia or death in extremely low birth weight infants. Pediatrics 2009;123(4):1132–41.
26. Bose C, Laughon M, Allred EN, et al, Elgan Study Investigators. Blood protein concentrations in the first two postnatal weeks that predict bronchopulmonary dysplasia among infants born before the 28th week of gestation. Pediatr Res 2011;69(4):347–53.
27. Bhattacharya S, Go D, Krenitsky DL, et al. Genome-wide transcriptional profiling reveals connective tissue mast cell accumulation in bronchopulmonary dysplasia. Am J Respir Crit Care Med 2012;186(4):349–58.
28. Cheah FC, Winterbourn CC, Darlow BA, et al. Nuclear factor kappaB activation in pulmonary leukocytes from infants with hyaline membrane disease: associations with chorioamnionitis and *Ureaplasma urealyticum* colonization. Pediatr Res 2005;57(5 Pt 1):616–23.
29. Blackwell TS, Hipps AN, Yamamoto Y, et al. NF-kappaB signaling in fetal lung macrophages disrupts airway morphogenesis. J Immunol 2011;187(5):2740–7.
30. Benjamin JT, Carver BJ, Plosa EJ, et al. NF-kappaB activation limits airway branching through inhibition of Sp1-mediated fibroblast growth factor-10 expression. J Immunol 2010;185(8):4896–903.
31. Jobe AH, Ikegami M. Antenatal infection/inflammation and postnatal lung maturation and injury. Respir Res 2001;2(1):27–32.
32. Le Cras TD, Hardie WD, Deutsch GH, et al. Transient induction of TGF-alpha disrupts lung morphogenesis, causing pulmonary disease in adulthood. Am J Physiol Lung Cell Mol Physiol 2004;287(4):L718–29.
33. Kallapur SG, Bachurski CJ, Le Cras TD, et al. Vascular changes after intra-amniotic endotoxin in preterm lamb lungs. Am J Physiol Lung Cell Mol Physiol 2004;287(6):L1178–85.
34. Combs CA, Gravett M, Garite TJ, et al. Amniotic fluid infection, inflammation, and colonization in preterm labor with intact membranes. Am J Obstet Gynecol 2014;210(2):125.e1–15.
35. Wang X, Buhimschi CS, Temoin S, et al. Comparative microbial analysis of paired amniotic fluid and cord blood from pregnancies complicated by preterm birth and early-onset neonatal sepsis. PLoS One 2013;8(2):e56131.

36. Ardissone AN, de la Cruz DM, Davis-Richardson AG, et al. Meconium microbiome analysis identifies bacteria correlated with premature birth. PLoS One 2014;9(3):e90784.
37. Wassenaar TM, Panigrahi P. Is a foetus developing in a sterile environment? Lett Appl Microbiol 2014;59(6):572–9.
38. Payne MS, Bayatibojakhi S. Exploring preterm birth as a polymicrobial disease: an overview of the uterine microbiome. Front Immunol 2014;5:595.
39. Antony KM, Ma J, Mitchell KB, et al. The preterm placental microbiome varies in association with excess maternal gestational weight gain. Am J Obstet Gynecol 2015;212(5):653.e1–16.
40. Aagaard K, Ma J, Antony KM, et al. The placenta harbors a unique microbiome. Sci Transl Med 2014;6(237):237ra265.
41. Romero R, Miranda J, Kusanovic JP, et al. Clinical chorioamnionitis at term I: microbiology of the amniotic cavity using cultivation and molecular techniques. J Perinat Med 2015;43(1):19–36.
42. Smulian JC, Shen-Schwarz S, Vintzileos AM, et al. Clinical chorioamnionitis and histologic placental inflammation. Obstet Gynecol 1999;94(6):1000–5.
43. Kim SM, Romero R, Park JW, et al. The relationship between the intensity of intra-amniotic inflammation and the presence and severity of acute histologic chorioamnionitis in preterm gestation. J Matern Fetal Neonatal Med 2014;1–10.
44. Romero R, Miranda J, Chaemsaithong P, et al. Sterile and microbial-associated intra-amniotic inflammation in preterm prelabor rupture of membranes. J Matern Fetal Neonatal Med 2014;1–16.
45. Katzman PJ. Chronic inflammatory lesions of the placenta. Semin Perinatol 2015;39(1):20–6.
46. Watterberg KL, Demers LM, Scott SM, et al. Chorioamnionitis and early lung inflammation in infants in whom bronchopulmonary dysplasia develops. Pediatrics 1996;97:210–5.
47. Viscardi RM, Hasday JD. Role of *Ureaplasma* species in neonatal chronic lung disease: epidemiologic and experimental evidence. Pediatr Res 2009;65(5 Pt 2):84R–90R.
48. Kallapur SG, Moss JTM, Newnham JP, et al. Recruited inflammatory cells mediate endotoxin-induced lung maturation in preterm fetal lambs. Am J Respir Crit Care Med 2005;172:1315–21.
49. Moss TJM, Knox CL, Kallapur SG, et al. Experimental amniotic fluid infection in sheep; effects of *Ureaplasma parvum*. Am J Obstet Gynecol 2008;198(1):122.e1–8.
50. Willet KE, Jobe AH, Ikegami M, et al. Antenatal endotoxin and glucocorticoid effects on lung morphometry in preterm lambs. Pediatr Res 2000;48:782–8.
51. Ikegami M, Jobe A. Postnatal lung inflammation increased by ventilation of preterm lambs exposed antenatally to *E. coli* endotoxin. Pediatr Res 2002;52:356–62.
52. Van Marter LJ, Dammann O, Allred EN, et al. Chorioamnionitis, mechanical ventilation, and postnatal sepsis as modulators of chronic lung disease in preterm infants. J Pediatr 2002;140(2):171–6.
53. Lowe J, Watkins WJ, Edwards MO, et al. Association between pulmonary *Ureaplasma* colonization and bronchopulmonary dysplasia in preterm infants: updated systematic review and meta-analysis. Pediatr Infect Dis J 2014;33(7):697–702.
54. Kallapur SG, Kramer BW, Jobe AH. Ureaplasma and BPD. Semin Perinatol 2013;37(2):94–101.

55. Viscardi RM, Kallapur SG. Role of Ureaplasma Respiratory Tract Colonization in Bronchopulmonary Dysplasia Pathogenesis-Current Concepts and Update. Clin Perinatol 2015, in press.
56. Lacaze-Masmonteil T. That chorioamnionitis is a risk factor for bronchopulmonary dysplasia–the case against. Paediatr Respir Rev 2014;15(1):53–5.
57. Thomas W, Speer CP. Chorioamnionitis is essential in the evolution of bronchopulmonary dysplasia–the case in favour. Paediatr Respir Rev 2014;15(1):49–52.
58. Laughon M, Allred EN, Bose C, et al. Patterns of respiratory disease during the first 2 postnatal weeks in extremely premature infants. Pediatrics 2009;123(4):1124–31.
59. Soraisham AS, Singhal N, McMillan DD, et al. A multicenter study on the clinical outcome of chorioamnionitis in preterm infants. Am J Obstet Gynecol 2009;200(4):372.e1–6.
60. Lahra MM, Beeby PJ, Jeffery HE. Intrauterine inflammation, neonatal sepsis, and chronic lung disease: a 13-year hospital cohort study. Pediatrics 2009;123(5):1314–9.
61. Goldenberg RL, Hauth JC, Andrews WW. Intrauterine infection and preterm delivery. N Engl J Med 2000;342(20):1500–7.
62. Stimac M, Juretic E, Vukelic V, et al. Effect of chorioamnionitis on mortality, early onset neonatal sepsis and bronchopulmonary dysplasia in preterm neonates with birth weight of <1,500 grams. Coll Antropol 2014;38(1):167–71.
63. Watterberg KL, Scott SM, Naeye RL. Chorioamnionitis, cortisol, and acute lung disease in very low birth weight infants. Pediatrics 1997;99:E6.
64. Kramer BW, Ikegami M, Moss TJ, et al. Endotoxin-induced chorioamnionitis modulates innate immunity of monocytes in preterm sheep. Am J Respir Crit Care Med 2005;171(1):73–7.
65. Maitre NL, Ballard RA, Ellenberg JH, et al, Prematurity and Respiratory Outcomes Program Investigators. Respiratory consequences of prematurity: evolution of a diagnosis and development of a comprehensive approach. J Perinatol 2015;35(5):313–21.
66. Vinnars MT, Nasiell J, Holmstrom G, et al. Association between placental pathology and neonatal outcome in preeclampsia: a large cohort study. Hypertens Pregnancy 2014;33(2):145–58.
67. Yen TA, Yang HI, Hsieh WS, et al, Taiwan Premature Infant Developmental Collaborative Study Group. Preeclampsia and the risk of bronchopulmonary dysplasia in VLBW infants: a population based study. PLoS One 2013;8(9):e75168.
68. Lees C, Marlow N, Arabin B, et al. Perinatal morbidity and mortality in early-onset fetal growth restriction: cohort outcomes of the trial of randomized umbilical and fetal flow in Europe (TRUFFLE). Ultrasound Obstet Gynecol 2013;42(4):400–8.
69. Eriksson L, Haglund B, Odlind V, et al. Prenatal inflammatory risk factors for development of bronchopulmonary dysplasia. Pediatr Pulmonol 2014;49(7):665–72.
70. Ozkan H, Cetinkaya M, Koksal N. Increased incidence of bronchopulmonary dysplasia in preterm infants exposed to preeclampsia. J Matern Fetal Neonatal Med 2012;25(12):2681–5.
71. O'Shea JE, Davis PG, Doyle LW, Victorian Infant Collaborative Study Group. Maternal preeclampsia and risk of bronchopulmonary dysplasia in preterm infants. Pediatr Res 2012;71(2):210–4.
72. Mestan KK, Check J, Minturn L, et al. Placental pathologic changes of maternal vascular underperfusion in bronchopulmonary dysplasia and pulmonary hypertension. Placenta 2014;35(8):570–4.

73. Ahn HM, Park EA, Cho SJ, et al. The association of histological chorioamnionitis and antenatal steroids on neonatal outcome in preterm infants born at less than thirty-four weeks' gestation. Neonatology 2012;102(4):259–64.

74. Jonsson B, Tullus K, Brauner A, et al. Early increase of TNF alpha and IL-6 in tracheobronchial aspirate fluid indicator of subsequent chronic lung disease in preterm infants. Arch Dis Child Fetal Neonatal Ed 1997;77(3):F198–201.

75. Lorch SA, Banks BA, Christie J, et al. Plasma 3-nitrotyrosine and outcome in neonates with severe bronchopulmonary dysplasia after inhaled nitric oxide. Free Radic Biol Med 2003;34(9):1146–52.

76. Varsila E, Pesonen E, Andersson S. Early protein oxidation in the neonatal lung is related to development of chronic lung disease. Acta Paediatr 1995;84(11): 1296–9.

77. Schlenzig JS, Bervoets K, von Loewenich V, et al. Urinary malondialdehyde concentration in preterm neonates: is there a relationship to disease entities of neonatal intensive care? Acta Paediatr 1993;82(2):202–5.

78. Shah J, Jefferies AL, Yoon EW, et al, Canadian Neonatal Network. Risk factors and outcomes of late-onset bacterial sepsis in preterm neonates born at <32 weeks' gestation. Am J Perinatol 2015;32(7):675–82.

79. Landry JS, Menzies D. Occurrence and severity of bronchopulmonary dysplasia and respiratory distress syndrome after a preterm birth. Paediatr Child Health 2011;16(7):399–403.

80. Klinger G, Levy I, Sirota L, et al, Israel Neonatal Network. Outcome of early-onset sepsis in a national cohort of very low birth weight infants. Pediatrics 2010; 125(4):e736–40.

81. Lardon-Fernandez M, Uberos J, Molina-Oya M, et al. Epidemiological factors involved in the development of bronchopulmonary dysplasia in very low birth-weight preterm infants. Minerva Pediatr 2015. [Epub ahead of print].

82. Ivarsson M, Schollin J, Bjorkqvist M. *Staphylococcus epidermidis* and *Staphylococcus aureus* trigger different interleukin-8 and intercellular adhesion molecule-1 in lung cells: implications for inflammatory complications following neonatal sepsis. Acta Paediatr 2013;102(10):1010–6.

83. Ohlsson A, Lacy JB. Intravenous immunoglobulin for preventing infection in preterm and/or low-birth-weight infants. Cochrane Database Syst Rev 2004;(1):CD000361.

84. Faden H, Wynn RJ, Campagna L, et al. Outbreak of adenovirus type 30 in a neonatal intensive care unit. J Pediatr 2005;146(4):523–7.

85. Verboon-Maciolek MA, Krediet TG, Gerards LJ, et al. Clinical and epidemiologic characteristics of viral infections in a neonatal intensive care unit during a 12-year period. Pediatr Infect Dis J 2005;24(10):901–4.

86. Maniscalco WM, Watkins RH, Pryhuber GS, et al. Angiogenic factors and alveolar vasculature: development and alterations by injury in very premature baboons. Am J Physiol Lung Cell Mol Physiol 2002;282(4):L811–23.

87. Gagneur A, Sizun J, Vallet S, et al. Coronavirus-related nosocomial viral respiratory infections in a neonatal and paediatric intensive care unit: a prospective study. J Hosp Infect 2002;51(1):59–64.

88. Meier J, Lienicke U, Tschirch E, et al. Human cytomegalovirus reactivation during lactation and mother-to-child transmission in preterm infants. J Clin Microbiol 2005;43(3):1318–24.

89. Morgan MA, el-Ghany el-SM, Khalifa NA, et al. Prevalence of cytomegalovirus (CMV) infection among neonatal intensive care unit (NICU) and healthcare workers. Egypt J Immunol 2003;10(2):1–8.

90. Maschmann J, Hamprecht K, Dietz K, et al. Cytomegalovirus infection of extremely low-birth weight infants via breast milk. Clin Infect Dis 2001;33(12): 1998–2003.

91. Prosch S, Lienicke U, Priemer C, et al. Human adenovirus and human cytomegalovirus infections in preterm newborns: no association with bronchopulmonary dysplasia. Pediatr Res 2002;52(2):219–24.

92. Neuberger P, Hamprecht K, Vochem M, et al. Case-control study of symptoms and neonatal outcome of human milk-transmitted cytomegalovirus infection in premature infants. J Pediatr 2006;148(3):326–31.

93. Capretti MG, Lanari M, Lazzarotto T, et al. Very low birth weight infants born to cytomegalovirus-seropositive mothers fed with their mother's milk: a prospective study. J Pediatr 2009;154(6):842–8.

94. Coclite E, Di Natale C, Nigro G. Congenital and perinatal cytomegalovirus lung infection. J Matern Fetal Neonatal Med 2013;26(17):1671–5.

95. Kuijpers TW, Vossen MT, Gent MR, et al. Frequencies of circulating cytolytic, CD45RA+CD27-, CD8+ T lymphocytes depend on infection with CMV. J Immunol 2003;170(8):4342–8.

96. Miles DJ, van der Sande M, Jeffries D, et al. Cytomegalovirus infection in Gambian infants leads to profound CD8 T-cell differentiation. J Virol 2007;81(11):5766–76.

97. Hassan J, Dooley S, Hall W. Immunological response to cytomegalovirus in congenitally infected neonates. Clin Exp Immunol 2007;147(3):465–71.

98. Saurwein-Teissl M, Lung TL, Marx F, et al. Lack of antibody production following immunization in old age: association with CD8(+)CD28(-) T cell clonal expansions and an imbalance in the production of Th1 and Th2 cytokines. J Immunol 2002;168(11):5893–9.

99. Lemanske RF Jr, Dick EC, Swenson CA, et al. Rhinovirus upper respiratory infection increases airway hyperreactivity and late asthmatic reactions. J Clin Invest 1989;83(1):1–10.

100. Simoes EA, Carbonell-Estrany X, Rieger CH, et al. The effect of respiratory syncytial virus on subsequent recurrent wheezing in atopic and nonatopic children. J Allergy Clin Immunol 2010;126(2):256–62.

101. Stein RT, Martinez FD. Respiratory syncytial virus and asthma: still no final answer. Thorax 2010;65(12):1033–4.

102. Broughton S, Thomas MR, Marston L, et al. Very prematurely born infants wheezing at follow-up: lung function and risk factors. Arch Dis Child 2007; 92(9):776–80.

103. Lee KK, Hegele RG, Manfreda J, et al. Relationship of early childhood viral exposures to respiratory symptoms, onset of possible asthma and atopy in high risk children: the Canadian Asthma Primary Prevention Study. Pediatr Pulmonol 2007;42(3):290–7.

104. Broughton S, Roberts A, Fox G, et al. Prospective study of healthcare utilisation and respiratory morbidity due to RSV infection in prematurely born infants. Thorax 2005;60(12):1039–44.

105. Jacob SV, Coates AL, Lands LC, et al. Long-term pulmonary sequelae of severe bronchopulmonary dysplasia. J Pediatr 1998;133(2):193–200.

106. Greenough A, Alexander J, Boit P, et al. School age outcome of hospitalisation with respiratory syncytial virus infection of prematurely born infants. Thorax 2009;64(6):490–5.

107. Sigurs N, Aljassim F, Kjellman B, et al. Asthma and allergy patterns over 18 years after severe RSV bronchiolitis in the first year of life. Thorax 2010; 65(12):1045–52.

108. Collins PL, Graham BS. Viral and host factors in human respiratory syncytial virus pathogenesis. J Virol 2008;82(5):2040–55.
109. Graham BS. Biological challenges and technological opportunities for respiratory syncytial virus vaccine development. Immunol Rev 2011;239(1): 149–66.
110. Genc MR, Onderdonk A. Endogenous bacterial flora in pregnant women and the influence of maternal genetic variation. BJOG 2011;118(2):154–63.
111. Kerk J, Dordelmann M, Bartels DB, et al. Multiplex measurement of cytokine/receptor gene polymorphisms and interaction between interleukin-10 (-1082) genotype and chorioamnionitis in extreme preterm delivery. J Soc Gynecol Investig 2006;13(5):350–6.
112. Bhandari V, Bizzarro MJ, Shetty A, et al, Neonatal Genetics Study Group. Familial and genetic susceptibility to major neonatal morbidities in preterm twins. Pediatrics 2006;117(6):1901–6.
113. Floros J, Londono D, Gordon D, et al. IL-18R1 and IL-18RAP SNPs may be associated with bronchopulmonary dysplasia in African-American infants. Pediatr Res 2012;71(1):107–14.
114. Ali S, Hirschfeld AF, Mayer ML, et al. Functional genetic variation in NFKBIA and susceptibility to childhood asthma, bronchiolitis, and bronchopulmonary dysplasia. J Immunol 2013;190(8):3949–58.
115. Wang H, St Julien KR, Stevenson DK, et al. A genome-wide association study (GWAS) for bronchopulmonary dysplasia. Pediatrics 2013;132(2):290–7.
116. Hagood JS. Beyond the genome: epigenetic mechanisms in lung remodeling. Physiology (Bethesda) 2014;29(3):177–85.
117. Park J, Wick HC, Kee DE, et al. Finding novel molecular connections between developmental processes and disease. PLoS Comput Biol 2014;10(5):e1003578.
118. Hoffmann TJ, Shaw GM, Stevenson DK, et al. Copy number variation in bronchopulmonary dysplasia. Am J Med Genet A 2014;164A(10):2672–5.
119. Stouch AN, Zaynagetdinov R, Barham WJ, et al. IkappaB kinase activity drives fetal lung macrophage maturation along a non-M1/M2 paradigm. J Immunol 2014;193(3):1184–93.
120. Lingappan K, Srinivasan C, Jiang W, et al. Analysis of the transcriptome in hyperoxic lung injury and sex-specific alterations in gene expression. PLoS One 2014;9(7):e101581.
121. Sorensen GL, Dahl M, Tan Q, et al. Surfactant protein-D-encoding gene variant polymorphisms are linked to respiratory outcome in premature infants. J Pediatr 2014;165(4):683–9.
122. Bhattacharya S, Zhou Z, Yee M, et al. The genome-wide transcriptional response to neonatal hyperoxia identifies Ahr as a key regulator. Am J Physiol Lung Cell Mol Physiol 2014;307(7):L516–23.
123. Ambalavanan N, Cotten CM, Page GP, et al. Integrated genomic analyses in bronchopulmonary dysplasia. J Pediatr 2015;166(3):531–7.e13.
124. Carrera P, Di Resta C, Volonteri C, et al. Exome sequencing and pathway analysis for identification of genetic variability relevant for bronchopulmonary dysplasia (BPD) in preterm newborns: a pilot study. Clin Chim Acta 2015. [Epub ahead of print].
125. Li J, Yu KH, Oehlert J, et al. Exome sequencing of neonatal blood spots identifies genes implicated in bronchopulmonary dysplasia. Am J Respir Crit Care Med 2015;192(5):589–96.
126. Dowling DJ, Levy O. Ontogeny of early life immunity. Trends Immunol 2014; 35(7):299–310.

127. Levy O. Innate immunity of the newborn: basic mechanisms and clinical correlates. Nat Rev Immunol 2007;7(5):379–90.

128. Hillman NH, Moss TJ, Nitsos I, et al. Toll-like receptors and agonist responses in the developing fetal sheep lung. Pediatr Res 2008;63(4):388–93.

129. Ivarsson MA, Loh L, Marquardt N, et al. Differentiation and functional regulation of human fetal NK cells. J Clin Invest 2013;123(9):3889–901.

130. Bruder D, Srikiatkhachorn A, Enelow RI. Cellular immunity and lung injury in respiratory virus infection. Viral Immunol 2006;19(2):147–55.

131. Adkins B, Leclerc C, Marshall-Clarke S. Neonatal adaptive immunity comes of age. Nat Rev Immunol 2004;4(7):553–64.

132. Marchant A, Goldman M. T cell-mediated immune responses in human newborns: ready to learn? Clin Exp Immunol 2005;141(1):10–8.

133. Zhao Y, Dai ZP, Lv P, et al. Phenotypic and functional analysis of human T lymphocytes in early second- and third-trimester fetuses. Clin Exp Immunol 2002;129(2):302–8.

134. Schultz C, Reiss I, Bucsky P, et al. Maturational changes of lymphocyte surface antigens in human blood: comparison between fetuses, neonates and adults. Biol Neonate 2000;78(2):77–82.

135. Ballow M, Cates KL, Rowe JC, et al. Peripheral blood T-cell subpopulations in the very low birth weight (less than 1,500-g) infant. Am J Hematol 1987;24(1):85–92.

136. Series IM, Pichette J, Carrier C, et al. Quantitative analysis of T and B cell subsets in healthy and sick premature infants. Early Hum Dev 1991;26(2):143–54.

137. Kotiranta-Ainamo A, Apajasalo M, Pohjavuori M, et al. Mononuclear cell subpopulations in preterm and full-term neonates: independent effects of gestational age, neonatal infection, maternal pre-eclampsia, maternal betamethason therapy, and mode of delivery. Clin Exp Immunol 1999;115(2):309–14.

138. Suursalmi P, Kopeli T, Korhonen P, et al. Very low birthweight bronchopulmonary dysplasia survivors show no substantial association between lung function and current inflammatory markers. Acta Paediatr 2015;104(3):264–8.

139. Kuypers E, Collins JJ, Kramer BW, et al. Intra-amniotic LPS and antenatal betamethasone: inflammation and maturation in preterm lamb lungs. Am J Physiol Lung Cell Mol Physiol 2012;302(4):L380–9.

140. Rosen D, Lee JH, Cuttitta F, et al. Accelerated thymic maturation and autoreactive T cells in bronchopulmonary dysplasia. Am J Respir Crit Care Med 2006; 174(1):75–83.

141. Ryan RM, Ahmed Q, D'Angelis CA, et al. CD8+ T-lymphocytes in infants with bronchopulmonary dysplasia (BPD). Pediatric Academic Society; 2009. E-PAS2009: 3858.137. Available at: http://www.abstracts2view.com/pasall/index.php. Accessed September 9, 2015.

142. Ballabh P, Simm M, Kumari J, et al. Lymphocyte subpopulations in bronchopulmonary dysplasia. Am J Perinatol 2003;20(8):465–75.

143. Turunen R, Vaarala O, Nupponen I, et al. Activation of T cells in preterm infants with respiratory distress syndrome. Neonatology 2009;96(4):248–58.

144. Berrington JE, Barge D, Fenton AC, et al. Lymphocyte subsets in term and significantly preterm UK infants in the first year of life analysed by single platform flow cytometry. Clin Exp Immunol 2005;140(2):289–92.

145. Luciano AA, Yu H, Jackson LW, et al. Preterm labor and chorioamnionitis are associated with neonatal T cell activation. PLoS One 2011;6(2):e16698.

146. Scheible KM, Emo J, Yang H, et al. Developmentally determined reduction in CD31 during gestation is associated with CD8+ T cell effector differentiation in preterm infants. Clin Immunol 2015. [Epub ahead of print].

147. Duggan PJ, Maalouf EF, Watts TL, et al. Intrauterine T-cell activation and increased proinflammatory cytokine concentrations in preterm infants with cerebral lesions. Lancet 2001;358(9294):1699–700.
148. Misra RS, Shah S, Fowell DJ, et al. Preterm cord blood CD4(+) T cells exhibit increased IL-6 production in chorioamnionitis and decreased CD4(+) T cells in bronchopulmonary dysplasia. Hum Immunol 2015;76(5):329–38.
149. Kallapur SG, Presicce P, Senthamaraikannan P, et al. Intra-amniotic IL-1beta induces fetal inflammation in rhesus monkeys and alters the regulatory T cell/IL-17 balance. J Immunol 2013;191(3):1102–9.
150. Sunday ME, Yoder BA, Cuttitta F, et al. Bombesin-like peptide mediates lung injury in a baboon model of bronchopulmonary dysplasia. J Clin Invest 1998; 102(3):584–94.
151. Scher H, Miller YE, Aguayo SM, et al. Urinary bombesin-like peptide levels in infants and children with bronchopulmonary dysplasia and cystic fibrosis. Pediatr Pulmonol 1998;26(5):326–31.
152. Culley FJ, Pollott J, Openshaw PJ. Age at first viral infection determines the pattern of T cell-mediated disease during reinfection in adulthood. J Exp Med 2002;196(10):1381–6.
153. Tregoning JS, Yamaguchi Y, Harker J, et al. The role of T cells in the enhancement of respiratory syncytial virus infection severity during adult reinfection of neonatally sensitized mice. J Virol 2008;82(8):4115–24.
154. Tasker L, Lindsay RW, Clarke BT, et al. Infection of mice with respiratory syncytial virus during neonatal life primes for enhanced antibody and T cell responses on secondary challenge. Clin Exp Immunol 2008;153(2):277–88.
155. You D, Ripple M, Balakrishna S, et al. Inchoate CD8+ T cell responses in neonatal mice permit influenza-induced persistent pulmonary dysfunction. J Immunol 2008;181(5):3486–94.
156. Gern JE, Brooks GD, Meyer P, et al. Bidirectional interactions between viral respiratory illnesses and cytokine responses in the first year of life. J Allergy Clin Immunol 2006;117(1):72–8.
157. Friedlander SL, Jackson DJ, Gangnon RE, et al. Viral infections, cytokine dysregulation and the origins of childhood asthma and allergic diseases. Pediatr Infect Dis J 2005;24(11 Suppl):S170–6 [discussion: S174–5].
158. Wang EE, Law BJ, Robinson JL, et al. PICNIC (Pediatric Investigators Collaborative Network on Infections in Canada) study of the role of age and respiratory syncytial virus neutralizing antibody on respiratory syncytial virus illness in patients with underlying heart or lung disease. Pediatrics 1997;99(3):E9.
159. DeVincenzo JP, Wilkinson T, Vaishnaw A, et al. Viral load drives disease in humans experimentally infected with respiratory syncytial virus. Am J Respir Crit Care Med 2010;182(10):1305–14.
160. Houben ML, Coenjaerts FE, Rossen JW, et al. Disease severity and viral load are correlated in infants with primary respiratory syncytial virus infection in the community. J Med Virol 2010;82(7):1266–71.
161. Bosis S, Esposito S, Osterhaus AD, et al. Association between high nasopharyngeal viral load and disease severity in children with human metapneumovirus infection. J Clin Virol 2008;42(3):286–90.
162. Utokaparch S, Marchant D, Gosselink JV, et al. The relationship between respiratory viral loads and diagnosis in children presenting to a pediatric hospital emergency department. Pediatr Infect Dis J 2011;30(2):e18–23.
163. Barnes MJ, Powrie F. Regulatory T cells reinforce intestinal homeostasis. Immunity 2009;31(3):401–11.

164. Biswas A, Wilmanski J, Forsman H, et al. Negative regulation of Toll-like receptor signaling plays an essential role in homeostasis of the intestine. Eur J Immunol 2011;41(1):182–94.
165. Jacquot A, Neveu D, Aujoulat F, et al. Dynamics and clinical evolution of bacterial gut microflora in extremely premature patients. J Pediatr 2011;158(3):390–6.
166. Namba K, Hatano M, Yaeshima T, et al. Effects of *Bifidobacterium longum* BB536 administration on influenza infection, influenza vaccine antibody titer, and cell-mediated immunity in the elderly. Biosci Biotechnol Biochem 2010; 74(5):939–45.
167. Warner BB, Hamvas A. Lungs, microbes and the developing neonate. Neonatology 2015;107(4):337–43.
168. Tracy M, Cogen J, Hoffman LR. The pediatric microbiome and the lung. Curr Opin Pediatr 2015;27(3):348–55.
169. Bisgaard H, Hermansen MN, Bonnelykke K, et al. Association of bacteria and viruses with wheezy episodes in young children: prospective birth cohort study. BMJ 2010;341:c4978.
170. Lohmann P, Luna RA, Hollister EB, et al. The airway microbiome of intubated premature infants: characteristics and changes that predict the development of bronchopulmonary dysplasia. Pediatr Res 2014;76(3):294–301.
171. Mourani PM, Harris JK, Sontag MK, et al. Molecular identification of bacteria in tracheal aspirate fluid from mechanically ventilated preterm infants. PLoS One 2011;6(10):e25959.

Role of *Ureaplasma* Respiratory Tract Colonization in Bronchopulmonary Dysplasia Pathogenesis

Current Concepts and Update

CrossMark

Rose Marie Viscardi, MD[a],*, Suhas G. Kallapur, MD[b]

KEYWORDS

- *Ureaplasma parvum* • *Ureaplasma urealyticum* • Prematurity
- Bronchopulmonary dysplasia • Macrolide antibiotics

KEY POINTS

- Meta-analyses of clinical studies over the past 30 years have confirmed ureaplasma respiratory colonization as an independent risk factor for bronchopulmonary dysplasia (BPD) but have not established causality.
- Experimental infection models in sheep and nonhuman primates have demonstrated that *Ureaplasma* can establish a chronic infection with inflammation in the intrauterine compartment and alter fetal lung development.
- Although *U parvum* serovars are the most commonly isolated serovars from clinical samples, no specific serovar or virulence factor has been identified in association with BPD.
- There is currently insufficient data concerning the benefit/risk ratio of antibiotic therapy to recommend treatment guidelines to prevent BPD in preterm infants at risk for or with confirmed ureaplasma infection.

INTRODUCTION

The mycoplasma species *Ureaplasma parvum* and *U urealyticum* are genitourinary tract commensals in adults but are associated with adverse pregnancy outcomes[1] and neonatal morbidities of prematurity, including bronchopulmonary dysplasia

Conflicts of Interest: None.
Funding: Supported by grants from the Eunice Kennedy Shriver National Institute of Child Health and Human Development R01HD067126 (R.M. Viscardi) and R01HD57869, R01HL97064 (S.G. Kallapur).

[a] Department of Pediatrics, University of Maryland School of Medicine, 110 South Paca Street, 8th Floor, Baltimore, MD 21093, USA; [b] Division of Neonatology, Cincinnati Children's Hospital Medical Center, University of Cincinnati, 3333, Burnet Avenue, Cincinnati, OH 45229, USA
* Corresponding author.
E-mail address: rviscard@umaryland.edu

Clin Perinatol 42 (2015) 719–738
http://dx.doi.org/10.1016/j.clp.2015.08.003
0095-5108/15/$ – see front matter

(BPD),[2] necrotizing enterocolitis,[3] and severe intraventricular hemorrhage.[4] These organisms are the most commonly isolated organisms from infected placentas and amniotic fluid.[1,5] They have been detected in cord blood,[4,6] cerebrospinal fluid,[4] respiratory secretions,[2,7] gastric aspirates,[8] and brain[9] and lung tissue[10] of preterm infants. This review focuses on the epidemiologic and experimental evidence for a causal role of *Ureaplasma* species in BPD pathogenesis and implications for therapeutic interventions.

UREAPLASMA SPECIES

The 14 *Ureaplasma* serovars are grouped in 2 species, *U parvum* (serovars 1, 3, 6, and 14) and *U urealyticum* (serovars 2, 4, 5, and 7–13) (**Box 1**). These organisms are among the smallest free-living, self-replicating cells. They lack cell walls, hydrolyze urea to generate ATP, have limited biosynthetic functions, and adhere to human mucosal surfaces of the genitourinary tract in adults and respiratory tract in newborns.[11] The authors' group and others have recently demonstrated that most *Ureaplasma* isolates from neonatal and adult clinical specimens as well as American Type Culture Collection (ATCC) reference strains have the capacity to form biofilms in vitro.[12,13] If biofilm formation is confirmed in vivo, it may be another mechanism by which *Ureaplasmas* evade the host immune response and increase resistance to antibiotics.

U parvum serovars are the most common serovars detected in neonatal respiratory samples at all gestational ages. In a prospective preterm cohort in a single institution, *U parvum* was detected in 63% of respiratory isolates.[7] Serovars 3 and 6 alone and in combination accounted for 96% of *U parvum* respiratory isolates in this cohort.[7] *U urealyticum* isolates were commonly a mixture of multiple serovars, with serovar 11 alone or combined with other serovars (59%) as the most common serovar. Most studies have not observed differences in prevalence of either species or specific serovars

---

Box 1
Characteristics of genital mycoplasmas isolated from preterm infants

- Two species
  - *U parvum* (serovar 1, 3, 6, and 14)
  - *U urealyticum* (serovars 2, 4, 5, 7–13)
- Small genomes (limited biosynthetic abilities)
- Lack cell walls (susceptible to desiccation and heat)
- Hydrolyze urea to generate ATP
- Biofilm-forming capacity demonstrated in vitro and in vivo[12,13,95]
- *U parvum* serovars most common in clinical specimens (70%)[7]
- Require special transport and culture media to support growth
- Virulence factors
  - Urease production of ammonia
  - IgA protease (degrading mucosal IgA)
  - Hydrogen peroxide (membrane peroxidation)
  - Phospholipases A and C (membrane phospholipid degradation)
  - Inhibition of host cell antimicrobial peptide expression[22]
  - Serine//threonine kinase and protein phosphatase (cytotoxicity)[20]
  - Multiple-banded antigen, major pathogen-associated molecular pattern of *Ureaplasma* serovars recognized by host immune system: size variations evade immune detection[24,53,96]

Abbreviation: IgA, immunoglobulin A.

---

between infants with and without BPD.[7,14] Biofilm-forming capacity of clinical isolates also did not differ between infants with and without BPD.[13] For clinical diagnostic purposes, it is not necessary to determine the species or serovar.

Ureaplasma Species Virulence Factors

Before the advent of genomics, potential ureaplasmal virulence factors including immunoglobulin A protease and phospholipase A1, A2, and C were identified by functional and enzymatic assays.[15,16] However, no matches were found to known sequences for these proteins in any of the 14 ATCC reference *Ureaplasma* serovar genomes (ATCC)[17] or clinical *U parvum* serovar 3 genome.[18] Although not confirmed experimentally to date, ammonia generated by urea hydrolysis may react with water in tissues to form ammonium hydroxide that may contribute to mucosal injury and inflammation.[19] Recently, the sequence of a *U parvum* serovar 3 clinical strain SV3F4 revealed a putative new virulence factor serine/threonine kinase and serine/threonine protein phosphatase (STP).[20] In *Mycoplasma genitalium*, an STP protein is required for host cell cytotoxicity and mutant strains lacking the STP gene produce less hydrogen peroxide than wild-type strains.[21] Recently, Xiao and colleagues[22] demonstrated that *Ureaplasma* spp suppress expression of antimicrobial peptides genes *DEFB1, DEFA5, DEFA6,* and *CAMP* in vitro that may be an additional mechanism by which these organisms avoid the host immune response.

The proposed major ureaplasma virulence factor is the multiple banded antigen (MBA), a surface lipoprotein that is the predominant pathogen-associated molecular pattern (PAMP) detected by the host immune system.[23] The organism may evade host recognition by varying the MBA size.[19,23] In the sheep intrauterine infection model, MBA protein/*mba* gene size variants were detected in infected amniotic fluid and fetal lung with increasing duration of gestation, suggesting that the size variants escaped eradication.[19] However, the MBA size variation did not correlate with chorioamnionitis severity in the sheep model, suggesting that difference in the host immune response may be important in ureaplasma pathogenicity.[24]

Host Response to Ureaplasma Infection

Microbial recognition by innate immune systems can be mediated by a variety of germline-encoded receptors, including Toll-like receptors (TLRs), RIG-like receptors, Nod-like receptors, and cytosolic DNA sensors, such as the HIN200 family member AIM2.[25] *Ureaplasma* spp lack a gram-negative or gram-positive bacterial cell wall, thus are devoid of lipopolysaccharides (LPSs) or peptidoglycans, the microbial products that are potent activators of TR4 (LPS) and the TLR2 or NOD1/2 (peptidoglycan) pathways. Nevertheless, placental leukocytes or neonatal monocytes exposed in vitro to *Ureaplasma* spp induce the release of inflammatory cytokines.[26,27] Shimizu and colleagues[28] showed that *U parvum* lipoproteins, including the MBA, activate nuclear factor-kappa B in reporter cell lines via TLR1, TLR2, and TLR6 signaling. Peltier and colleagues[29] found that the macrophage-stimulating activity from *U urealyticum* is mainly due to lipoproteins, and signaling involves TLR2 or TLR4 receptors. Mechanisms of immune alterations induced by *Ureaplasma* spp in vivo have not been identified. However, ureaplasmas do induce antibody production in both humans and animals.[24,30]

Ureaplasma clearance in the lung depends on local mediators of the host immune response. Surfactant protein A (SP-A) enhances ureaplasmal phagocytosis and killing in vitro.[31] Compared with wild-type mice, SP-A–deficient mice had delayed clearance of *Ureaplasma* from the lungs, increased inflammatory cells, and proinflammatory cytokine expression.[32] This observation may be relevant to preterm fetuses and neonates who will have low levels of SP-A and other innate host defense factors in the lungs.

Observed differences in host susceptibility may be due, in part, to variants in genes regulating the innate immune response, thus altering the risk for *Ureaplasma* spp respiratory colonization and BPD in preterm infants. In a study of single nucleotide polymorphisms (SNP) of TLR genes in a cohort of preterm infants with known ureaplasma respiratory colonization status, 4 SNPs in *TLR2* and *TLR6* were significantly associated with ureaplasma respiratory tract colonization.[33] Interestingly, a *TLR6* SNP (rs5743827) was associated with both a decreased risk for ureaplasma respiratory tract colonization and decreased risk for BPD (odds ratio [OR] = 0.54 [0.34–0.86] and OR = 0.54 [0.31–0.95], respectively). This variant may alter the susceptibility to ureaplasma infection and the severity of the inflammatory response that contributes to the development of BPD.

Another factor that may explain the variability in pathogenicity is immune modulation. Chronic intra-amniotic ureaplasma infection in sheep profoundly diminished the responses to intra-amniotic LPS in the preterm fetal sheep.[34] A benefit of endotoxin tolerance is decreased inflammation in the host and, therefore, decreased organ injury. However, endotoxin tolerance also can increase susceptibility to infections due to suppression of innate immune responses. Thus, several potential microbial factors may play in role in the variability of host responses; but none are known to play a role in clinical infection.

Ureaplasma Species as Perinatal Pathogens Causing Preterm Birth

Intrauterine inflammation is a common cause of preterm labor,[35] and *Ureaplasma* spp are the most common organisms isolated in the amniotic fluid either alone or as a part of a polymicrobial flora.[36,37] Presence of *Ureaplasma* spp in the amniotic fluid is associated with a shorter time from the amniocentesis to delivery time compared with cases whereby *Ureaplasma* was not isolated.[38] At the time of genetic amniocentesis at 15 to 17 weeks' gestation, *Ureaplasma* species were identified in 11% pregnancies with subsequent preterm labor in 59% of *Ureaplasma*-positive women compared with 4% *Ureaplasma*-negative women.[39] Intra-amniotic inoculation of Rhesus macaques with *U parvum* or the related organism *Mycoplasma hominis* induced chorioamnionitis, fetal inflammation, and preterm labor.[40] Thus, perinatal infections from *Ureaplasma* spp are an important cause of preterm labor and delivery. These data also demonstrate the difficulties of reversing ureaplasma-induced pathologies by postnatal treatment because many preterm infants may have been exposed to these organisms antenatally often for prolonged durations.

EPIDEMIOLOGIC EVIDENCE FOR ROLE OF *UREAPLASMA* SPECIES IN BRONCHOPULMONARY DYSPLASIA PATHOGENESIS
Characteristics of Infants with Ureaplasma Respiratory Tract Colonization

The reported incidence of ureaplasma respiratory tract colonization rate in infants with less than 1501-g birthweight ranges from 28% to 33%.[41] In a prospective study, the authors observed that the risk of *Ureaplasma* spp respiratory colonization decreased with increasing gestational age (OR, 0.821; confidence interval [CI], 0.720–0.934).[7] Sixty-five percent of infants less than 26 weeks' gestation were culture or polymerase chain reaction (PCR) positive one or more times during the first month of life compared with 31% of infants 26 or more weeks' or gestational age. As summarized in **Box 2**, infants with respiratory colonization are more likely to be born extremely preterm by vaginal delivery to women with pregnancies complicated by chorioamnionitis and

---

Box 2
Characteristics of infants with *Ureaplasma* spp respiratory tract colonization

- Extreme prematurity
  - Respiratory colonization rate inversely related to gestational age[2]
  - Respiratory colonization rate 65% less than 26 weeks' versus 31% 26 or greater weeks' gestational age[7]
  - Immature innate immune responses
    - SP-A deficiency[31,32]
    - Low expression of relevant TLRs?[97]
- Preterm premature rupture of membreanes[5]
  - Increased vertical transmission with longer-duration ROM[45]
- Evidence for fetal inflammatory response syndrome
  - Histologic chorioamnionitis and fetal vasculitis[43,44]
  - Elevated admission white blood cell count[98]
- Less severe respiratory distress syndrome[47]
- Early radiographic BPD changes[48,99]
- Early lung fibrosis and disordered elastin distribution[49,50,60]

---

preterm labor or preterm premature rupture of membranes.[42–44] The vertical transmission rate increases with a longer duration of membrane rupture.[45] Infants delivered for maternal indications have the lowest rate of respiratory tract colonization.

Postnatally, ureaplasma-colonized infants frequently exhibit peripheral blood leukocytosis[46] and less severe respiratory distress syndrome (RDS)[47] but early radiographic emphysematous changes of BPD.[42,48] In archived autopsy specimens of colonized infants, the authors observed early lung fibrosis, increased number of myofibroblasts, disordered elastin accumulation, and increased number of immunoreactive cells expressing inflammatory mediators tumor necrosis factor alpha and transforming growth factor β1.[49,50]

Association of Ureaplasma Respiratory Tract Colonization and Bronchopulmonary Dysplasia

As summarized in **Table 1**, 3 meta-analyses that include data from more than 4000 infants and more than 40 individual studies have been published to date at approximately 10-year intervals that have assessed the association of ureaplasma respiratory tract colonization and BPD. In the first meta-analysis in 1995, BPD at 28 days (BPD28) was the outcome for all studies, and only 4 of 17 studies were done after exogenous surfactant was available.[51] In 2005, Schelonka and colleagues[52] demonstrated a significant association between ureaplasma respiratory colonization and both BPD28 and 36 weeks' postmenstrual age (BPD36) but noted significant heterogeneity among the studies primarily due to the inclusion of studies with a small sample size. Lowe and colleagues[2] extended the analyses in 2014 to more recent studies and demonstrated persistence of the ureaplasma-BPD association over time and no significant effect of differences in gestational ages between colonized and noncolonized infants on the strength of the association. Interestingly, the studies included in the latest meta-analysis were published over a 25-year span of considerable changes in neonatal care; but there has been no decrease in odds over time in the ureaplasma-BPD association. However, no study to date has used physiologic BPD as an outcome.

Table 1
Association of *Ureaplasma* spp respiratory colonization and BPD28 and BPD36: summary of 3 meta-analyses

Meta-analysis	Years Included in Database Search	Outcomes	Number of Publications	Number of Subjects	RR (95% CI)	What Study Added
Wang et al,[51] 1995	1988–1994	BPD28	17	1479	1.75 (1.5–1.99)	Only 4 out of 17 studies after surfactant available, none with BPD36 outcome
		BPD36	0	N/A	N/A	—
Schelonka et al,[52] 2005	1966–2004	BPD28	23	2216	2.8 (2.3–3.5)	Includes 15 studies 1995–2004
		BPD36	8	751	1.6 (1.1–2.3)	Earlier publication year, sample size <100, reported surfactant use >90%, and endotracheal culture only diagnostic method were associated with higher reported odds of ureaplasma-BPD association
Lowe et al,[2] 2014	1947–2013	BPD28	31	2421	3.04 (2.4–3.8)	Used meta-regression to demonstrate that ureaplasma-BPD28 association persists despite difference in gestational age of colonized and noncolonized infants
		BPD36	17	1599	2.2 (1.4–3.5)	Demonstrates persistence of ureaplasma-BPD36 association over time; no studies reported testing for severity of BPD

Abbreviations: BPD28, BPD at 28 days; BPD36, BPD at 36 weeks' postmenstrual age; N/A, not applicable; RR, relative risk.

Ureaplasma Species and Lung Inflammation in the Developing Lung: Animal Studies

Animal studies lend support to the hypothesis that ureaplasma colonization can lead to lung injury similar to BPD. Intra-amniotic injection of *Ureaplasma* in early gestation sheep resulted in efficient colonization with persistent infection for 3 months to term with very little overt adverse effects in the ewe, consistent with a commensal-like host response[24] (**Fig. 1**). The severity of chorioamnionitis following intra-amniotic injection of *Ureaplasma* was variable, with 10% of sheep not demonstrating any chorioamnionitis despite efficient colonization.[53] These experiments illustrate the complexities in understanding the host response to a ureaplasma exposure.

Recruitment to and activation of inflammatory cells in the fetal lung could be detected as early as 3 days after intra-amniotic injection of live *Ureaplasma* in sheep[54] (**Fig. 2A**). Both monocytes and neutrophils increased, and MHCII expression in the monocytes increased 14 days after intra-amniotic ureaplasma injection, consistent with the maturation of the monocytic cells.[54] The inflammatory cell infiltration was focal in nature, and no areas of consolidation or pneumonia were detected. The inflammatory infiltrate was accompanied by modest increases in the pulmonary expression of the proinflammatory cytokines/chemokines interleukin (IL)-1ß, IL-6, and IL-8 within 1 week that persisted for at least 6 weeks.[55,56]

The modest lung inflammation was followed by the counterintuitive observation of significant increases in lung gas volumes and surfactant lipids in the preterm fetal sheep. This early lung maturation was first detected in the preterm fetal lungs 3 weeks after intra-amniotic ureaplasma injection and persisted for 10 weeks despite continuous exposures[57] (see **Fig. 2B**). Although these striking effects on lung physiology are consistent with clinical lung maturation, they probably represent dysmaturation because the improved lung physiology was accompanied by evidence of impaired lung development.[54] Fourteen days after intra-amniotic ureaplasma injection, preterm fetal sheep delivered at 80% gestation had decreased elastic foci and increased smooth muscle around bronchioles and pulmonary artery/arterioles.[54] These changes in elastin and smooth muscle are similar to those reported for infants with BPD and

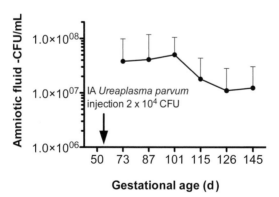

Gestational age (d)

Fig. 1. *Persistent colonization of Ureaplasma in the sheep amniotic compartment.* Pregnant ewes (n = 20) were given intra-amniotic injection of *Ureaplasma parvum* (UP) (2×10^4 colony-forming unit [CFU]) at 55 days' gestational age (term = 150 d). Amniocentesis was done at regular intervals until term gestation, and the amniotic fluid titers of *Ureaplasma* were determined. There was a rapid growth of UP, and the titers persisted until term gestation demonstrating poor clearance of UP. IA, intraamniotic. (*Data from* Dando SJ, Nitsos I, Kallapur SG, et al. The role of the multiple banded antigen of Ureaplasma parvum in intra-amniotic infection: major virulence factor or decoy? PLoS One 2012;7:e29856.)

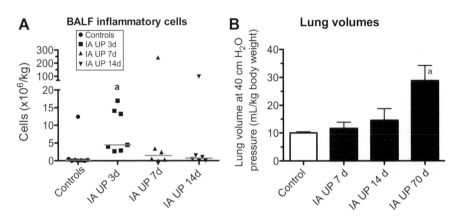

Fig. 2. Lung inflammation and increased lung maturation after intra-amniotic injection of *Ureaplasma parvum* (UP) in sheep. Pregnant ewes were given intra-amniotic injection of UP 3 days, 7 days, 14 days, or 70 days before delivery at 125 days' gestation (term = 150 days). (*A*) Inflammatory cells (neutrophils + monocytes) in the bronchoalveolar lavage fluid (BALF) normalized to body weight. (*B*) Lung volumes measured at 40 cm H_2O pressure normalized to body weight. Intra-amniotic injection of UP caused an initial lung inflammation followed by improved static compliance. [a]$P<.05$ vs controls. IA, intraamniotic. (*Data from* Kallapur SG, Kramer BW, Knox CL, et al. Chronic fetal exposure to Ureaplasma parvum suppresses innate immune responses in sheep. J Immunol 2011;187:2688–95; and Collins JJ, Kallapur SG, Knox CL, et al. Inflammation in fetal sheep from intra-amniotic injection of Ureaplasma parvum. Am J Physiol Lung Cell Mol Physiol 2010;299:L852–60.)

those dying with ureaplasma infection.[49,50,58] Overall, the sheep studies lend support to the clinical observation of less RDS but more BPD after ureaplasma exposure.

In Rhesus macaques, intra-amniotic injection of *Ureaplasma* caused chorioamnionitis, preterm labor, and delivery within 15 days and fetal pneumonia characterized by increased neutrophils and macrophages and alveolar type II cell proliferation indicating injury.[40] In preterm baboons delivered at 65% gestation 2 to 3 days after intra-amniotic inoculation with *Ureaplasma* and exposed to mechanical ventilation for 14 days, half of the neonatal baboons cleared *Ureaplasma* from their airways, whereas the remaining half had persistent ureaplasma colonization of the lungs.[59] The neonatal baboons with persistent ureaplasma colonization demonstrated lung inflammation and fibrosis and worse lung function compared with those animals that cleared the *Ureaplasma* from the lungs.[59,60] In general, the lung pathology after intrauterine ureaplasma exposure was more severe in nonhuman primates compared with sheep, suggesting species differences in susceptibility to *Ureaplasma*.

DIAGNOSTIC METHODS
Culture Methods

Although new diagnostic methods are currently available, culture remains the gold standard for *Ureaplasma* spp detection (**Table 2**). Proper sample collection is essential to avoid false-negative results. Because the organisms lack a cell wall and are susceptible to drying and heat, tracheal or nasopharyngeal (NP) aspirates or NP swabs should be directly inoculated in10B broth, Copan's Universal transport media, or routine Bacteriology Transport media for transport on ice to the laboratory. Once inoculated in urea-containing media, such as 10B broth, organism growth is indicated by color change from yellow to pink, indicating a pH change due to urease activity in the absence of turbidity.[61] The *Ureaplasma* colonies are identified by their characteristic brown appearance in the presence of the calcium chloride indicator in A8 agar. Although ureaplasmas can be detected after 24 to 48 hours' incubation, results may take up to 7 days; there are few laboratories with ureaplasma culture expertise.

Colorimetric Assays

To facilitate *Ureaplasma* spp detection, commercially available diagnostic kits have been developed that require less skilled personnel and more rapid detection time. The diagnostic kits listed in **Table 2** have reported sensitivities and specificities comparable with culture and PCR methods.[62–64] These kits also allow organism quantitation and antimicrobial susceptibility testing but do not differentiate between species, and only the Mycoplasma Duo Kit (Sanofi Diagnostics Pasteur, Marnes la Coquette, France) has been tested in preterm infants.[62]

Molecular Diagnostic Methods

Both conventional gel-based PCR and real-time PCR methods have been developed to improve ureaplasma detection. Real-time PCR can differentiate serovars and detects 15% more positive samples than culture and 6% more positive samples than conventional PCR.[65] PCR does not distinguish between viable and nonviable organisms. Although real-time PCR provides for rapid detection, often samples are batched for cost-effectiveness. Recently a DNA chip assay (STDetect Chip, LabGenomics, Korea) has been developed that allows rapid simultaneous detection of 13 major genitourinary pathogens, including *Ureaplasma* spp.[66] It has not been tested with infant respiratory samples.

THERAPEUTIC CONSIDERATIONS
Macrolide Antibiotics

Azithromycin, an azalide antibiotic and clarithromycin, a macrolide, have immunomodulatory properties,[67–69] are preferentially concentrated in lung epithelial lining fluid and alveolar macrophages,[70,71] and have antimicrobial activity against *Ureaplasma* spp in vitro[72–74] and in in vivo experimental models.[75–78] Treatment with these antibiotics may enhance ureaplasma clearance in infected infants and inhibit the pulmonary inflammatory response possibly contributing to a decreased risk for BPD. A new fluoroketolide antimicrobial, Solithromycin, has shown promising efficacy in sheep models.[79]

Efficacy Studies

Table 3 summarizes clinical studies of macrolides in eradicating *Ureaplasma* spp from the respiratory tract and prevention of BPD in colonized infants. There are significant methodological issues with each study, such as appropriate controls, lack of blinding, low colonization rate, suggesting false-negatives included in comparison group, and lack of adequate pharmacokinetic data to inform dose selection. However, when post-dosing cultures were obtained, erythromycin therapy was effective in eradicating respiratory tract colonization in 3 of 4 studies[80–83] but did not alter the BPD rates. In a single-center study by Ballard and colleagues,[84] 10 mg/kg/d azithromycin for 1 week followed by up to 5 weeks of 5 mg/kg/d was no different than placebo in eradication rates determined by PCR but reduced the risk for BPD in colonized infants. The BPD36 rate was high (70%–90%), so these results may not be replicated in centers with lower incidences of BPD. Ozdemir and colleagues,[85] who conducted a trial of a 10-day course of clarithromycin 20 mg/kg/d, observed 68.5% eradication based on follow-up cultures 2 days after the last dose and greatly reduced BPD rate in

Table 2
Diagnostic tests for *Ureaplasma* spp detection in clinical specimens

Diagnostic Method	Test	Source	Detection Time	Advantages	Disadvantages
Culture[11]	10B broth A8 agar	Remel, Lenexa, KS	1–7 d, A8 agar morphology confirmation	Detects live organisms; quantitation; is gold standard	Requires special transport media; unable to speciate; requires laboratory skilled in organism detection
Colorimetric assays[62–64]	Mycofast Revolution Mycoplasma Duo Kit MycoView MycoIST2	Elitech Diagnostic, Puteaux, France Sanofi Diagnostics Pasteur, Marnes la Coquette, France Fumouze Diagnostics, Cedex, France BioMérieux, Marcy l'Etoile, France	24–48 h	Detects live organism (>10^3 CCU/mL), organism enumeration, antimicrobial susceptibility; does not require skilled personnel	Requires special transport media; unable to speciate; less sensitive than PCR
Molecular assays[11]					
Gel-based conventional PCR	Targets sequences of 16S rRNA and 16S rRNA to 23S rRNA intergenic spacer regions and the urease and *mba* genes	—	1–2 d	More sensitive than culture; provides speciation; detects nonviable organisms; does not require use of transport media	Does not distinguish between live and dead organisms; no antibiotic susceptibility

Real-time PCR	Targets conserved sequences specific to either U parvum or U urealyticum; urease gene subunits; 16S rRNA	—	Hours, but often samples batched for cost-effectiveness	More sensitive than culture; provides speciation; detects nonviable organisms; does not require use of transport media; provides quantitation of bacterial load	High cost of equipment and reagents
Multiplex PCR	See earlier entry	—	1–2 d	Detects multiple organisms in same specimen	—
DNA chip assay[66]	STDetectChip	LabGenomics, Korea	6 h	Simultaneous detection of 13 GU pathogens; high sensitivity and specificity compared with multiplex PCR	Not trialed with infant samples; no antibiotic susceptibility testing

Abbreviation: GU, genitourinary.

Table 3
Impact of macrolides on ureaplasma respiratory colonization and BPD prevention in infected preterm infants: summary of clinical studies

Source	Macrolide Study Design	Dose and Duration	N	Inclusion Criteria	Age Drug Initiated	Ureaplasma Detection Method and Colonization Rate	Rate Ureaplasma Clearance	BPD 36-wk Rate
Waites et al,[80] 1994	Erythromycin, open-label PK study	25 or 40 mg/kg/d IV × 10 d	14	BW <1500 g with TA *Ureaplasma* positive; no noncolonized comparisons	Median 7 d (2–15 d)	TA culture only; colonization rate not reported	9 of 10 (90%) posttreatment cultures negative	Not reported
Lyon et al,[86] 1998	Erythromycin, randomized, no placebo, not blinded	45 mg/kg/d IV × 7 vs no therapy	75 (34 treated and 41 controls)	<30 wk mechanically ventilated	Day of birth	TA culture and conventional PCR; 9 of 60 (15%) positive pre-Rx (3 of 34 [9%] treatment group vs 6 of 41 [15%])	Not reported	Controls 27%, erythromycin 38%
Jonsson et al,[81] 1998	Erythromycin, randomized, no placebo, not blinded	40 mg/kg/d oral or IV × 10 d	28 (14 treated and 14 not treated)	<30 wk mechanically ventilated, TA/NP culture positive	Mean 7 d	TA and NP culture; 29 of 155 (19%)	Erythromycin-treated: 12 of 14 (86%) Nontreated: 0 of 14 (0%)	*Ureaplasma*+/ nontreated (71%) *Ureaplasma*+/ treated (64%)

Study	Description	Dose	N	Inclusion criteria	Timing	Culture method	Treatment outcome	Ureaplasma outcome
Bowman et al,[82] 1998	Erythromycin, comparison with noncolonized infants	20 mg/kg/d IV × 7 d	124 (22 UU positive)	<1000 g BW; IMV >6 h; TA culture positive	Median 7 d (1–31 d)	TA culture only; 22 of 124 (18%)	Erythromycin-treated: 18 of 22 (82%)	Ureaplasma+/treated (32%) Ureaplasma-/nontreated (48%)
Baier et al,[83] 2003	Erythromycin, dose-duration comparison	40 mg/kg/d IV × 5 d vs 10 d	17	<1500 g BW, mechanically ventilated	Median 7 d (2–33 d)	TA culture only; colonization rate not reported	5-d Rx: 25% 10-d Rx: 57%	Not reported
Ballard et al,[84] 2011	Azithromycin, RCT	10 mg/kg/d IV × 7 d & 5 mg/kg/d IV up to 5 wk	220 (111 Azithromycin vs 109 placebo)	<1250 g BW, mechanically ventilated	Within 72 h birth and 12 h start mechanical ventilation	TA conventional PCR only 31% AZI group 40% controls	5 subjects each group (AZI and placebo) still PCR positive ≥5 wk	Ureaplasma+/AZI treated: 19 of 26 (73%) Ureaplasma+/placebo: 33 of 35 (94%)
Ozdemir, et al,[85] 2011	Clarithromycin, RCT, blinded?	20 mg/kg/d IV × 10 d	74 (37 CLAR vs 37 placebo)	750–1250 g BW; NP culture positive first 72 h	1–5 d age	NP swab culture only: 33% positive	Follow-up cultures once 2 d after last dose in clarithromycin-treated subjects: 68.5% eradication; no follow-up cultures on placebo group	Ureaplasma+/CLAR-treated: 1 of 33 (3%)[a] Ureaplasma+/placebo: 12 of 33 (36.4%)

Abbreviations: BW, birth weight; CLAR, clarithromycin; IMV, intermittent manditory ventilation; IV, intravenous; NP, nasopharyngeal; PK, pharmacokinetic; RCT, randomized clinical trials; Rx, prescription; TA, tracheal aspirate; UU, U. urealyticum.

Ureaplasma+ indicates culture positive.

[a] Physiologic BPD at 36 weeks by timed oxygen reduction test.[100]

colonized infants compared with the treatment group. However, infants less than 750 g with the highest ureaplasma colonization rate and risk for BPD were excluded; the duration of mechanical ventilation was brief in all subjects. The culture status was based on NP cultures, so they did not distinguish between upper and lower respiratory tract infection; organism clearance was not assessed in the placebo group. In most studies, treatment was started at a median age of 7 days, suggesting that antibiotic therapy in colonized infants needs to be started soon after birth to prevent BPD. However, treatment started on the day of birth in one randomized trial of erythromycin did not affect the BPD rate.[86] Because the sample size of this study was small and the ureaplasma colonization rate was lower than expected, repeat studies of adequate sample size with early treatment with appropriate antibiotic dose determined in initial dose-response studies should be conducted.

Pharmacokinetics Studies

Only 7 (16%) randomized clinical trials (RCTs) included in a systematic review of pharmacologic interventions to prevent BPD were preceded by early phase studies evaluating pharmacokinetics and/or safety and efficacy.[87] In addition, despite the large number of RCTs to prevent BPD, no drugs are currently labeled by the Food and Drug Administration (FDA) for the prevention of BPD. Under an FDA Investigational New Drug application, the authors have completed a phase I open-label, pharmacokinetic (PK) study characterizing the population PK, safety, tolerability, and bacterial clearance of a single dose of 10 and 20 mg/kg intravenous azithromycin and multi-dose 20 mg/kg/d $\times$ 3 days in preterm neonates 24^0 to 28^6 weeks' gestation who are at high-risk for *Ureaplasma* spp respiratory tract colonization and BPD.[88–90] Inclusion of drug concentration data from the combined 40 subjects showed that the disposition of azithromycin in plasma was biphasic suggesting that azithromycin pharmacokinetics follows a 2-compartment model and the inclusion of body weight as a covariate for clearance and volume of the peripheral compartment improved the model fit to the data and explained some of the intersubject variability. The single 10-mg/kg and 20-mg/kg dose regimens were safe but did not completely eradicate *Ureaplasma* or suppress pulmonary inflammatory responses. The multi-dose eradicated respiratory colonization in all culture-positive subjects and decreased IL-17A but not other tracheal aspirate cytokines (IL-1ß, IL-8, IL-6) associated with BPD.

BEST PRACTICES: CURRENT RECOMMENDATIONS AND THE FUTURE

Azithromycin is increasingly used in neonatal intensive care units in the United States and Europe,[91,92] but its safety in the preterm population has not been adequately assessed. The FDA added a warning in 2013 to the drug label concerning its proarrhythmic potential. Azithromycin has been associated with an increased risk for cardiovascular death in older adults, primarily those with coexisting risk factors.[41,93,94] The authors are currently conducting a phase IIb, placebo-controlled, randomized trial of the multi-dose azithromycin regimen in a larger sample of preterm infants (clinicaltrials.gov NCT01778634) that will include assessments of long-term pulmonary and neurodevelopmental outcomes.

REFERENCES

1. Murtha AP, Edwards JM. The role of mycoplasma and ureaplasma in adverse pregnancy outcomes. Obstet Gynecol Clin North Am 2014;41:615–27.

2. Lowe J, Watkins WJ, Edwards MO, et al. Association between pulmonary urea-plasma colonization and bronchopulmonary dysplasia in preterm infants: updated systematic review and meta-analysis. Pediatr Infect Dis J 2014;33: 697–702.

3. Okogbule-Wonodi AC, Gross GW, Sun CC, et al. Necrotizing enterocolitis is associated with ureaplasma colonization in preterm infants. Pediatr Res 2011; 69:442–7.

4. Viscardi RM, Hashmi N, Gross GW, et al. Incidence of invasive ureaplasma in VLBW infants: relationship to severe intraventricular hemorrhage. J Perinatol 2008;28:759–65.

5. Romero R, Miranda J, Chaemsaithong P, et al. Sterile and microbial-associated intra-amniotic inflammation in preterm prelabor rupture of membranes. J Matern Fetal Neonatal Med 2014;1–16.

6. Goldenberg RL, Andrews WW, Goepfert AR, et al. The Alabama Preterm Birth Study: umbilical cord blood Ureaplasma urealyticum and Mycoplasma hominis cultures in very preterm newborn infants. Am J Obstet Gynecol 2008;198: 43.e1–5.

7. Sung TJ, Xiao L, Duffy L, et al. Frequency of ureaplasma serovars in respiratory secretions of preterm infants at risk for bronchopulmonary dysplasia. Pediatr Infect Dis J 2011;30:379–83.

8. Payne MS, Goss KC, Connett GJ, et al. Molecular microbiological characteriza-tion of preterm neonates at risk of bronchopulmonary dysplasia. Pediatr Res 2010;67:412–8.

9. Rao RP, Ghanayem NS, Kaufman BA, et al. Mycoplasma hominis and Urea-plasma species brain abscess in a neonate. Pediatr Infect Dis J 2002;21: 1083–5.

10. Madan E, Meyer MP, Amortegui AJ. Isolation of genital mycoplasmas and Chla-mydia trachomatis in stillborn and neonatal autopsy material. Arch Pathol Lab Med 1988;112:749–51.

11. Waites KB, Xiao L, Paralanov V, et al. Molecular methods for the detection of My-coplasma and ureaplasma infections in humans: a paper from the 2011 William Beaumont Hospital Symposium on molecular pathology. J Mol Diagn 2012;14: 437–50.

12. Garcia-Castillo M, Morosini MI, Galvez M, et al. Differences in biofilm develop-ment and antibiotic susceptibility among clinical Ureaplasma urealyticum and Ureaplasma parvum isolates. J Antimicrob Chemother 2008;62:1027–30.

13. Pandelidis K, McCarthy A, Chesko KL, et al. Role of biofilm formation in Urea-plasma antibiotic susceptibility and development of bronchopulmonary dysplasia in preterm neonates. Pediatr Infect Dis J 2013;32:394–8.

14. Katz B, Patel P, Duffy L, et al. Characterization of ureaplasmas isolated from pre-term infants with and without bronchopulmonary dysplasia. J Clin Microbiol 2005;43:4852–4.

15. Kilian M, Brown MB, Brown TA, et al. Immunoglobulin A1 protease activity in strains of Ureaplasma urealyticum. Acta Pathol Microbiol Immunol Scand B 1984;92:61–4.

16. DeSilva NS, Quinn PA. Characterization of phospholipase A_1, A_2, C activity in *Ureaplasma urealyticum* membranes. Mol Cell Biochem 1999;201:159–67.

17. Paralanov V, Lu J, Duffy LB, et al. Comparative genome analysis of 19 Urea-plasma urealyticum and Ureaplasma parvum strains. BMC Microbiol 2012;12:88.

18. Glass JI, Lefkowitz EJ, Glass JS, et al. The complete sequence of the mucosal pathogen Ureaplasma urealyticum. Nature 2000;407:757–62.

19. Robinson JW, Dando SJ, Nitsos I, et al. Ureaplasma parvum serovar 3 multiple banded antigen size variation after chronic intra-amniotic infection/colonization. PLoS One 2013;8:e62746.

20. Wu HN, Nakura Y, Motooka D, et al. Complete genome sequence of ureaplasma parvum serovar 3 strain SV3F4, isolated in Japan. Genome Announc 2014;2(3): e00256-14.

21. Martinez MA, Das K, Saikolappan S, et al. A serine/threonine phosphatase encoded by MG_207 of Mycoplasma genitalium is critical for its virulence. BMC Microbiol 2013;13:44.

22. Xiao L, Crabb DM, Dai Y, et al. Suppression of antimicrobial peptide expression by ureaplasma species. Infect Immun 2014;82:1657-65.

23. Zheng X, Teng L-J, Watson HL, et al. Small repeating units within the *Ureaplasma urealyticum* MB antigen gene encode serovar specificity and are associated with antigen size variation. Infect Immun 1995;63:891-8.

24. Dando SJ, Nitsos I, Kallapur SG, et al. The role of the multiple banded antigen of Ureaplasma parvum in intra-amniotic infection: major virulence factor or decoy? PLoS One 2012;7:e29856.

25. Kumar H, Kawai T, Akira S. Pathogen recognition by the innate immune system. Int Rev Immunol 2011;30:16-34.

26. Estrada-Gutierrez G, Gomez-Lopez N, Zaga-Clavellina V, et al. Interaction between pathogenic bacteria and intrauterine leukocytes triggers alternative molecular signaling cascades leading to labor in women. Infect Immun 2010;78:4792-9.

27. Manimtim WM, Hasday JD, Hester L, et al. Ureaplasma urealyticum modulates endotoxin-induced cytokine release by human monocytes derived from preterm and term newborns and adults. Infect Immun 2001;69:3906-15.

28. Shimizu T, Kida Y, Kuwano K. Ureaplasma parvum lipoproteins, including MB antigen, activate NF-{kappa}B through TLR1, TLR2 and TLR6. Microbiology 2008;154:1318-25.

29. Peltier MR, Freeman AJ, Mu HH, et al. Characterization of the macrophage-stimulating activity from Ureaplasma urealyticum. Am J Reprod Immunol 2007;57:186-92.

30. Quinn PA. Evidence of an immune response to Ureaplasma urealyticum in perinatal morbidity and mortality. Pediatr Infect Dis 1986;5:S282-7.

31. Okogbule-Wonodi AC, Chesko KL, Famuyide ME, et al. Surfactant protein-A enhances ureaplasmacidal activity in vitro. Innate Immun 2011;17:145-51.

32. Famuyide ME, Hasday JD, Carter HC, et al. Surfactant protein-A limits Ureaplasma-mediated lung inflammation in a murine pneumonia model. Pediatr Res 2009;66:162-7.

33. Winters AH, Levan TD, Vogel SN, et al. Single nucleotide polymorphism in toll-like receptor 6 is associated with a decreased risk for ureaplasma respiratory tract colonization and bronchopulmonary dysplasia in preterm infants. Pediatr Infect Dis J 2013;32:898-904.

34. Kallapur SG, Kramer BW, Knox CL, et al. Chronic fetal exposure to Ureaplasma parvum suppresses innate immune responses in sheep. J Immunol 2011;187:2688-95.

35. Romero R, Dey SK, Fisher SJ. Preterm labor: one syndrome, many causes. Science 2014;345:760-5.

36. DiGiulio DB. Diversity of microbes in amniotic fluid. Semin Fetal Neonatal Med 2012;17:2-11.

37. Combs CA, Gravett M, Garite TJ, et al. Amniotic fluid infection, inflammation, and colonization in preterm labor with intact membranes. Am J Obstet Gynecol 2014;210:125.e1-15.

38. Yoon BH, Romero R, Lim JH, et al. The clinical significance of detecting Ureaplasma urealyticum by the polymerase chain reaction in the amniotic fluid of patients with preterm labor. Am J Obstet Gynecol 2003;189:919–24.
39. Gerber S, Vial Y, Hohlfeld P, et al. Detection of Ureaplasma urealyticum in second-trimester amniotic fluid by polymerase chain reaction correlates with subsequent preterm labor and delivery. J Infect Dis 2003;187:518–21.
40. Novy MJ, Duffy L, Axthelm MK, et al. Ureaplasma parvum or Mycoplasma hominis as sole pathogens cause chorioamnionitis, preterm delivery, and fetal pneumonia in rhesus macaques. Reprod Sci 2009;16:56–70.
41. Albert RK, Schuller JL. Macrolide antibiotics and the risk of cardiac arrhythmias. Am J Respir Crit Care Med 2014;189(10):1173–80.
42. Theilen U, Lyon AJ, Fitzgerald T, et al. Infection with Ureaplasma urealyticum: is there a specific clinical and radiological course in the preterm infant? Arch Dis Child Fetal Neonatal Ed 2004;89:F163–7.
43. Olomu IN, Hecht JL, Onderdonk AO, et al. Perinatal correlates of Ureaplasma urealyticum in placenta parenchyma of singleton pregnancies that end before 28 weeks of gestation. Pediatrics 2009;123:1329–36.
44. Namba F, Hasegawa T, Nakayama M, et al. Placental features of chorioamnionitis colonized with Ureaplasma species in preterm delivery. Pediatr Res 2010;67:166–72.
45. Grattard F, Soleihac B, De Barbeyrac B, et al. Epidemiologic and molecular investigations of genital mycoplasmas from women and neonates at delivery. Pediatr Infect Dis J 1995;14:853–8.
46. Panero A, Pacifico L, Roggini M, et al. *Ureaplasma urealyticum* as a cause of pneumonia in preterm infants: analysis of the white cell response. Arch Dis Child 1995;73:F37–40.
47. Hannaford K, Todd DA, Jeffrey H, et al. Role of *Ureaplasma urealyticum* in lung disease of prematurity. Arch Dis Child Fetal Neonatal Ed 1999;81:F162–7.
48. Pacifico L, Panero A, Roggini M, et al. *Ureaplasma urealyticum* and pulmonary outcome in a neonatal intensive care population. Pediatr Infect Dis 1997;16:579–86.
49. Viscardi RM, Manimtim WM, Sun CC, et al. Lung pathology in premature infants with Ureaplasma urealyticum infection. Pediatr Dev Pathol 2002;5:141–50.
50. Viscardi R, Manimtim W, He JR, et al. Disordered pulmonary myofibroblast distribution and elastin expression in preterm infants with Ureaplasma urealyticum pneumonitis. Pediatr Dev Pathol 2006;9:143–51.
51. Wang EL, Ohlsson A, Kellner JD. Association of *Ureaplasma urealyticum* colonization with chronic lung disease of prematurity: results of a meta-analysis. J Pediatr 1995;127:640–4.
52. Schelonka RL, Katz B, Waites KB, et al. Critical appraisal of the role of Ureaplasma in the development of bronchopulmonary dysplasia with meta-analytic techniques. Pediatr Infect Dis J 2005;24:1033–9.
53. Knox CL, Dando SJ, Nitsos I, et al. The severity of chorioamnionitis in pregnant sheep is associated with in vivo variation of the surface-exposed multiple-banded antigen/gene of Ureaplasma parvum. Biol Reprod 2010;83:415–26.
54. Collins JJ, Kallapur SG, Knox CL, et al. Inflammation in fetal sheep from intra-amniotic injection of Ureaplasma parvum. Am J Physiol Lung Cell Mol Physiol 2010;299:L852–60.
55. Moss TJ, Knox CL, Kallapur SG, et al. Experimental amniotic fluid infection in sheep: effects of Ureaplasma parvum serovars 3 and 6 on preterm or term fetal sheep. Am J Obstet Gynecol 2008;198(122):e1–8.

56. Moss TJ, Nitsos I, Knox CL, et al. Ureaplasma colonization of amniotic fluid and efficacy of antenatal corticosteroids for preterm lung maturation in sheep. Am J Obstet Gynecol 2009;200(96):e1–6.

57. Moss TJ, Nitsos I, Ikegami M, et al. Experimental intrauterine Ureaplasma infection in sheep. Am J Obstet Gynecol 2005;192:1179–86.

58. Husain AN. Pathology of arrested acinar development in postsurfactant bronchopulmonary dysplasia. Hum Pathol 1998;29:710–7.

59. Yoder BA, Coalson JJ, Winter VT, et al. Effects of antenatal colonization with Ureaplasma urealyticum on pulmonary disease in the immature baboon. Pediatr Res 2003;54:797–807.

60. Viscardi RM, Atamas SP, Luzina IG, et al. Antenatal Ureaplasma urealyticum respiratory tract infection stimulates proinflammatory, profibrotic responses in the preterm baboon lung. Pediatr Res 2006;60:141–6.

61. Waites KB, Duffy LB, Bebear CM, et al. Standardized methods and quality control limits for agar and broth microdilution susceptibility testing of Mycoplasma pneumoniae, Mycoplasma hominis, and Ureaplasma urealyticum. J Clin Microbiol 2012;50:3542–7.

62. Cheah FC, Anderson TP, Darlow BA, et al. Comparison of the Mycoplasma Duo test with PCR for detection of ureaplasma species in endotracheal aspirates from premature infants. J Clin Microbiol 2005;43:509–10.

63. Redelinghuys MJ, Ehlers MM, Dreyer AW, et al. Comparison of the new Mycofast Revolution assay with a molecular assay for the detection of genital mycoplasmas from clinical specimens. BMC Infect Dis 2013;13:453.

64. Machado Ldel P, Molinari MA, dos Santos L, et al. Performance of four commercial kits for laboratory diagnosis of urogenital mollicute infection. Can J Microbiol 2014;60:613–7.

65. Xiao L, Glass JI, Paralanov V, et al. Detection and characterization of human ureaplasma species and serovars by real-time PCR. J Clin Microbiol 2010;48: 2715–23.

66. Kweon OJ, Choi J, Song UH, et al. Performance evaluation of a DNA chip assay in the identification of major genitourinary pathogens. J Microbiol Methods 2014; 109C:117–22.

67. Amsden GW. Anti-inflammatory effects of macrolides–an underappreciated benefit in the treatment of community-acquired respiratory tract infections and chronic inflammatory pulmonary conditions? J Antimicrob Chemother 2005;55: 10–21.

68. Beigelman A, Gunsten S, Mikols CL, et al. Azithromycin attenuates airway inflammation in a noninfectious mouse model of allergic asthma. Chest 2009; 136:498–506.

69. Parnham MJ, Erakovic Haber V, Giamarellos-Bourboulis EJ, et al. Azithromycin: mechanisms of action and their relevance for clinical applications. Pharmacol Ther 2014;143:225–45.

70. Patel KB, Xuan D, Tessier PR, et al. Comparison of bronchopulmonary pharmacokinetics of clarithromycin and azithromycin. Antimicrob Agents Chemother 1996;40:2375–9.

71. Rodvold KA, Danziger LH, Gotfried MH. Steady-state plasma and bronchopulmonary concentrations of intravenous levofloxacin and azithromycin in healthy adults. Antimicrob Agents Chemother 2003;47:2450–7.

72. Matlow A, Th'ng C, Kovach D, et al. Susceptibilities of neonatal respiratory isolates of Ureaplasma urealyticum to antimicrobial agents. Antimicrob Agents Chemother 1998;42:1290–2.

73. Duffy LB, Crabb D, Searcey K, et al. Comparative potency of gemifloxacin, new quinolones, macrolides, tetracycline and clindamycin against Mycoplasma spp. J Antimicrob Chemother 2000;45(Suppl 1):29–33.

74. Waites KB, Crabb DM, Duffy LB. Comparative in vitro susceptibilities of human mycoplasmas and ureaplasmas to a new investigational ketolide, CEM-101. Antimicrob Agents Chemother 2009;53:2139–41.

75. Walls SA, Kong L, Leeming HA, et al. Antibiotic prophylaxis improves Ureaplasma-associated lung disease in suckling mice. Pediatr Res 2009;66: 197–202.

76. Grigsby PL, Novy MJ, Sadowsky DW, et al. Maternal azithromycin therapy for Ureaplasma intraamniotic infection delays preterm delivery and reduces fetal lung injury in a primate model. Am J Obstet Gynecol 2012;207:475.e1–14.

77. Acosta EP, Grigsby PL, Larson KB, et al. Transplacental transfer of Azithromycin and its use for eradicating intra-amniotic ureaplasma infection in a primate model. J Infect Dis 2014;209:898–904.

78. Miura Y, Payne MS, Keelan JA, et al. Maternal intravenous treatment with either azithromycin or solithromycin clears Ureaplasma parvum from the amniotic fluid in an ovine model of intrauterine infection. Antimicrob Agents Chemother 2014; 58:5413–20.

79. Keelan JA, Kemp MW, Payne MS, et al. Maternal administration of solithromycin, a new, potent, broad-spectrum fluoroketolide antibiotic, achieves fetal and intra-amniotic antimicrobial protection in a pregnant sheep model. Antimicrob Agents Chemother 2014;58:447–54.

80. Waites KB, Sims PJ, Crouse DT, et al. Serum concentrations of erythromycin after intravenous infusion in preterm neonates treated for Ureaplasma urealyticum infection. Pediatr Infect Dis J 1994;13:287–93.

81. Jonsson B, Rylander M, Faxelius G. *Ureaplasma urealyticum*, erythromycin and respiratory morbidity in high-risk preterm neonates. Acta Paediatr 1998;87: 1079–84.

82. Bowman ED, Dharmalingam A, Fan WQ, et al. Impact of erythromycin on respiratory colonization of *Ureaplasma urealyticum* and the development of chronic lung disease in extremely low birth weight infants. Pediatr Infect Dis J 1998;17:615–20.

83. Baier RJ, Loggins J, Kruger TE. Failure of erythromycin to eliminate airway colonization with ureaplasma urealyticum in very low birth weight infants. BMC Pediatr 2003;3:10.

84. Ballard HO, Shook LA, Bernard P, et al. Use of azithromycin for the prevention of bronchopulmonary dysplasia in preterm infants: a randomized, double-blind, placebo controlled trial. Pediatr Pulmonol 2011;46:111–8.

85. Ozdemir R, Erdeve O, Dizdar EA, et al. Clarithromycin in preventing bronchopulmonary dysplasia in Ureaplasma urealyticum-positive preterm infants. Pediatrics 2011;128:e1496–501.

86. Lyon AJ, McColm J, Middlemist L, et al. Randomised trial of erythromycin on the development of chronic lung disease in preterm infants. Arch Dis Child Fetal Neonatal Ed 1998;78:F10–4.

87. Beam KS, Aliaga S, Ahlfeld SK, et al. A systematic review of randomized controlled trials for the prevention of bronchopulmonary dysplasia in infants. J Perinatol 2014;34:705–10.

88. Hassan HE, Othman AA, Eddington ND, et al. Pharmacokinetics, safety, and biologic effects of azithromycin in extremely preterm infants at risk for ureaplasma colonization and bronchopulmonary dysplasia. J Clin Pharmacol 2011;51:1264–75.

89. Viscardi RM, Othman AA, Hassan HE, et al. Azithromycin to prevent broncho-pulmonary dysplasia in ureaplasma-infected preterm infants: pharmacokinetics, safety, microbial response, and clinical outcomes with a 20-milligram-per-kilo-gram single intravenous dose. Antimicrob Agents Chemother 2013;57:2127–33.

90. Merchan LM, Hassan HE, Terrin ML, et al. Pharmacokinetics, microbial response, and pulmonary outcomes of multidose intravenous azithromycin in preterm infants at risk for ureaplasma respiratory colonization. Antimicrob Agents Chemother 2015;59:570–8.

91. Hsieh EM, Hornik CP, Clark RH, et al. Medication use in the neonatal intensive care unit. Am J Perinatol 2014;31(9):811–21.

92. Pansieri C, Pandolfini C, Elie V, et al. Ureaplasma, bronchopulmonary dysplasia, and azithromycin in European neonatal intensive care units: a survey. Sci Rep 2014;4:4076.

93. Ray WA, Murray KT, Hall K, et al. Azithromycin and the risk of cardiovascular death. N Engl J Med 2012;366:1881–90.

94. Giudicessi JR, Ackerman MJ. Azithromycin and risk of sudden cardiac death: guilty as charged or falsely accused? Cleve Clin J Med 2013;80:539–44.

95. Romero R, Schaudinn C, Kusanovic JP, et al. Detection of a microbial biofilm in intraamniotic infection. Am J Obstet Gynecol 2008;198:135.e1–5.

96. Uchida K, Nakahira K, Mimura K, et al. Effects of Ureaplasma parvum lipopro-tein multiple-banded antigen on pregnancy outcome in mice. J Reprod Immunol 2013;100:118–27.

97. Harju K, Glumoff V, Hallman M. Ontogeny of Toll-like receptors Tlr2 and Tlr4 in mice. Pediatr Res 2001;49:81–3.

98. Ohlsson A, Wang E, Vearncombe M. Leukocyte counts and colonization with *Ureaplasma urealyticum* in preterm neonates. Clin Infect Dis 1993;17(Suppl 1):S144–7.

99. Crouse DT, Odrezin GT, Cutter GR, et al. Radiographic changes associated with tracheal isolation of *Ureaplasma urealyticum* from neonates. Clin Infect Dis 1993;17(Suppl 1):S122–30.

100. Walsh MC, Yao Q, Gettner P, et al. Impact of a physiologic definition on broncho-pulmonary dysplasia rates. Pediatrics 2004;114:1305–11.

Biomarkers, Early Diagnosis, and Clinical Predictors of Bronchopulmonary Dysplasia

CrossMark

Charitharth Vivek Lal, MD, Namasivayam Ambalavanan, MD*

KEYWORDS

- Bronchopulmonary dysplasia • Biomarkers • Prognosis • Early diagnosis • Infant
- Premature • Systems biology • Pulmonary hypertension

KEY POINTS

- Bronchopulmonary dysplasia (BPD) is a disease with a clinical operational definition and multiple different clinical subphenotypes.
- Most clinical prediction models of BPD do not have a high predictive accuracy.
- Various biofluid biomarkers have been studied over the years, but none are currently used in routine clinical care.
- Newer omic strategies are promising for the discovery of novel biomarkers of BPD diagnosis, prognosis, and therapeutic response.

INTRODUCTION

Bronchopulmonary dysplasia (BPD) is a common morbidity in extremely preterm infants. However, BPD defined by oxygen requirement even when more precisely assessed by the physiologic definition of BPD[1] is only an operational definition, which does not indicate the magnitude of lung disease or the underlying disease process. Lung disease process in BPD is variable, as certain infants with BPD have pulmonary hypertension (PH) as a major component of their pathophysiology,[2] whereas others have severe tracheobronchomalacia,[3] and many have patchy atelectasis or cystic

Disclosures: recent funding from Pfizer, Ikaria (Dr N. Ambalavanan).
Funding: NIH funding (U01 HL122626; R01 HD067126; R01 HD066982; U10 HD34216) (Dr N. Ambalavanan).
Division of Neonatology, Department of Pediatrics, Women and Infants Center, University of Alabama at Birmingham, 176F Suite 9380, 619 South 19th Street, Birmingham, AL 35249-7335, USA
* Corresponding author.
E-mail address: nambalavanan@peds.uab.edu

Clin Perinatol 42 (2015) 739–754
http://dx.doi.org/10.1016/j.clp.2015.08.004
0095-5108/15/$ – see front matter © 2015 Elsevier Inc. All rights reserved.

lesions in their lung parenchyma.[4] It has increasingly become evident that severe BPD may be a different entity from mild or moderate BPD, both in terms of clinical operational definition as well as in terms of genetic predisposition.[5] This genetic predisposition is very different by race/ethnicity, indicating that biological pathways (and resulting biomarkers) contributing to BPD in different infants are probably dissimilar.[5] Therefore, it is likely that what is now termed *BPD* is not a single entity, or even a spectrum of disease resulting from a single pathophysiologic process, but a combination of several chronic lung diseases characterized by a common at-risk population of infants in the saccular or early alveolar stage of lung development with varying magnitudes of impairment of alveolar septation, lung fibrosis, and abnormal vascular development and remodeling. To modify Leo Tolstoy's quote on happy families from *Anna Karenina*, all normally developed preterm lungs are alike; each BPD lung is abnormal in its own way. The natural corollary is that the clinical predictors and biomarkers of each of these subphenotypes of BPD may be different, depending on the pathophysiology.

In this article, the authors first discuss the predictors and biomarkers starting from the clinical arena and then move on to progressively more sophisticated investigations and research esoterica (which may be at the bedside in the near future).

WHY DO WE NEED BIOMARKERS OR PREDICTORS?

Many interventions to reduce the risk of BPD have been tested in randomized clinical trials, but only a few have shown significant treatment effects.[6] Hence, earlier disease predictors are warranted to initiate preventive strategies in select patients. A biomarker has been defined as "a characteristic that is, measured and evaluated as an indicator of normal biologic processes, pathogenic processes, or pharmacologic responses to a therapeutic intervention."[7,8] Biomarkers are any clinical features, radiological findings, or laboratory-based test markers that characterize disease activity, which are useful for early diagnosis, prediction of disease severity, and monitoring disease processes and response to therapy. Biomarkers are valuable for earlier diagnosis; it is possible that detection of BPD at an earlier stage may enable initiation of therapies when they may be more effective (a window of opportunity). It is also possible that nondetection of risk for BPD may enable the avoidance of therapies and their potential hazards.

Prognosis (risk prediction for the development of BPD or risk prediction for outcome of BPD in infants diagnosed with BPD) can also be evaluated using appropriate biomarkers. Similar to earlier diagnosis, the determination of a very high risk for BPD may enable the use of targeted therapy (eg, the use of vitamin A supplementation in extremely low-birth-weight [ELBW] infants[9]) and determination of a very low risk for BPD may enable the avoidance of therapies. As mentioned earlier, BPD has much heterogeneity with many subphenotypes in clinical presentation. The use of biomarkers may enable targeting specific therapies to specific subphenotypes (eg, use of inhaled nitric oxide in infants with biomarkers indicating early elevations in pulmonary arterial pressure).

Biomarkers may also be useful for following the efficacy of therapy as a surrogate measure. For example, the rate of the decrease of blood b-type natriuretic peptide (BNP) may possibly enable a clinician to determine the efficacy of a therapy for PH in BPD. The search for reliable biomarkers in BPD is ongoing and remains a challenge. Important issues to be addressed include the accuracy and reliability of biomarkers for the clinical state of interest, evaluation of clinical utility and cost-effectiveness, and real-world effectiveness compared with other biomarkers.[10]

BIOMARKERS

Traditionally, risk prediction was done using clinical variables. Clinical variables can usually be obtained without difficulty. Other biomarkers include those based on imaging, lung function measures, and measurements of various analytes in different body fluids (blood, tracheal aspirates, exhaled breath condensates, urine, and so forth) that have been determined to be associated with BPD either in a targeted manner (eg, specific cytokines) or by unbiased omic (eg, genomic/proteomic/metabonomic/microbiomic) profiling (**Fig. 1**).

Clinical Predictors as Biomarkers of Bronchopulmonary Dysplasia

Many clinical prediction models have been developed to predict the development of BPD.[11–17] However, some of these models were developed many years ago, a few even before the routine use of surfactant therapy or antenatal steroids. These models may not be generalizable to the current era with survival of many infants at the threshold of viability (22–24 weeks' gestation). The models have also had a moving

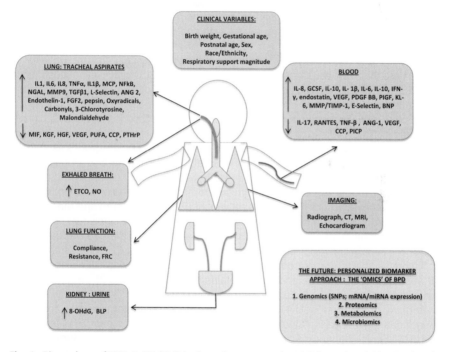

Fig. 1. Biomarkers of BPD. 8-OHdG, 8-hydroxydeoxyguanosine; ANG, angiopoietin; BLP, bombesinlike peptide; CCP, Clara cell proteins; CT, computed tomography; ETCO, end tidal carbon monoxide; FGF, fibroblast growth factor; FRC, functional residual capacity; GCSF, granulocyte-colony stimulating factor; HGF, hepatocyte growth factor; IFN, interferon; IL, interleukin; KGF, keratinocyte growth factor; KL-6, Kerbs von Lungren 6; MCP, Monocyte Chemoattractant Protein; MIF, macrophage migration inhibitory factor; MMP, matrix metalloproteinase; NFkB, nuclear factor kappa B; NGAL, neutrophil-gelatinase-associated lipocalin; NO, nitric oxide; PDGF BB, platelet derived growth factor BB; PICP, C-terminal fragment of type I procollagen; PIGF, placental growth factor; PTHrP, parathyroid hormone-related protein; PUFA, polyunsaturated fatty acid; RANTES, Regulated on Activation, Normal T Expressed and Secreted; SNP, single-nucleotide polymorphism; TGF, transforming growth factor; TIMP-1, tissue inhibitor of metalloproteinase-1; TNF, tumor necrosis factor; VEGF, vascular endothelial growth factor.

target, as the definition of BPD has changed with time, with a transition from the initial definition of oxygen requirement at 28 days to the more recent National Institutes of Health consensus definition[18] and the physiologic BPD definition.[19] A common problem with most prediction models is that they are often based on statistical analyses that provide odds ratios and risk factors but not an easy way for a clinician at the bedside to precisely and accurately determine the risk of BPD for an individual infant.

In a recent systematic review, Onland and colleagues[20] evaluated 26 published prediction models on BPD in premature infants. Onland and colleagues[20] also did external validation on a relatively recent cohort of infants (the PreVILIG [Prevention of Ventilator Induced Lung Injury Group] dataset)[21] and reported that most existing clinical prediction models are at best only moderate predictors for BPD, as none had an area under the curve (AUC) of the receiver operating characteristic (ROC) curve (AUROC) of greater than 0.80.[20] The authors describe 4 models that had fair performance (AUC >0.70) for predicting BPD in the analysis by Onland and colleagues.[20]

In the mid 1990s, Ryan and colleagues[22] developed models to predict chronic lung disease (CLD) in very-low-birth-weight (VLBW) neonates using clinical and radiological variables.[22] Logistic regression analysis was used to identify independent risk factors for CLD, and the AUROC was used to determine the discriminatory capacity of the models. The AUC was similar in a model with and without radiographic information (0.926 vs 0.913) and was 0.937 in a validation cohort.

In 1999, Yoder and colleagues[12] developed a respiratory failure score (RFS) for infants of less than 32 weeks' gestation to predict neonatal CLD at 36 weeks' postmenstrual age (PMA) and compared it with the Sinkin and colleagues'[11] and Ryan and colleagues' models.[22] Five clinical parameters reflecting the severity of pulmonary dysfunction were selected for the development of the scoring system and were assessed at 12, 24, 48, 72, and 168 hours of age. The RFS method at 72 hours demonstrated the greatest AUROC for the prediction of neonatal CLD in the groups as a whole. A limitation of this study is that this model was developed in infants born during 1990 to 1992 and included preterm infants who are at lower risk of BPD during the current era.

A predictive model was created by Kim and colleagues[23] based on their findings that peak inspiratory pressure (PIP) over birth weight (PIP per kilogram) and mean airway pressure (MAP) over birth weight (MAP per kilogram) were more significant risk factors for the development of CLD than PIP and MAP per se. A scoring method was developed using clinical data and modified respiratory variables to predict CLD on postnatal days 4, 7, and 10.[23] The primary outcome variable for this study was CLD diagnosed at 36 weeks of corrected age, and AUCs obtained (0.92 on day 4, 0.95 on day 10) were comparable with those obtained by the Yoder and colleagues'[12] model.

As most of these models typically do not include postnatal age and, therefore, cannot quantify the variable contribution of neonatal exposures over time, investigators at the Eunice Kennedy Shriver National Institute of Child Health and Human Development Neonatal Research Network (NICHD NRN) recently introduced a Web-based BPD estimator to determine a risk estimate for BPD and the competing outcome of death by postnatal day.[24] This study was a secondary analysis of the data from a benchmarking trial on BPD.[25] This online tool can be found at https://neonatal.rti.org/index.cfm?fuseaction=BPDCalculator.start.

Imaging Biomarkers of Bronchopulmonary Dysplasia

Chest radiographs

Studies in the 1970s first described an association between the presence of fibrosis/interstitial shadows on chest radiographs (CXRs) and respiratory morbidity.[26] Mortensson and colleagues[27] described that focal or general hyperinflation or both were associated with a greater risk of airway obstruction in newborn infants, whereas infants with only interstitial abnormalities were at a higher risk to develop general hyperinflation and increased airway obstruction even at 8 to 10 years of age, as compared with infants with a normal chest examination.[27] In a study of scoring CXRs of premature infants at 1 month of age, radiographs with cystic elements or interstitial changes were scored the highest and a high score was associated with oxygen dependency at 28 days and an abnormal airway resistance at 6 months of age.[28] Greenough and colleagues[29] formulated an objective scoring system for the assessment of CXRs at 1 month and concluded that scoring only for the presence of fibrosis/interstitial shadows, cystic elements, and degree of hyperinflation predicts oxygen dependency at 36 weeks' postmenstrual age.[29] The same group later reported that CXR appearance on postnatal day 7 facilitates the prediction of outcome of infants born very prematurely.[30] CXRs, however, have significant limitations in the evaluation of children with BPD, as there is a poor correlation between CXRs' appearance and clinical status.[31]

Chest computed tomography scans

Chest radiography has a drawback of superimposition of structures, and there is controversy on the reliability of CXR in preterm infants.[32] Computed tomography (CT) scans can potentially provide more objective and definitive evidence of pulmonary structural damage in preterm infants with BPD.[33,34] Tracheobronchomalacia is commonly seen in children with BPD; hence, advanced CT techniques are often useful. In 1994, Oppenheim and colleagues[33] systematically described the chest CT findings of BPD.[33] Kubota and colleagues[34] and Ochiai and coworkers[35] have described CT-based scoring systems. Recently, Shin and colleagues[36] developed a high-resolution CT scoring system for BPD for both evaluation of the disease status and the prediction of clinical severity.[36] In all the aforementioned studies, CT scans were performed at late PMA when the disease is well established; hence, these models do not aid in predicting the development of BPD but may help in forecasting the outcome of established BPD. The utility of CT scans as a predictor of BPD in premature infants remains to be fully defined. Moreover, the risks of irradiation during CT should not be underestimated despite recent efforts at reducing irradiation.

Chest MRI

MRI of the lung is technically challenging because of the low proton density and fast signal decay of the lung parenchyma itself.[37] However, pathologic changes resulting in an increase of tissue density, such as atelectasis, nodules, infiltrates, mucus, or pleural effusion, are readily identified. Adams and colleagues[38] used MRI to assess lung water content and tissue injury in infants of 23 to 33 weeks' gestational age. Proton density was significantly higher in dependent regions of the lungs; average proton density, proton density gradient, and severity of lung damage were greater in infants with severe BPD.[38]

Newer MRI technologies can facilitate measurements of perfusion, blood flow, ventilation, gas exchange, as well as respiratory motion and mechanics.[39] In addition, hyperpolarized gas MRI is particularly sensitive to early changes in emphysema.[40] The technique of helium-3 MRI has been used to compare alveolar structure in term-born and preterm-born schoolchildren (including survivors of neonatal BPD).[41] Such advanced techniques complemented by the nonionizing nature of the method could potentially help BPD evaluation in premature infants, although the current duration of the procedure and the requirement of sedation are limitations.

Echocardiogram for the diagnosis of pulmonary hypertension in bronchopulmonary dysplasia

PH is relatively common, affecting at least 1 in 6 ELBW infants, and persists to discharge in most survivors.[2] There are limited studies on this subject. A large prospective study from a single center by Bhat and colleagues[2] found that around 18% of ELBW infants were diagnosed with PH before discharge from the neonatal intensive care unit, and routine screening of ELBW infants with echocardiography at 4 weeks of age identifies only one-third of the infants with PH.[2] In another recent study by Mourani and colleagues,[42] it was found that early PH was a risk factor for increased BPD severity and late PH.

Although echocardiography is widely used in the determination of PH in BPD, estimates of pulmonary artery pressure are not obtained consistently and are not reliable for determining the severity of PH.[43] A major limitation of echocardiographic evaluation of tricuspid regurgitant jet velocity (TRJV) is that it relies on a TR regurgitant jet, which might not be present in all patients. The TRJV is also rarely of sufficient quality to adequately estimate right ventricular systolic pressure as in a recent study; 58% of children without a measureable TRJV had PH by cardiac catheterization, and overall echocardiogram was accurate in determining the severity of PH in just 47% of cases.[42] Hill and colleagues[44] also found a poor correlation between transthoracic echocardiographic estimates of right ventricular systolic pressure based on TRJV and cardiac catheterization. In essence, the lack of a measurable TRJV on echocardiogram should not be interpreted as absence of PH.

Lung Function Biomarkers

Lung compliance and resistance have been demonstrated to differ between infants with and without BPD,[13,45,46] but most of these studies were undertaken before the routine use of surfactant. Recent studies suggest that BPD survivors continue to have airway obstruction and lower forced expiratory volume in 1 second even as late as young adult life.[47]

Freezer and Sly[46] observed that the dynamic compliance of the respiratory system in intubated premature infants was significantly lower on day 1 and during the first week of life in the infants who went on to develop BPD. Lung compliance on day 1 and birth weight or gestational age were significant independent predictors for the development of BPD.[46] May and colleagues[48] found that airway resistance, compliance, functional residual capacity, and end-tidal carbon monoxide (ETCO) differed significantly on day 3 between infants who did and did not develop BPD. On day 14, however, only a higher ETCO and none of the pulmonary function parameters were predictive of BPD.[48] Van Lierde and colleagues[49] found that gestational age and the ventilatory index (ventilator frequency × maximal inspiratory pressure) on day 3 were the best early predictors of poor outcome, but pulmonary function tests were not helpful.

Biofluid Biomarkers

Various cytokines and growth factors mediate lung development or may be involved in lung injury.[50] Hence, various investigators have explored the biomarker potential of various cytokines and growth factors in premature infants.

Blood

Limitations of systemic cytokine or growth factor measurement are that they may not accurately reflect the concentrations of the mediator in the lung and it is not possible to identify if pulmonary cells are producing or releasing them. Nevertheless, blood biomarker measurement for BPD has been frequently studied mainly because blood is relatively easily accessible.

Inflammatory markers Chorioamnioitis,[51] ureaplasma infection,[52] and postnatal sepsis[53] have all been associated with the development of BPD, presumably because of the proinflammatory environment resulting from these conditions. In one of the larger studies in this field, investigators of the NICHD NRN developed a multivariate logistic regression model for the outcome of BPD and/or the competing outcome of death at PMA of 36 weeks by using a repository of prospectively collected clinical and cytokine data.[54] Higher serum concentrations of certain cytokines (Interleukin [IL]-1β, IL-6, IL-8, IL-10, and interferon-γ) and lower concentrations of other cytokines (IL-17, RANTES [Regulated on Activation, Normal T Expressed and Secreted], and tumor necrosis factor [TNF]-β) were associated with the development of BPD/death in ELBW infants, after adjustment for other clinical variables and concentrations of other cytokines. However, the addition of cytokine data did not add much predictive ability to models using only clinical data, which suggests that clinical variables (eg, mechanical ventilation or its duration) may drive changes in cytokine concentrations, rather than vice versa.

Angiogenic growth factors Abnormal angiogenesis may contribute to the development of BPD.[50,55] Investigators have, therefore, explored the biomarker potentials of proangiogenic and antiangiogenic factors. The angiopoietin (ANG)/Tie-2 ligand/receptor system interacts with the vascular endothelial growth factor (VEGF) pathway to determine the fate of blood vessels during angiogenesis. Low concentrations of the proangiogenic ANG-1 and high concentration of the antiangiogenic endostatin in cord blood have been found to be predictive of subsequent BPD.[56,57] VEGF and the proangiogenic factor platelet-derived growth factor BB were significantly elevated in blood at 5 days of life in infants who later developed the new BPD.[58,59] Tsao and colleagues[60] found that a higher level of placental growth factor in cord blood was associated with a higher risk of BPD.[60] Similarly, the potent antiangiogenic endothelial monocyte activating polypeptide II (EMAP II), which downregulates VEGFR2 phosphorylation, has been speculated to play a role in BPD pathogenesis.[50]

Epithelial and fibrotic markers Pulmonary epithelial cell markers as well as extracellular matrix molecules may serve as biomarkers of alveolar hypoplasia in preterm infants. Members of the transforming growth factor (TGF) family, including TGFβ, activins, and bone morphogenetic proteins, are crucial factors during normal lung development as well as in the response to lung injury.[61] Clara cells are epithelial cells that line respiratory and terminal bronchioles and secrete Clara cell proteins (CCP). The levels of CCP in cord blood and serum have been reported to be low in infants who developed BPD,[62] whereas conflicting results were noted in another study in which serum CCP levels within 2 hours of life and on postnatal day 14 were higher in preterm neonates who later developed BPD.[63] Elevated cord blood levels of KL-6 (Kerbs von Lungren 6), which is a lung injury marker, and ratios of matrix metalloproteinase-9 (MMP9) to tissue inhibitor of metalloproteinase-1 have also been found to be predictors of moderate to severe BPD.[64,65]

Markers of pulmonary hypertension in bronchopulmonary dysplasia PH is common in BPD and is associated with increased mortality and morbidity.[66] BNP or N-terminal-pro-BNP is being increasingly used for the evaluation of PH in BPD.[67] However, BNP could be elevated in the absence of echocardiographic signs of PH or vice versa. It is important to remember that BNP is a marker of cardiac ventricular strain that is not specific to the right ventricle. Infants with systemic hypertension, persistent ductus arteriosus,[68] or left ventricular dysfunction for other reasons may also have elevations of BNP.

Tracheal aspirate or bronchoalveolar lavage

Tracheal aspirate analysis has historically served as a surrogate to analyze biological processes in the pulmonary compartment, in the absence of fresh neonatal lung tissue being readily available. One of the major advantages of tracheal aspirate evaluation is the ease of sample collection through the endotracheal tube, although this leads to a lack of sampling of initially nonintubated infants who may later develop BPD. In addition, the quantities of analytes in tracheal aspirate may have to be adjusted for dilution using an internal standard, such as secretory immunoglobulin A, urea, or total protein.[69] In the presence of severe lung inflammation, there is a possibility of influx of protein due to epithelial disruption making total protein a less useful internal standard. Despite its shortcomings, tracheal aspirate evaluation may provide useful information about the status of lung disease.

Inflammatory, fibrotic and epithelial markers Various cytokines and chemokines are synthesized by neutrophils and other inflammatory cells in the airway and interstitium in addition to a variety of cells of the lung parenchyma (eg, airway and alveolar epithelial cells, endothelium, and fibroblasts). The proinflammatory cytokines IL-1, IL-6, IL-8, TNF-α, and IL-1β in tracheal aspirates have been shown to predict adverse pulmonary outcomes in preterm infants and increased IL-1β concentrations; IL-1β/IL-6 ratios are associated with an increased risk for BPD, especially when infants are colonized with *Ureaplasma urealyticum*.[70–72] Increased IL-1, TNF-α, IL-6, and IL-8 correlate with the duration of supplemental oxygen and mechanical ventilation and are increased in infants who develop BPD compared with infants of similar gestational age who do not develop BPD.[71] In addition, tracheal aspirate monocyte chemoattractant protein (MCP)-1, -2, and -3 were increased in infants developing BPD.[73] Nuclear factor-kappa B, which is a critical component of the inflammasome, was increased, whereas parathyroid hormone-related protein levels were decreased in the tracheal aspirates of infants at higher risk of BPD.[74] Lower levels of CCP (CC10) have been associated with an increased risk of BPD similar to studies using blood, as mentioned earlier.[74] Among fibrotic markers, TGF-β1 is increased in tracheal aspirates of infants who go on to develop BPD.[74] Neutrophil-gelatinase-associated lipocalin (NGAL) included in a large macromolecular complex together with MMP9 is considered a marker of infectious/inflammatory processes and induction of apoptosis. In a study by Capoluongo and colleagues,[75] NGAL was increased both in infants developing BPD and in those with a patent ductus arteriosus even after adjustment for possible confounders.

Oxidant injury markers Reactive oxygen species (ROS) may cause tissue damage in lungs via multiple mechanisms.[76] Premature infants may be particularly vulnerable to oxidant injury because they have a relative deficiency of these antiproteases and deficient quantities of enzymes responsible for scavenging ROS, including superoxide dismutase and glutathione peroxidase.[77,78] Contreras and colleagues[79] established the presence of oxyradical constituents in tracheal aspirates, such as epithelial lining fluid leukocytes, elastase, myeloperoxidase, xanthine oxidase, catalase, and total sulfhydryls, as one aspect of the pulmonary inflammatory responses in infants who progressed to develop BPD.[79] Also, increased concentrations of epithelial lining fluid carbonyls, an indicator of protein oxidation, have been linked to an increased risk of BPD.[80] Increased levels of 3-chlorotyrosine and malondialdehyde are seen in oxidant injury and correlated with BPD.[81]

Angiogenic growth factors A recent study speculated that low levels of VEGF in tracheal aspirate fluid, concurrent with elevated soluble VEGF receptor 1 (VEGFR1) levels on the first day of life, are biological markers for the development of BPD.[82] EMAP II is a mediator of pulmonary vascular and alveolar formation, and its expression is inversely related to the periods of vascularization and alveolarization in the developing lung.[50] Its role as a tracheal aspirate biomarker of BPD is being investigated in ongoing studies.

Other factors Polyunsaturated fatty acids (PUFAs) and plasmalogens are the two main substrates for lipid peroxidation in the pulmonary surfactant. Rudiger and colleagues[83] found that higher levels of PUFA and plasmalogens are initially associated with a reduced risk of developing BPD and are reduced during the first day of ventilation.[83]

Urine

Joung and colleagues[84] compared urinary inflammatory and oxidative stress markers between infants with no/mild BPD group and moderate/severe BPD and between BPD cases with significant early respiratory distress syndrome (classic BPD) and with minimal early lung disease (atypical BPD). The 8-hydroxydeoxyguanosine (8-OHdG) levels on day 7 of life were an independent risk factor for developing moderate/severe BPD. In classic BPD, the 8-OHdG values on the third day of life were higher than those of atypical BPD. In atypical BPD, leukotriene E4 values on day 7 of life were higher than the values in classic BPD.[84] In other studies, high urinary concentrations of bombesinlike peptide, which are stimulated by hyperoxic exposure, were associated with an increased BPD.[85] Further studies for the prediction of BPD by analyzing proteomic signatures in the urine or blood are ongoing.

Exhaled Breath Condensates as Biomarkers

Advances in technology have produced small portable electronic noses that use a variety of technologies to emulate the human nose, with volatile organic compounds adsorbing onto sensors to produce a change in conductivity, color, or oscillation of a crystal, leading to readouts that are analyzed. Similar to how the human nose can tell the difference between different scents without needing to know the chemical constituents of the vapor, the electronic nose is able to discriminate between 2 vapor mixtures without needing to characterize the exact molecules responsible. In a recent study, Rogosch and colleagues[86] showed that smell prints of volatile organic compounds measured with an electronic nose differ between tracheal aspirates from preterm infants with or without subsequent BPD.[86]

BPD is marked by lung inflammation, and exhaled breath condensates may be a useful technique for noninvasive assessment of markers of airway inflammation.[87] Exhaled breath condensate collected from ventilated infants can be used for diagnostic purposes using gas chromatography and mass spectrometry.[88] Increased ETCO[48] and exhaled nitric oxide[89] were also found to be higher in infants with BPD on postnatal day 14 and 28, respectively.

Genomic Biomarkers

Advances in molecular genetics have enabled improvement of knowledge in pathogenesis and diagnosis of either monogenic or multifactorial neonatal lung diseases. Recent studies have indicated a major genetic contribution to BPD susceptibility.[90,91] Genetic variants predisposing to BPD may be single-nucleotide polymorphisms that may increase susceptibility to the disease. Identification of infants at higher risk of this disease by genomic analyses may be useful to provide them individualized therapies in the future.[92]

Differences in the genome

In a genome-wide association study, Hadchouel and colleagues[93] identified SPOCK2 as a new possible candidate susceptibility gene; but this target was not confirmed by Wang and colleagues.[94] As single marker approaches might not explain more than a small fraction of heritability of BPD, an integrated genomic analysis was conducted recently by the NICHD NRN.[5] Genome-wide association and gene set analysis were performed for BPD or death, severe BPD or death, and severe BPD in survivors. Specific targets were validated via the use of gene expression in BPD lung tissue and in a mouse model. Pathway analyses confirmed involvement of known pathways of lung development and repair (CD44, phosphorus oxygen lyase activity) and indicated novel molecules and pathways (adenosine deaminase, targets of miR-219) involved in genetic predisposition to BPD. In addition, this study observed marked differences in pathways by race/ethnicity suggesting that, although the clinical phenotype of BPD may be similar, the underlying genetic predisposition may differ significantly. An additional major finding was that the pathways associated with mild/moderate BPD were very different from those associated with severe BPD, suggesting that the pathophysiology and potential therapies of severe BPD may be substantially different from those for mild/moderate BPD.

Differences in gene expression

Using a biorepository of autopsy tissues, Bhattacharya and colleagues[95] performed a genome-wide transcriptional profiling to comprehensively define gene expression changes from the lung tissue of premature babies who died with a diagnosis of BPD. This study identified both general mast cell (tryptase) and mucosal-type mast cell specific (CPA3) markers increased in BPD tissue. Pietrzyk and colleagues[96] carried out genome-wide transcriptional profiling of RNA extracted from peripheral blood mononuclear cells of BPD subjects and non-BPD controls followed by pathway enrichment analysis. They found that the expression of nearly 10% of the genome was altered in infants with BPD, mostly in the cell cycle pathway and T-cell signaling pathway.

Recently discovered microRNAs regulating target mRNAs have been seen to be dysregulated in multiple disorders. Because miRNAs have the ability to modify gene expression rapidly and reversibly, they are ideal mediators for sensing and responding to hypoxic or hyperoxic stress and may, therefore, be associated with alveolar dysplasias. In a recent analysis by Yang and colleagues,[97] 4 upregulated miRNAs (miRNA-21, miRNA-34a, miRNA-431, and Let-7f) and one downregulated miRNA (miRNA-335) were differentially expressed in BPD lung tissues compared with normal lungs. In addition, 8 miRNAs (miRNA-146b, miRNA-29a, miRNA-503, miRNA-411, miRNA-214, miRNA-130b, miRNA-382, and miRNA-181a-1) were found to show differential expression in the process of normal lung development and during the progress of BPD. Finally, several meaningful target genes (such as the HPGD and NTRK genes) of common miRNAs (such as miRNA-21 and miRNA-141) were systematically predicted. Also, as mentioned previously, in the integrated genomic analyses conducted by the NICHD NRN, the pathway with the lowest false discovery rate for BPD/death was the targets of miR-219.

Respiratory Microbiome as a Biomarker of Bronchopulmonary Dysplasia

Microbiota can be defined as the microbes associated with a particular context; unlike traditional microbiological approaches that aim to identify individual pathogens, microbiota analysis characterizes all of the bacterial species present, both in terms of their identities and relative abundance.[98] High-throughput sequencing of the 16S rRNA gene generated from bacteria-containing samples yields a large number of short sequences that can be subsequently aligned and sorted according to a predefined level of homology and classified according to taxonomic databases. To date, there are few studies that use culture-independent methods for detection of airway organisms in preterm infants. Recently in a small study of 25 preterm infants, Lohmann and colleagues[99] demonstrated that the airways of premature infants are not sterile at birth. They speculated that reduced diversity of the microbiome may be an associated factor in the development of BPD. In a small study of 10 infants, Mourani and colleagues[100] demonstrated by newer techniques that early bacterial colonization with diverse species are present in the airways of intubated preterm infants and can be characterized by bacterial load and species diversity. None of the aforementioned small studies used a control population for comparison; hence, a much larger study in this field is warranted to evaluate the biomarker potential of the respiratory microbiome.

THE FUTURE OF BRONCHOPULMONARY DYSPLASIA DIAGNOSTICS AND BIOMARKERS

BPD is a disease, which has many different subphenotypes with a common operational definition. Hence, better phenotyping of the disease and more detailed data collection of clinical variables, in addition to careful determination of specific and temporal biomarkers are warranted. Novel systems biology approaches are required for evaluating the multiple interacting cellular and molecular networks that control lung development and regeneration or remodeling in response to injury and in chronic diseases. These approaches are the newer omic strategies that supplement or expand on the genomic, proteomic, and microbiomic approaches that were discussed earlier. State-of-the-art prediction tools involving an amalgamation of clinical predictors with systems biology analysis might provide better insight to understanding the pathogenesis of the disease and could facilitate novel biomarker development for early detection and treatment of BPD.

REFERENCES

1. Walsh MC, Yao Q, Gettner P, et al. Impact of a physiologic definition on bronchopulmonary dysplasia rates. Pediatrics 2004;114(5):1305–11.
2. Bhat R, Salas AA, Foster C, et al. Prospective analysis of pulmonary hypertension in extremely low birth weight infants. Pediatrics 2012;129(3):e682–9.
3. Doull IJ, Mok Q, Tasker RC. Tracheobronchomalacia in preterm infants with chronic lung disease. Arch Dis Child Fetal Neonatal Ed 1997;76(3):F203–5.
4. Northway WH Jr, Rosan RC, Porter DY. Pulmonary disease following respirator therapy of hyaline-membrane disease. Bronchopulmonary dysplasia. N Engl J Med 1967;276(7):357–68.
5. Ambalavanan N, Cotten CM, Page GP, et al. Integrated genomic analyses in bronchopulmonary dysplasia. J Pediatr 2014;166:531–7.e13.
6. Tin W, Wiswell TE. Adjunctive therapies in chronic lung disease: examining the evidence. Semin Fetal Neonatal Med 2008;13(1):44–52.
7. Woodcock J. Chutes and ladders on the critical path: comparative effectiveness, product value, and the use of biomarkers in drug development. Clin Pharmacol Ther 2009;86(1):12–4.
8. Biomarkers Definitions Working Group. Biomarkers and surrogate endpoints: preferred definitions and conceptual framework. Clin Pharmacol Ther 2001; 69(3):89–95.

9. Darlow BA, Graham PJ. Vitamin A supplementation to prevent mortality and short- and long-term morbidity in very low birthweight infants. Cochrane Database Syst Rev 2011;(10):CD000501.

10. Woodcock J. Assessing the clinical utility of diagnostics used in drug therapy. Clin Pharmacol Ther 2010;88(6):765–73.

11. Sinkin RA, Cox C, Phelps DL. Predicting risk for bronchopulmonary dysplasia: selection criteria for clinical trials. Pediatrics 1990;86(5):728–36.

12. Yoder BA, Anwar MU, Clark RH. Early prediction of neonatal chronic lung disease: a comparison of three scoring methods. Pediatr Pulmonol 1999;27(6):388–94.

13. Goldman SL, Gerhardt T, Sonni R, et al. Early prediction of chronic lung disease by pulmonary function testing. J Pediatr 1983;102(4):613–7.

14. Bhutani VK, Abbasi S. Relative likelihood of bronchopulmonary dysplasia based on pulmonary mechanics measured in preterm neonates during the first week of life. J Pediatr 1992;120(4 Pt 1):605–13.

15. Corcoran JD, Patterson CC, Thomas PS, et al. Reduction in the risk of bronchopulmonary dysplasia from 1980-1990: results of a multivariate logistic regression analysis. Eur J Pediatr 1993;152(8):677–81.

16. Farstad T, Bratlid D. Incidence and prediction of bronchopulmonary dysplasia in a cohort of premature infants. Acta Paediatr 1994;83(1):19–24.

17. Hentschel J, Friedel C, Maier RF, et al. Predicting chronic lung disease in very low birthweight infants: comparison of 3 scores. J Perinat Med 1998;26(5):378–83.

18. Jobe AH, Bancalari E. Bronchopulmonary dysplasia. Am J Respir Crit Care Med 2001;163(7):1723–9.

19. Walsh MC, Wilson-Costello D, Zadell A, et al. Safety, reliability, and validity of a physiologic definition of bronchopulmonary dysplasia. J Perinatol 2003;23(6):451–6.

20. Onland W, Debray TP, Laughon MM, et al. Clinical prediction models for bronchopulmonary dysplasia: a systematic review and external validation study. BMC Pediatr 2013;13:207.

21. Cools F, Askie LM, Offringa M, Prevention of Ventilator Induced Lung Injury Collaborative Study Group. Elective high-frequency oscillatory ventilation in preterm infants with respiratory distress syndrome: an individual patient data meta-analysis. BMC Pediatr 2009;9:33.

22. Ryan SW, Wild NJ, Arthur RJ, et al. Prediction of chronic neonatal lung disease in very low birthweight neonates using clinical and radiological variables. Arch Dis Child Fetal Neonatal Ed 1994;71(1):F36–9.

23. Kim YD, Kim EA, Kim KS, et al. Scoring method for early prediction of neonatal chronic lung disease using modified respiratory parameters. J Korean Med Sci 2005;20(3):397–401.

24. Laughon MM, Langer JC, Bose CL, et al. Prediction of bronchopulmonary dysplasia by postnatal age in extremely premature infants. Am J Respir Crit Care Med 2011;183(12):1715–22.

25. Walsh M, Laptook A, Kazzi SN, et al. A cluster-randomized trial of benchmarking and multimodal quality improvement to improve rates of survival free of bronchopulmonary dysplasia for infants with birth weights of less than 1250 grams. Pediatrics 2007;119(5):876–90.

26. Edwards DK, Colby TV, Northway WH Jr. Radiographic-pathologic correlation in bronchopulmonary dysplasia. J Pediatr 1979;95(5 Pt 2):834–6.

27. Mortensson W, Andreasson B, Lindroth M, et al. Potential of early chest roentgen examination in ventilator treated newborn infants to predict future lung function and disease. Pediatr Radiol 1989;20(1–2):41–4.

28. Yuksel B, Greenough A, Karani J, et al. Chest radiograph scoring system for use in pre-term infants. Br J Radiol 1991;64(767):1015–8.
29. Greenough A, Kavvadia V, Johnson AH, et al. A simple chest radiograph score to predict chronic lung disease in prematurely born infants. Br J Radiol 1999; 72(858):530–3.
30. Greenough A, Thomas M, Dimitriou G, et al. Prediction of outcome from the chest radiograph appearance on day 7 of very prematurely born infants. Eur J Pediatr 2004;163(1):14–8.
31. Fitzgerald DA, Van Asperen PP, Lam AH, et al. Chest radiograph abnormalities in very low birthweight survivors of chronic neonatal lung disease. J Paediatr Child Health 1996;32(6):491–4.
32. Moya MP, Bisset GS 3rd, Auten RL Jr, et al. Reliability of CXR for the diagnosis of bronchopulmonary dysplasia. Pediatr Radiol 2001;31(5):339–42.
33. Oppenheim C, Mamou-Mani T, Sayegh N, et al. Bronchopulmonary dysplasia: value of CT in identifying pulmonary sequelae. AJR Am J Roentgenol 1994; 163(1):169–72.
34. Kubota J, Ohki Y, Inoue T, et al. Ultrafast CT scoring system for assessing bronchopulmonary dysplasia: reproducibility and clinical correlation. Radiat Med 1998;16(3):167–74.
35. Ochiai M, Hikino S, Yabuuchi H, et al. A new scoring system for computed tomography of the chest for assessing the clinical status of bronchopulmonary dysplasia. J Pediatr 2008;152(1):90–5, 95.e1–3.
36. Shin SM, Kim WS, Cheon JE, et al. Bronchopulmonary dysplasia: new high resolution computed tomography scoring system and correlation between the high resolution computed tomography score and clinical severity. Korean J Radiol 2013;14(2):350–60.
37. Wielputz M, Kauczor HU. MRI of the lung: state of the art. Diagn Interv Radiol 2012;18(4):344–53.
38. Adams EW, Harrison MC, Counsell SJ, et al. Increased lung water and tissue damage in bronchopulmonary dysplasia. J Pediatr 2004;145(4):503–7.
39. Hopkins SR, Levin DL, Emami K, et al. Advances in magnetic resonance imaging of lung physiology. J Appl Physiol 2007;102(3):1244–54.
40. Yablonskiy DA, Sukstanskii AL, Woods JC, et al. Quantification of lung microstructure with hyperpolarized 3He diffusion MRI. J Appl Physiol 2009;107(4): 1258–65.
41. Narayanan M, Beardsmore CS, Owers-Bradley J, et al. Catch-up alveolarization in ex-preterm children: evidence from (3)He magnetic resonance. Am J Respir Crit Care Med 2013;187(10):1104–9.
42. Mourani PM, Sontag MK, Younoszai A, et al. Early pulmonary vascular disease in preterm infants at risk for bronchopulmonary dysplasia. Am J Respir Crit Care Med 2015;191(1):87–95.
43. Mourani PM, Sontag MK, Younoszai A, et al. Clinical utility of echocardiography for the diagnosis and management of pulmonary vascular disease in young children with chronic lung disease. Pediatrics 2008;121(2):317–25.
44. Hill KD, Lim DS, Everett AD, et al. Assessment of pulmonary hypertension in the pediatric catheterization laboratory: current insights from the Magic registry. Catheter Cardiovasc Interv 2010;76(6):865–73.
45. Graff MA, Novo RP, Diaz M, et al. Compliance measurement in respiratory distress syndrome: the prediction of outcome. Pediatr Pulmonol 1986;2(6):332–6.
46. Freezer NJ, Sly PD. Predictive value of measurements of respiratory mechanics in preterm infants with HMD. Pediatr Pulmonol 1993;16(2):116–23.

47. Gibson AM, Reddington C, McBride L, et al. Lung function in adult survivors of very low birth weight, with and without bronchopulmonary dysplasia. Pediatr Pulmonol 2014. [Epub ahead of print].
48. May C, Patel S, Kennedy C, et al. Prediction of bronchopulmonary dysplasia. Arch Dis Child Fetal Neonatal Ed 2011;96(6):F410–6.
49. Van Lierde S, Smith J, Devlieger H, et al. Pulmonary mechanics during respiratory distress syndrome in the prediction of outcome and differentiation of mild and severe bronchopulmonary dysplasia. Pediatr Pulmonol 1994;17(4):218–24.
50. Lal CV, Schwarz MA. Vascular mediators in chronic lung disease of infancy: role of endothelial monocyte activating polypeptide II (EMAP II). Birth Defects Res A Clin Mol Teratol 2014;100(3):180–8.
51. Watterberg KL, Demers LM, Scott SM, et al. Chorioamnionitis and early lung inflammation in infants in whom bronchopulmonary dysplasia develops. Pediatrics 1996;97(2):210–5.
52. Schelonka RL, Katz B, Waites KB, et al. Critical appraisal of the role of Ureaplasma in the development of bronchopulmonary dysplasia with meta-analytic techniques. Pediatr Infect Dis J 2005;24(12):1033–9.
53. Stoll BJ, Hansen N, Fanaroff AA, et al. Changes in pathogens causing early-onset sepsis in very-low-birth-weight infants. N Engl J Med 2002;347(4):240–7.
54. Ambalavanan N, Carlo WA, D'Angio CT, et al. Cytokines associated with bronchopulmonary dysplasia or death in extremely low birth weight infants. Pediatrics 2009;123(4):1132–41.
55. Thebaud B, Abman SH. Bronchopulmonary dysplasia: where have all the vessels gone? Roles of angiogenic growth factors in chronic lung disease. Am J Respir Crit Care Med 2007;175(10):978–85.
56. Mohamed WA, Niyazy WH, Mahfouz AA. Angiopoietin-1 and endostatin levels in cord plasma predict the development of bronchopulmonary dysplasia in preterm infants. J Trop Pediatr 2011;57(5):385–8.
57. Janer J, Andersson S, Kajantie E, et al. Endostatin concentration in cord plasma predicts the development of bronchopulmonary dysplasia in very low birth weight infants. Pediatrics 2009;123(4):1142–6.
58. Vento G, Capoluongo E, Matassa PG, et al. Serum levels of seven cytokines in premature ventilated newborns: correlations with old and new forms of bronchopulmonary dysplasia. Intensive Care Med 2006;32(5):723–30.
59. Jobe AH. The new bronchopulmonary dysplasia. Curr Opin Pediatr 2011;23(2):167–72.
60. Tsao PN, Wei SC, Su YN, et al. Placenta growth factor elevation in the cord blood of premature neonates predicts poor pulmonary outcome. Pediatrics 2004;113(5):1348–51.
61. Ambalavanan N, Nicola T, Hagood J, et al. Transforming growth factor-beta signaling mediates hypoxia-induced pulmonary arterial remodeling and inhibition of alveolar development in newborn mouse lung. Am J Physiol Lung Cell Mol Physiol 2008;295(1):L86–95.
62. Schrama AJ, Bernard A, Poorthuis BJ, et al. Cord blood Clara cell protein CC16 predicts the development of bronchopulmonary dysplasia. Eur J Pediatr 2008;167(11):1305–12.
63. Sarafidis K, Stathopoulou T, Diamanti E, et al. Clara cell secretory protein (CC16) as a peripheral blood biomarker of lung injury in ventilated preterm neonates. Eur J Pediatr 2008;167(11):1297–303.
64. Ogihara T, Hirano K, Morinobu T, et al. Plasma KL-6 predicts the development and outcome of bronchopulmonary dysplasia. Pediatr Res 2006;60(5):613–8.

65. Fukunaga S, Ichiyama T, Maeba S, et al. MMP-9 and TIMP-1 in the cord blood of premature infants developing BPD. Pediatr Pulmonol 2009;44(3): 267–72.
66. Ambalavanan N, Mourani P. Pulmonary hypertension in bronchopulmonary dysplasia. Birth Defects Res A Clin Mol Teratol 2014;100(3):240–6.
67. Kim GB. Pulmonary hypertension in infants with bronchopulmonary dysplasia. Korean J Pediatr 2010;53(6):688–93.
68. Sanjeev S, Pettersen M, Lua J, et al. Role of plasma B-type natriuretic peptide in screening for hemodynamically significant patent ductus arteriosus in preterm neonates. J Perinatol 2005;25(11):709–13.
69. Truog WE, Ballard PL, Norberg M, et al. Inflammatory markers and mediators in tracheal fluid of premature infants treated with inhaled nitric oxide. Pediatrics 2007;119(4):670–8.
70. Kotecha S, Wilson L, Wangoo A, et al. Increase in interleukin (IL)-1 beta and IL-6 in bronchoalveolar lavage fluid obtained from infants with chronic lung disease of prematurity. Pediatr Res 1996;40(2):250–6.
71. Jonsson B, Tullus K, Brauner A, et al. Early increase of TNF alpha and IL-6 in tracheobronchial aspirate fluid indicator of subsequent chronic lung disease in preterm infants. Arch Dis Child Fetal Neonatal Ed 1997;77(3):F198–201.
72. Patterson AM, Taciak V, Lovchik J, et al. Ureaplasma urealyticum respiratory tract colonization is associated with an increase in interleukin 1-beta and tumor necrosis factor alpha relative to interleukin 6 in tracheal aspirates of preterm infants. Pediatr Infect Dis J 1998;17(4):321–8.
73. Bose CL, Dammann CE, Laughon MM. Bronchopulmonary dysplasia and inflammatory biomarkers in the premature neonate. Arch Dis Child Fetal Neonatal Ed 2008;93(6):F455–61.
74. Bhandari A, Bhandari V. Biomarkers in bronchopulmonary dysplasia. Paediatr Respir Rev 2013;14(3):173–9.
75. Capoluongo E, Vento G, Lulli P, et al. Epithelial lining fluid neutrophil-gelatinase-associated lipocalin levels in premature newborns with bronchopulmonary dysplasia and patency of ductus arteriosus. Int J Immunopathol Pharmacol 2008;21(1):173–9.
76. Saugstad OD. Oxidative stress in the newborn–a 30-year perspective. Biol Neonate 2005;88(3):228–36.
77. Frank L, Sosenko IR. Development of lung antioxidant enzyme system in late gestation: possible implications for the prematurely born infant. J Pediatr 1987;110(1):9–14.
78. Autor AP, Frank L, Roberts RJ. Developmental characteristics of pulmonary superoxide dismutase: relationship to idiopathic respiratory distress syndrome. Pediatr Res 1976;10(3):154–8.
79. Contreras M, Hariharan N, Lewandoski JR, et al. Bronchoalveolar oxyradical inflammatory elements herald bronchopulmonary dysplasia. Crit Care Med 1996; 24(1):29–37.
80. Gladstone IM Jr, Levine RL. Oxidation of proteins in neonatal lungs. Pediatrics 1994;93(5):764–8.
81. Thompson A, Bhandari V. Pulmonary biomarkers of bronchopulmonary dysplasia. Biomark Insights 2008;3:361–73.
82. Hasan J, Beharry KD, Valencia AM, et al. Soluble vascular endothelial growth factor receptor 1 in tracheal aspirate fluid of preterm neonates at birth may be predictive of bronchopulmonary dysplasia/chronic lung disease. Pediatrics 2009;123(6):1541–7.

83. Rudiger M, von Baehr A, Haupt R, et al. Preterm infants with high polyunsaturated fatty acid and plasmalogen content in tracheal aspirates develop bronchopulmonary dysplasia less often. Crit Care Med 2000;28(5):1572–7.

84. Joung KE, Kim HS, Lee J, et al. Correlation of urinary inflammatory and oxidative stress markers in very low birth weight infants with subsequent development of bronchopulmonary dysplasia. Free Radic Res 2011;45(9):1024–32.

85. Cullen A, Van Marter LJ, Allred EN, et al. Urine bombesin-like peptide elevation precedes clinical evidence of bronchopulmonary dysplasia. Am J Respir Crit Care Med 2002;165(8):1093–7.

86. Rogosch T, Herrmann N, Maier RF, et al. Detection of bloodstream infections and prediction of bronchopulmonary dysplasia in preterm neonates with an electronic nose. J Pediatr 2014;165(3):622–4.

87. Rosias PP, Dompeling E, Hendriks HJ, et al. Exhaled breath condensate in children: pearls and pitfalls. Pediatr Allergy Immunol 2004;15(1):4–19.

88. Kushch I, Schwarz K, Schwentner L, et al. Compounds enhanced in a mass spectrometric profile of smokers' exhaled breath versus non-smokers as determined in a pilot study using PTR-MS. J Breath Res 2008;2(2):026002.

89. May C, Williams O, Milner AD, et al. Relation of exhaled nitric oxide levels to development of bronchopulmonary dysplasia. Arch Dis Child Fetal Neonatal Ed 2009;94(3):F205–9.

90. Bhandari V, Bizzarro MJ, Shetty A, et al. Familial and genetic susceptibility to major neonatal morbidities in preterm twins. Pediatrics 2006;117(6):1901–6.

91. Lavoie PM, Pham C, Jang KL. Heritability of bronchopulmonary dysplasia, defined according to the consensus statement of the national institutes of health. Pediatrics 2008;122(3):479–85.

92. Somaschini M, Castiglioni E, Presi S, et al. Genetic susceptibility to neonatal lung diseases. Acta Biomed 2012;83(Suppl 1):10–4.

93. Hadchouel A, Durrmeyer X, Bouzigon E, et al. Identification of SPOCK2 as a susceptibility gene for bronchopulmonary dysplasia. Am J Respir Crit Care Med 2011;184(10):1164–70.

94. Wang H, St Julien KR, Stevenson DK, et al. A genome-wide association study (GWAS) for bronchopulmonary dysplasia. Pediatrics 2013;132(2):290–7.

95. Bhattacharya S, Go D, Krenitsky DL, et al. Genome-wide transcriptional profiling reveals connective tissue mast cell accumulation in bronchopulmonary dysplasia. Am J Respir Crit Care Med 2012;186(4):349–58.

96. Pietrzyk JJ, Kwinta P, Wollen EJ, et al. Gene expression profiling in preterm infants: new aspects of bronchopulmonary dysplasia development. PLoS one 2013;8(10):e78585.

97. Yang Y, Qiu J, Kan Q, et al. MicroRNA expression profiling studies on bronchopulmonary dysplasia: a systematic review and meta-analysis. Genet Mol Res 2013;12(4):5195–206.

98. Rogers GB, Shaw D, Marsh RL, et al. Respiratory microbiota: addressing clinical questions, informing clinical practice. Thorax 2015;70(1):74–81.

99. Lohmann P, Luna RA, Hollister EB, et al. The airway microbiome of intubated premature infants: characteristics and changes that predict the development of bronchopulmonary dysplasia. Pediatr Res 2014;76(3):294–301.

100. Mourani PM, Harris JK, Sontag MK, et al. Molecular identification of bacteria in tracheal aspirate fluid from mechanically ventilated preterm infants. PLoS one 2011;6(10):e25959.

Evidence-Based Pharmacologic Therapies for Prevention of Bronchopulmonary Dysplasia

Application of the Grading of Recommendations Assessment, Development, and Evaluation Methodology

Erik A. Jensen, MD, Elizabeth E. Foglia, MD,
Barbara Schmidt, MD, MSc*

KEYWORDS

- Bronchopulmonary dysplasia • Chronic lung disease • Azithromycin • Caffeine
- Dexamethasone • Vitamin A

KEY POINTS

- Caffeine and vitamin A are the only pharmacologic therapies with high-quality evidence to support routine use for prevention of bronchopulmonary dysplasia (BPD) in extremely preterm infants.
- Dexamethasone is effective for the prevention of BPD but can increase the risk for neurodevelopmental impairment.
- Among extremely preterm infants at high risk for BPD, the net balance of benefits and harms may favor the use of dexamethasone after the first week of life; however, the optimal dose and duration of therapy is unknown.

INTRODUCTION

Bronchopulmonary dysplasia (BPD) occurs in approximately 50% of extremely low-birth-weight infants, affecting 10,000 to 15,000 infants per year in the United States and accounting for more than $2.4 billion in annual health care costs.[1–3] BPD is

Funding Source: No funding was secured for this study.
Disclosures: The authors have no conflicts of interest or relevant financial interests to disclose.
Division of Neonatology, Department of Pediatrics, The Children's Hospital of Philadelphia, The University of Pennsylvania, Philadelphia, PA 19104, USA
* Corresponding author. Division of Neonatology, Hospital of the University of Pennsylvania, 3400 Spruce Street, 8 Ravdin, Philadelphia, PA 19104.
E-mail address: barbara.schmidt@uphs.upenn.edu

Clin Perinatol 42 (2015) 755–779
http://dx.doi.org/10.1016/j.clp.2015.08.005
0095-5108/15/$ – see front matter © 2015 Elsevier Inc. All rights reserved.

associated with higher mortality rates and predisposes survivors to chronic respiratory and cardiovascular impairments, growth failure, and neurodevelopmental delay.[4–10]

The increased use of antenatal corticosteroids, surfactant therapy, and noninvasive ventilation has changed the course of lung disease associated with prematurity.[11] Once a common problem in all mechanically ventilated preterm infants, BPD is rarely seen today in bigger and more mature preterm babies with birth weights more than 1500 g.[11] In contrast, most studies suggest that BPD rates have remained stable or even increased among extremely preterm infants.[3,11–15]

Neonatal pharmacologic therapies are one important tool to reduce the burden of BPD among very immature infants. Four medications have been shown in meta-analyses or large individual randomized controlled trials (RCTs) to reduce the risk of BPD in infants born 32 weeks' gestation or earlier.[16] The authors' objective was to systematically review the evidence in support of these 4 medications (azithromycin, caffeine, dexamethasone, and vitamin A). The authors then applied the Grading of Recommendations Assessment, Development, and Evaluation (GRADE) framework to assess the quality of the evidence and formulate recommendations for the use of each medication.[17]

Grading of Recommendations Assessment, Development, and Evaluation Framework

The GRADE approach provides a "systematic and transparent" framework to develop clinical recommendations based on the quality of available evidence and the balance between the benefits and harms of a therapy.[17,18] The quality of the evidence in GRADE is rated as *high* to *very low* depending on the underlying study methodology and several key strengths and weaknesses that may affect the study validity.[18] RCTs begin with a *high* rating but can be downgraded because of study limitations (**Box 1**).[18] Observational studies begin with a *low* rating and can be downgraded to *very low* or upgraded to *moderate* or rarely *high* based on their strengths and weaknesses (see **Box 1**).[18]

Recommendations in GRADE are made as *strong* or *weak* and for or against the use of a therapy.[18] A strong recommendation in favor of a therapy indicates that guideline developers are confident that the desirable effects outweigh the undesirable effects.[18] In contrast, a weak recommendation in favor of a therapy implies that the guideline developers are less certain that the desirable effects outweigh the undesirable ones.[18] Most individuals should receive a therapy that is strongly recommended.[18] Much more individualized consideration of a patient's characteristics or disease state is needed when selecting the appropriate course of action in the case of a weak recommendation.[18]

METHODS
Search Strategy

The authors conducted a systematic search of PubMed from the inception of the database through 12/31/2014 for all meta-analyses, RCTs, and observational studies that assessed the efficacy of azithromycin, caffeine, dexamethasone, and vitamin A for the prevention of BPD. The search combined the individual therapy name with the following terms: *bronchopulmonary dysplasia* or *chronic lung disease*. The authors excluded case reports, editorials, letters, and non-English publications from their initial search. They reviewed the citation lists of the reviewed articles to identify additional publications for potential inclusion.

Box 1
Factors that may decrease or increase the GRADE quality of evidence

Factors that may decrease the quality of evidence

- Limitations in the design and implementation of RCTs suggesting a high likelihood of bias (−1 or 2 quality categories)
- Inconsistency of results, including problems with subgroup analyses (−1)
- Indirectness of the evidence (indirect population, intervention, control, outcomes) (−1 or −2)
- Sparse evidence, small sample size (−1)
- High probability of reporting bias (−1)

Factors that may increase the quality of evidence

- Large magnitude of effect from direct evidence
  - RR >2 or RR <0.5 with no plausible confounders (+1)
  - RR >5 or RR <0.2 with no threats to validity (+2)
- All plausible confounding would reduce a demonstrated effect (+1)
- Dose-response gradient (+1)

Numbers in parentheses indicate the levels of change in the quality of evidence.
Abbreviations: RCT, randomized controlled trial; RR, relative risk.
Adapted from Schünemann HJ, Jaeschke R, Cook DJ, et al. An official ATS statement: grading the quality of evidence and strength of recommendations in ATS guidelines and recommendations. Am J Respir Crit Care Med 2006;174:610.

Study Selection

Two reviewers independently conducted the search (EAJ, EEF). The authors selected meta-analyses, RCTs, and observational studies that assessed BPD, defined as a supplemental oxygen requirement at 36 weeks' postmenstrual age (PMA), as a primary or secondary outcome. For meta-analyses that have been updated, only the most recent version was reviewed. Individual RCTs were only included if the trial results had not been pooled in a meta-analysis. Studies that evaluated the composite outcome of death or BPD were excluded if the rates of BPD in survivors were not reported. Observational studies were included only if they used contemporary and not historical controls.

Clinical Trials Registry Search

To gain a better understanding of the ongoing research of therapeutic agents to prevent BPD, the authors queried the clinicaltrials.gov Web site on 1/19/2015 using the search terms *bronchopulmonary dysplasia* and *chronic lung disease*. The authors limited the search to interventional studies in the child age group. The authors excluded completed studies with published results and those with unknown status.

SUMMARY OF THE EVIDENCE FOR INDIVIDUAL THERAPIES
Azithromycin

Azithromycin belongs to a class of agents called macrolides, which have both antimicrobial and antiinflammatory properties.[19,20] In older children and adults, macrolides have been shown to be beneficial in inflammatory lung diseases, such as cystic fibrosis and chronic obstructive pulmonary disease.[21,22] In preterm infants, infection with

Ureaplasma species may play a role in the development of BPD.[23,24] Following this observation, investigators began to evaluate whether macrolides would benefit infants at risk for BPD. Three macrolides have been studied in RCTs, but only azithromycin has been shown to reduce the incidence of BPD.[25] A single RCT with clarithromycin and a Cochrane review of 2 small trials of erythromycin showed no benefit.[26,27]

Systematic search results

The authors' systematic search identified 6 articles for full review (**Fig. 1**). They excluded 2 pharmacokinetic studies that lacked a control group, leaving 3 RCTs summarized in a single meta-analysis by Nair and colleagues[25] (**Table 1**). None of the individual RCTs demonstrated a reduction in BPD.[25] However, a subgroup analysis of 61 surviving infants with tracheal aspirates that were positive for *Ureaplasma* in the trial by Ballard and colleagues[28] suggested that azithromycin may be most effective in colonized infants. In contrast, the meta-analysis found that prophylactic treatment of extremely preterm infants with azithromycin reduced the incidence of BPD regardless of known bacterial infection or colonization (see **Table 1**).[25]

Risk-to-benefit comparison

There are limited data available on the adverse effects of azithromycin to inform a proper assessment of the balance between potential benefits and harms in extremely preterm infants. Both trials by Ballard and colleagues[28,29] reported moderately higher rates of invasive fungal infections; however, the differences did not reach statistical significance. None of the trials observed clinically relevant differences in transaminase levels, rates of necrotizing enterocolitis, or hearing abnormalities before discharge.[25,28–30] Data on the impact of azithromycin use on microbial resistance patterns and long-term neurodevelopment are needed.

Overall quality of the evidence

The overall quality of the evidence was low. Beginning with an initial rating of *high* because the studies were RCTs, the authors downgraded the quality to *low* because it was unclear whether personnel were blinded to treatment allocation in 2 of the 3 RCTs (−1) and because the overall sample size was small (−1). The moderate study heterogeneity ($I^2 = 47\%$, $P = .15$) in the meta-analysis also raises concerns whether it is appropriate to pool the data.[25]

Recommendation

The combined data from the available published trials suggests that prophylactic use of azithromycin may reduce the incidence of BPD among high-risk infants, but the quality of the evidence is low. Additionally, high-quality safety and dosing data are not yet available; concerns for possible emergence of resistant organisms with widespread use remain. Therefore, pending the results of larger RCTs, the authors suggest that prophylactic azithromycin should not be used to prevent BPD in extremely preterm infants (**Box 2**).

Caffeine

Caffeine is a methylxanthine that reduces the effects of adenosine in the central nervous system.[31] Caffeine stimulates breathing by increasing minute ventilation, carbon dioxide sensitivity, and diaphragmatic activity.[32,33] The Caffeine for Apnea of Prematurity (CAP) trial showed that caffeine has several short- and long-term benefits, including a reduction in the risk of BPD.[34,35] Caffeine is now the most commonly prescribed medication after antibiotics in the neonatal intensive care unit.[36]

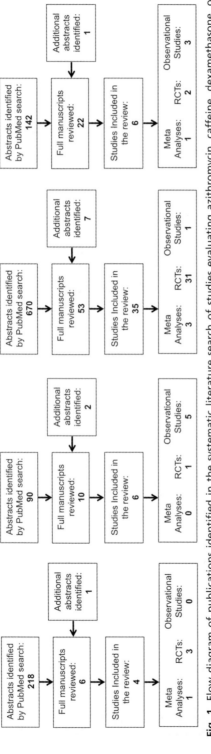

Fig. 1. Flow diagram of publications identified in the systematic literature search of studies evaluating azithromycin, caffeine, dexamethasone, or vitamin A for prevention of BPD.

Table 1
Placebo-controlled studies of prophylactic azithromycin for prevention of BPD

					Summary of Findings		GRADE Level of Evidence
Author/Year	Study Type	Study Comparison	Population	Limitations/Bias	Rates of BPD	Effect Size	

Prophylactic azithromycin vs placebo

| Nair et al,[25] 2014 | Meta-analysis | Azithromycin (10 mg/kg/d × 7 d initiated DOL 0–2 in 2 trials, 10 mg/kg/d × 7 d followed by 5 mg/kg/d × 7 d, initiated DOL 7 in 1 trial) vs placebo | 3 RCTs, all enrolled extremely preterm infants 2 RCTs enrolled only mechanically ventilated infants | Overall small sample size. Moderate study heterogeneity in the meta-analysis. Unclear blinding in 2 RCTs | Azithromycin 50.3% (81 of 161) vs placebo 60.4% (90 of 149) | RR 0.83 (95% CI 0.71–0.97) NNT 9.6 (95% CI 5.4–43.9)[a] | Low |

Abbreviations: DOL, day of life; NNT, number needed to treat; RR, relative risk.
[a] Estimates calculated with the use of the Woolf method because the data were pooled from multiple studies.[87]

> **Box 2**
> **Summary of the overall level of evidence and recommendations for therapies to prevent BPD in infants born less than 32 weeks' gestation**
>
> **Azithromycin**
>
> *Level of evidence:* low
>
> *Summary and recommendation:* A meta-analysis inclusive of 3 small RCTs demonstrated a reduction in BPD with early prophylactic azithromycin. However, the quality of evidence from these studies is low, and concerns remain regarding possible emergence of resistant organisms with widespread use. Pending the results of larger RCTs, *the authors suggest that prophylactic azithromycin should not be used to prevent BPD in extremely preterm infants (weak recommendation based on the low-quality evidence).*
>
> **Caffeine**
>
> *Level of evidence:* high
>
> *Summary and recommendation:* A large, multicenter RCT demonstrated a reduction in BPD among surviving infants born 500 to 1250 g. Multiple subsequent observational studies demonstrated a lower risk of BPD when caffeine therapy was initiated before the third day of life. *The authors strongly recommend the use of caffeine therapy for the prevention of BPD in extremely preterm infants and suggest initiation of therapy in most infants soon after birth.*
>
> **Dexamethasone**
>
> Level of evidence: *high*
>
> *Summary and recommendations:* Meta-analyses demonstrate a reduction in BPD when dexamethasone is initiated before or after the first week of life. However, dexamethasone may increase the risk of cerebral palsy (CP), hypertrophic cardiomyopathy, and gastrointestinal perforation. A meta-regression showed that the effect of corticosteroids on the composite outcome of death or CP varied depending on the risk of BPD in the enrolled patients. When the risk of BPD in the control population was less than approximately 33%, corticosteroid therapy significantly increased the risk of death or CP. When the risk of BPD exceeded approximately 60%, corticosteroids reduced the risk of death or CP. The authors suggest dexamethasone should not be routinely used to prevent BPD in all infants but may be indicated in some based on individual BPD risk *(weak recommendation based on the need to balance benefits and harms).*
>
> **Vitamin A**
>
> Level of evidence: *high*
>
> *Summary and recommendation:* A meta-analysis inclusive of 2 RCTs demonstrated a small but statistically significant reduction in BPD with intramuscular (IM) vitamin A supplementation. Recent observational studies suggest that vitamin A supplementation in the current era may not prevent BPD; however, these provide low-quality evidence. IM vitamin A supplementation in preterm infants carries high financial costs, and the IM route of administration may be painful. *The authors suggest vitamin A should be used to prevent BPD in extremely preterm infants (weak recommendation based on the small effect size).*

Systematic search results

The authors reviewed 10 full articles identified in their initial search. Six met their inclusion criteria: a single RCT (CAP trial), 4 observational studies, and 1 post hoc subgroup analysis of CAP trial data (see **Fig. 1**; **Table 2**).[37–41] The authors excluded one retrospective cohort study that evaluated the association between serum caffeine levels

Table 2
Placebo controlled and early versus late studies of caffeine therapy for prevention of BPD

Author/Year	Study Type	Study Comparison	Population	Limitations/Bias	Rates of BPD	Effect Size	GRADE Level of Evidence
					Summary of Findings		
Caffeine vs placebo							
Schmidt et al,[34] 2006	RCT	Caffeine citrate (20 mg/kg loading dose, 5–10 mg/kg/d maintenance dose) vs placebo. Therapy initiated DOL 0–10	BW 500–1250 g	No significant concerns for bias; BPD a priori specified secondary outcome	Caffeine 36.3% (350 of 963) vs placebo 46.9% (447 of 954)[a]	OR 0.63 (95% CI 0.52–0.76)[a,b] NNT 9.5 (95% CI 6.7–16.4)[47]	High
Early vs late initiation of caffeine therapy							
Dobson et al,[38] 2014	Multicenter propensity score matched retrospective cohort study	Early (DOL 0–2) vs late (≥DOL 3) Dose not specified	BW <1500 g Deaths before DOL 4 excluded	Possible residual confounding by unassessed prognostic factors	Early 23.1% vs late 30.7%[a,c]	OR 0.68 (95% CI 0.63–0.73)[a,d]	Moderate
Lodha et al,[39] 2015	Multicenter retrospective cohort study	Early (DOL 0–2) vs late (≥DOL 3) Usual practice to administer 20-mg/kg loading dose, 5- to 10-mg/kg/d maintenance dose	GA <31 wk	Possible residual confounding from greater respiratory disease severity in the late initiation group	Early 27.8% vs late 27.7%[a,e]	OR 0.79 (95% CI 0.64–0.96)[a,f]	Low
Taha et al,[41] 2014	Multicenter retrospective cohort study	Early (DOL 0–2) vs late (DOL 3–10) Dose not specified	BW ≤1250 g	Possible residual confounding by important prognostic factors; early respiratory disease severity not reported	Early 36.1% (716 of 1986) vs late 46.7% (451 of 965)	OR 0.69 (95% CI 0.58–0.83)[9]	Low

Study	Design	Intervention/dose	BW	Limitations	Outcomes	Effect estimate	Quality
Davis et al,[37] 2010	Post hoc subgroup analysis of Schmidt 2006	20-mg/kg loading dose, 5- to 10-mg/kg/d maintenance dose vs placebo. Therapy initiated early (DOL 0–2) or late (DOL 3–10)	BW 500–1250 g	Possible residual confounding by important prognostic factors; original RCT not powered for subgroup analyses	Early caffeine 28% (111 of 396) vs placebo 44.6% (190 of 426). Late caffeine 42.2% (239 of 567) vs placebo 48.8% (257 of 528)	Early caffeine vs placebo OR 0.48 (95% CI 0.36–0.65)[a,h]. Late caffeine vs placebo OR 0.77 (95% CI 0.61–0.98)[a,h]	Low
Patel et al,[40] 2013	Single-center retrospective cohort study	Early (DOL 0–2) vs late (≥DOL 3). Dose not specified	BW ≤1250 g	Possible residual confounding by important prognostic factors; small sample size	Early 24% vs late 51%[a,i]	Early caffeine vs placebo OR 0.33 (95% CI 0.11–0.98)[a,j]	Very low

Abbreviations: BW, birth weight; DOL, day of life; GA, gestational age; NNT, number needed to treat; OR, odds ratio.

a Determined for infants alive at 36 weeks' PMA.

b Odds ratoio adjusted for center.

c Unable to determine exact numerator and denominator from published data because of unclear timing of deaths. Total study sample size including deaths: early, n = 14,535; late, n = 14,535.

d Matched on gestational age, birth weight, sex, race, multiple gestation, small for gestational age, 5-minute Apgar score, antenatal corticosteroid exposure, outborn status, center, year, and the following day-of-life 1 variables: apnea, type of respiratory support, maximal fraction of inspired oxygen, and use of high-frequency mechanical ventilation.

e Unable to determine exact numerator and denominator from published data because of unclear timing of deaths. Total sample size including deaths: early, n = 3806; late, n = 1295.

f Odds ratio adjusted for gestational age, antenatal corticosteroid exposure, small for gestational age, endotracheal intubation on day 2, SNAP-II (Score of Neonatal Acute Physiology II) score, and surfactant administration.

g Odds ratio adjusted for gestational age, birth weight, antenatal corticosteroid exposure, and center.

h Odds ratio adjusted for gestational age, sex, level of maternal education, antenatal corticosteroid exposure, and multiple births.

i Unable to determine exact numerator and denominator from published data because of unclear timing of deaths. Total sample size including deaths: early, n = 83; late, n = 57.

j Odds ratio adjusted for gestational age, birth weight, sex, chorioamnionitis, surfactant administration, and antenatal corticosteroid exposure.

and BPD and the 3 most recent Cochrane reviews on methylxanthine use in preterm infants.[42–44] The Cochrane reviews were excluded because they divided safety and efficacy data into various subgroups based on the reported indication for caffeine therapy. However, participants in the CAP trial were not randomly assigned within those subgroups.[42–44] The authors present instead the full data from the CAP trial.[34]

Risk-to-benefit comparison
The CAP trial demonstrated that caffeine reduced rates of BPD (see **Table 2**) and improved neurodevelopmental outcomes at 18 to 21 months' corrected age.[34,35] Infants randomized to caffeine gained less weight during the first 3 weeks of therapy; but no significant differences in weight gain were observed thereafter, and catch-up growth was recorded.[34] Additional temporary side effects reported with caffeine include tachycardia, tachypnea, glucose instability, jitteriness, and feeding intolerance.[45]

Timing of caffeine initiation
The CAP trial enrolled infants in the first 10 days of life.[34] Recent studies evaluated the optimal timing for initiation of caffeine.[37–41] Four observational studies and a subgroup analysis from the CAP trial all suggest that initiation of caffeine therapy in the first 48 to 72 hours of life may be associated with the greatest reduction in BPD risk (see **Table 2**).[37–41] It is possible that these findings are explained by greater illness severity among the infants who were started on caffeine later. Mechanically ventilated infants with moderate to severe respiratory disease in the first days of life were unlikely to be considered eligible for enrollment in the CAP trial.[46] Therefore, it remains uncertain whether early initiation of caffeine in fully ventilated infants will confer benefit.[46]

Quality of the evidence
The overall quality of evidence to support the use of caffeine for the prevention of BPD in extremely preterm infants is high. There are no significant concerns for potential bias in the RCT data. Treatment allocation in the CAP trial was randomly selected, and the clinicians caring for the enrolled infants were blinded to treatment group during the trial and during all outcome assessments.[34] Moreover, the trial was powered to detect a 5% absolute risk reduction (ARR) in the composite outcome of death or neurodevelopmental impairment (based on a 20% baseline incidence), which provided more than adequate power to detect the observed ARR of 10.5% (95% confidence interval [CI] 6.1–14.9) for BPD.[35,47]

All 4 observational studies comparing early versus late initiation of caffeine therapy demonstrated a reduction in the risk of BPD with earlier use. However, the assessment of the quality of all these studies started at *low* because of their observational design.[38–41] The authors upgraded Dobson and colleagues[38] to *moderate* because propensity score matching was used to account for the differences in baseline illness severity between the infants started on caffeine in 2 different time periods (+1). Patel and colleagues[40] were downgraded to *very low* due to the small sample size (−1).

Recommendation
The available high-quality evidence indicates that treatment of extremely preterm infants with caffeine reduces the risk of BPD and improves neurodevelopmental outcomes at 18 to 21 months' corrected age. Initiation of caffeine therapy in the first 48 to 72 hours of life may confer additional benefit, particularly in infants without severe respiratory illness. The authors strongly recommend the use of caffeine therapy for the prevention of BPD and suggest initiation of therapy in most infants soon after birth (see **Box 2**).

Dexamethasone

Dexamethasone is a synthetic corticosteroid with potent glucocorticoid effects.[48] The first RCTs of dexamethasone in preterm infants demonstrated the short-term benefits of earlier weaning of respiratory support and successful endotracheal extubation.[49–51] These positive findings resulted in wide clinical adoption of high doses and often prolonged courses of dexamethasone.[52] It was not until after investigators reported follow-up data of study participants that the neonatal community recognized the adverse effects of high-dose dexamethasone on neurodevelopment.[53–56]

In an effort to find a regimen that would reduce BPD without harmful effects, investigators began to study lower doses of dexamethasone initiated after the first week of life. However, many clinicians were no longer willing to enroll infants in trials of corticosteroids. As a result, a large international RCT of low-dose dexamethasone (0.89 mg/kg over 10 days) in infants unable to extubate by 3 weeks of life with a primary outcome of death or disability was forced to close early because of poor recruitment.[57,58] At present, the neonatal community is left with the difficult task of weighing the potential risks and benefits of inadequately studied low-dose regimens of dexamethasone in selected infants at high risk of BPD against the long-term adverse effects that are known to be associated with BPD.

Systematic search results

The authors reviewed 51 full articles identified by their initial search (see **Fig. 1**). Of those, 35 met the inclusion criteria. Twenty-eight were RCTs included in one or more of the 2 Cochrane reviews by Doyle and colleagues[59,60] or meta-analysis by Onland and colleagues[61] (**Table 3**). We also included 1 observational study and 3 RCTs that were not incorporated into the meta-analyses.[62–66] We excluded 11 subsequently updated meta-analyses, 6 studies that did not include supplemental oxygen use at 36 weeks PMA as an outcome, and 1 observational study without a contemporary control group.

Risk-to-benefit comparison

Two recent Cochrane reviews confirmed that dexamethasone reduces the rate of BPD in mechanically ventilated extremely preterm infants, regardless of initiation of therapy during or after the first week of life.[59,60] Despite this benefit, the investigators concluded that the lower risk of BPD "may not outweigh" the actual or potential adverse effects of dexamethasone.[59,60] Early (<8 days of life) dexamethasone increases the risks of gastrointestinal perforation, hypertrophic cardiomyopathy, cerebral palsy (CP), and major neurosensory disability.[59] In contrast, it remains uncertain if late (>7 days of life) dexamethasone use results in similar long-term harm.[60] Short-term adverse effects of late dexamethasone include hyperglycemia, glycosuria, and hypertension.[60] Late dexamethasone may also increase the risk of severe retinopathy of prematurity.[60] The risk of CP at 1 to 3 years of age was not significantly increased among surviving infants treated with late dexamethasone (60 of 322, 18.6%) compared with controls (53 of 309, 17.2%) (relative risk [RR] 1.05, 95% CI 0.75–1.47).[60] However, the quality of evidence from several of these follow-up studies is low, and none were adequately powered to evaluate for differences in neurodevelopment.[60] Moreover, open-label corticosteroid use in many of the RCTs was common.[67] In some cases, this treatment crossover may have masked the actual treatment effects and resulted in smaller or nonsignificant observed differences between the treatment groups.[67]

In addition to age at initiation of dexamethasone therapy, the cumulative dose may also have implications for safety and efficacy. Onland and colleagues[61,68] evaluated

Table 3
Placebo-controlled studies and comparisons of different treatment regimens of dexamethasone for prevention of BPD

Author/Year	Study Type	Study Comparison	Population	Limitations/Bias	Rates of BPD	Effect Size	GRADE Level of Evidence
					Summary of Findings		
Dexamethasone vs placebo or no therapy							
Doyle et al,[59] 2014	Cochrane review	Dexamethasone (varying doses) vs placebo. Therapy initiated DOL 0–7	15 RCTs All enrolled mechanically ventilated, extremely preterm infants	Treatment allocation not blinded in 2 RCTs	Dexamethasone 19.8% (247 of 1249) vs placebo 28.3% (350 of 1235)	RR 0.70 (95% CI 0.61–0.81) NNT 12.2 (95% CI 8.9–19.6)[a]	High
Doyle et al,[60] 2014	Cochrane review	Dexamethasone (varying doses) vs placebo. Therapy initiated >DOL 8	9 RCTs All enrolled mechanically ventilated, extremely preterm infants	Treatment allocation not blinded in 2 RCTs Moderate study heterogeneity	Dexamethasone 47.1% (128 of 272) vs placebo 63.1% (166 of 263)	RR 0.76 (95% CI 0.66–0.88) NNT 6.5 (95% CI 4.3–13.2)[a]	Moderate
Yates & Newell,[66] 2011	Retrospective cohort study	Dexamethasone (0.05 mg/kg daily × 10 d then alternate day × 6 d) vs no steroid therapy	GA <30 wk or BW <1500 g	Small sample size; likely confounding by important prognostic factors	Dexamethasone 52% (26 of 50) vs placebo 42.3% (11 of 26)	OR 1.61 (95% CI 0.62–4.22)	Very low

Comparison of different dexamethasone treatment regimens vs active drug controls

Study	Type	Intervention	Population	Comments	Results	RR	Quality
Papile et al,[65] 1998	RCT	Dexamethasone (14-d course) started DOL 14 followed by placebo (14-d course) vs placebo started at DOL 14 (14-d course) followed by dexamethasone or continued placebo (infants with MAP × FiO2 ≥2.4 on DOL 28 received 14 d of dexamethasone, infants with MAP × FiO2 <2.4 received 14 d of placebo)	BW 501–1500 g, mechanically ventilated with MAP × FiO2 ≥2.4	Not powered to detect differences in BPD rates (a prior specified secondary outcome). Moderate number of infants with withheld doses	Dexamethasone-placebo 66.5% (121 of 182) vs placebo-dexamethasone or placebo 67.2% (127 of 189)	RR 0.99 (95% CI 0.86–1.14)[b]	Moderate
Onland et al,[61] 2008	Meta-analysis	RCTs of high dose vs low dose dexamethasone regimens. Comparison subdivided into RCTs with high dose >2.7 mg/kg and ≤2.7 mg/kg	2 RCTs compared high dose (>2.7 mg/kg) vs lower dose / 4 RCTs compared high dose (≤2.7 mg/kg) vs lower dose	Intervention not blinded in 1 trial, insufficient data to assess blinding in 1 trial; overall small size	Dexamethasone >2.7 mg/kg 51.7% (15 of 29) vs lower-dose dexamethasone 76.9% (20 of 26) / Dexamethasone ≤2.7 mg/kg 19.7% (15 of 76) vs lower-dose dexamethasone 21.8% (17 of 78)	RR 0.67 (95% CI 0.45–0.99) / RR 0.89 (95% CI 0.51–1.55)	Low
Odd et al,[64] 2004	RCT	Long dexamethasone course (42-d course, median total dose 6.5 mg/kg) vs Individual dexamethasone course (9 d + continued treatment while intubated, median total dose 3.8 mg/kg)	BW ≤1250 g. Infants ventilated between 1 and 3 wk of age	Treatment allocation not blinded; small sample size	Long course 69.2% (9 of 13) vs individual course 66.6% (8 of 12)[c]	RR 1.04 (95% CI 0.61–1.78)[b,c]	Low

(continued on next page)

Table 3
(continued)

Author/Year	Study Type	Study Comparison	Population	Limitations/Bias	Summary of Findings		GRADE Level of Evidence
					Rates of BPD	Effect Size	
Halliday et al,[62] 2001	4 group factorial RCT	Early (DOL 0–2) dexamethasone vs delayed selective dexamethasone (mechanical ventilation with FiO₂ >30% for >15 d) (both groups received a total dose of 2.7 mg/kg over 12 d) vs early budesonide vs delayed selective budesonide	GA <30 wk, enrolled DOL 0–2. Mechanically ventilated with >30% FiO₂	Not all centers blinded to treatment allocation; small sample size	Early 50% (32 of 64) vs delayed selective dexamethasone 85.7% (54 of 63)[c] Dexamethasone 67.7% (86 of 127) vs budesonide 90.5% (105 of 116)[c]	RR 0.58 (95% CI 0.45–0.76)[b,c] RR 0.75 (95% CI 0.65–0.86)[b,c]	Low
Merz et al,[63] 1999	RCT	Early dexamethasone (start DOL 7) vs late dexamethasone (start DOL 14). Both groups treated for 16 d total	BW ≤1250 g, mechanically ventilated	Unclear blinding of treatment allocation; small sample size	Early 6.7% (1 of 15) vs late 20% (3 of 15) dexamethasone	OR 0.29 (95% CI 0.03–3.12)	Low

Abbreviations: BW, birth weight; DOL, day of life; FiO₂, fraction of inspired oxygen; GA, gestational age; MAP, mean airway pressure; NNT, number needed to treat; OR, odds ratio; RR, relative risk.

a Estimates calculated with the use of the Woolf method because the data were pooled from multiple studies.[87]

b Summary estimate of effect not provided in the original publication, unadjusted relative risk calculated to facilitate comparison between studies.

c BPD determined for infants alive at 36 weeks' PMA.

the effects of different dosing regimens on rates of BPD and long-term neurodevelopment in a meta-analysis of placebo controlled RCTs. The authors reported a reduction in BPD only among RCTs that prescribed a cumulative dose of 4 mg/kg or greater.[68] Rates of neurodevelopmental impairment were similar between the treatment and control groups, regardless of dexamethasone dose.[68]

A meta-regression initially published in 2005 and updated in 2014 by Doyle and colleagues[69,70] shed important light on the need to balance the risks of neurodevelopmental impairment due to corticosteroids against those of BPD itself. These investigators showed that both the size and the direction of the effect of corticosteroids on the composite outcome of death or CP varied depending on the risk of BPD in the enrolled population (**Fig. 2**).[70] When the risk of BPD in the control population was less than approximately 33%, corticosteroid therapy significantly increased the risk of death or CP.[70] In contrast, when the risk of BPD exceeded approximately 60%, corticosteroids reduced the risk of death or CP.[70]

Quality of the evidence

The available high-quality evidence indicates that BPD is reduced when dexamethasone is initiated during the first week of life in mechanically ventilated extremely preterm infants.[59] However, the use of dexamethasone this early in life may result in adverse long-term effects.[59] The quality of evidence for the prevention of BPD with dexamethasone started after the first week of life is *moderate*.[60] The rating was downgraded from an initial *high* rating for RCTs due to sparseness of the data (−1). Nine trials evaluated late dexamethasone for the prevention of BPD, but all were small and underpowered to detect significant differences in the rates of BPD and long-term impairment.[60] In addition, 2 of the RCTs included in the Cochrane review did not blind providers to treatment allocation; there is evidence of moderate heterogeneity in the pooled analysis ($I^2 = 51\%$, $P = .04$).[60] The retrospective cohort study by Yates and Newell[66] was downgraded to *very low* from an initial rating of *low* for

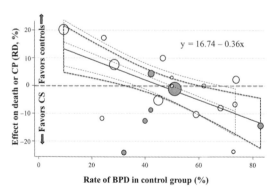

Fig. 2. Risk difference (RD) of corticosteroids (CS) versus control for death or cerebral palsy (CP) among all participants based on the rate of BPD in the control group. Studies included in the original (2005) meta-regression are shown in the open circles. Studies added to the updated meta-regression (2014) are shown in the shaded circles. The solid regression line and 95% CI represent the 20 studies included in the updated meta-regression. The dashed regression line and 95% CI represent the data for the 14 studies included in the original meta-regression. (*From* Doyle LW, Halliday HL, Ehrenkranz RA, et al. An update on the impact of postnatal systemic corticosteroids on mortality and cerebral palsy in preterm infants: effect modification by risk of bronchopulmonary dysplasia. J Pediatr 2014;165:1259; with permission.)

Table 4
Studies of vitamin A supplementation versus placebo or no therapy for prevention of BPD

Author/Year	Study Type	Study Comparison	Population	Limitations/Bias	Summary of Findings		GRADE Level of Evidence
					BPD Rates	Estimate of Effect	
Vitamin A supplementation vs no supplementation							
Darlow & Graham,[78] 2011	Cochrane review	Vitamin A (5000 IU IM injection 3 × per wk for 4 wk) vs sham in study 1. Vitamin A (1500–3000 IU IM injection on DOL 0, 2, and 6) vs no injection in study 2	2 RCTs Study 1: BW 400–1000 g, supplemental oxygen or mechanical ventilation on DOL 0 Study 2: BW 500–1500 g, <32 wk	Large difference in dosing regimens between RCTs; unclear blinding of intervention and small sample size in study 2	Vitamin A 46% (167 of 363) vs none 54.8% (198 of 361)	RR 0.84 (95% CI 0.73–0.97) NNT 11.5 (95% CI 6.3–68.0)[a]	High[b]
Tolia et al,[81] 2014	Multicenter retrospective cohort study	Vitamin A supplementation vs none; dose and route not specified	BW 401–1000 g infants who survived DOL 0–2 and were not transferred during the hospitalization	Possible residual confounding by illness severity; early respiratory disease severity not fully described	Vitamin A 43.7% (415 of 949) vs none 40.4% (1807 of 4472)[c]	RR 1.1 (95% CI 1.0–1.2)[c,d]	Low

Uberos et al,[82] 2014	Single-center retrospective cohort study	Vitamin A supplementation (5000 IU IM injection 3 × per week until DOL 28) vs none	BW <1500 g or GA <32 wk; excluded infants who died before 36 wk PMA or were transferred to another hospital	Incomplete description of early clinical characteristics, no adjustment for potential confounding characteristics, small sample size	Vitamin A 26.7% (16 of 60) vs none 12.8% (12 of 94)	RR 2.1 (95% CI 1.1–4.1)[d]	Very low
Gadhia et al,[79] 2014	Post hoc subgroup analysis of a multicenter RCT of iNO therapy	Vitamin A supplementation vs none; dose and route not specified	BW ≤1250 g and enrolled in an RCT of iNO therapy	Incomplete description of early clinical characteristics; no adjustment for potential confounding variables	Vitamin A 65% (132 of 203) vs none 67.4% (289 of 429)	RR 0.97 (95% CI 0.86–1.1)[d]	Very low

Abbreviations: BW, birth weight; DOL, day of life; iNO, inhaled nitric oxide; IU, international units; NNT, number needed to treat.

[a] Estimates calculated with the use of the Woolf method because the data were pooled from multiple studies.[87]

[b] High rating based on the quality of evidence from Tyson and colleagues,[77] which provided 95.7% of the patients included in the meta-analysis of IM vitamin A supplementation.

[c] Determined for infants alive at 36 weeks' PMA.

[d] Summary estimate of effect not provided in the original publication, unadjusted RR calculated to facilitate comparisons between studies.

observational studies due to the small sample size and lack of adjustment for potential confounders (−1).

The evidence that a cumulative dexamethasone dose of 4 mg/kg or greater is necessary to reduce the BPD risk is *moderate* in quality.[68] The authors downgraded the Onland and colleagues[68] meta-analysis on this topic from an initial rating of *high* due to the small sample sizes available for most of the dose comparisons (−1). Papile and colleagues[65] were downgraded to *moderate* from an initial *high* rating due to the small sample size and lack of power to detect differences in BPD rates between the study groups (−1). The remainder of the studies included in this review were rated as low quality of evidence due to the lack of blinding (−1) and small sample sizes (−1).[61–64]

Recommendation

The use of dexamethasone in mechanically ventilated extremely preterm infants reduces the risk of BPD. For many, but not all, the adverse long-term effects of dexamethasone will outweigh this benefit and treatment should not be used. Among those with an approximately 60% or greater probability of developing BPD, the balance may favor the use of corticosteroids. There are insufficient data at present to determine the optimal cumulative dexamethasone dose (see **Box 2**).

Vitamin A

Vitamin A is a group of fat-soluble organic compounds that includes retinol and the provitamin beta-carotene.[71] Vitamin A is involved in a variety of processes in the human body, such as formation of photosensitive visual pigment in the retina, immune regulation, and growth of epithelial cells in the respiratory tract.[72,73] Vitamin A deficiency may contribute to the development of BPD in preterm infants. Preliminary studies suggested that preterm infants who develop BPD have lower plasma vitamin A levels than infants who do not develop BPD.[74–76] In 1999, the National Institute of Child Health and Human Development Neonatal Research Network published a large, multicenter RCT that demonstrated a reduction in BPD among extremely low-birthweight infants treated with intramuscular (IM) injections of vitamin A during the first 4 weeks of life.[77]

Systematic search results

The authors reviewed 22 full articles identified in their initial search (see **Fig. 1**). Included in this review are 2 RCTs summarized in a meta-analysis by Darlow and Graham[78] and 3 observational studies (see **Fig. 1**; **Table 4**).[77,79–82] The authors excluded 3 subsequently updated meta-analyses, 1 RCT of enteral vitamin A that showed no benefit for BPD, 5 studies without a contemporary control group, 5 that did not include the use of supplemental oxygen at 36 weeks' PMA as an outcome, and 2 that only reported the composite of death or BPD.

Risk-to-benefit comparison

The available RCT data indicate that IM vitamin A supplementation during the first month of life reduces the risk of BPD in extremely preterm infants.[77,78] Two recent large observational studies, however, demonstrated similar rates of BPD among preterm infants treated with vitamin A and untreated controls.[79,81] Moreover, rates of BPD did not seem to increase during the US vitamin A shortage despite a precipitous decrease in usage.[81] Although these observational results should not supplant high-quality RCTs, they do raise questions about the efficacy of vitamin A to prevent BPD in the current era. A planned international RCT of oral vitamin A supplementation in extremely preterm infants may provide important, new, and contemporary data.[83]

Although vitamin A is potentially toxic when administered in high doses, the published RCTs did not demonstrate increased rates of any adverse events among vitamin A treated infants.[78] One RCT reported that IM vitamin A injections appeared to be painful.[84] When considering risks and benefits, the GRADE system recommends that the costs of a therapy may also be considered.[18] A single manufacturer produces injectable vitamin A in the United States. At approximately $1000 per dose (assuming administration of a single dose per vial), a full course of vitamin A for the prevention of BPD costs $12,000 per infant. Based on a number needed to treat of 11.5 (95% CI 6.3–68.0), vitamin A costs as much as $138,000 (95% CI $75,600–$816,000) per prevented case of BPD.

Quality of the evidence
The RCT by Tyson and colleagues[77] contributes most subjects to the Cochrane review and provides high-quality evidence that IM supplementation of vitamin A reduces the

Table 5
Ongoing or completed but not yet published RCTs of pharmacologic agents in preterm infants with BPD as a primary or secondary study outcome

Registry ID	Intervention	Control	Target Enrollment
Intrapulmonary Therapies			
NCT01895075	Budesonide	Placebo	50
NCT01035190	Budesonide	Placebo	850
NCT01022580	Calfactant	Sham	524
NCT00515281	iNO until 30 wk PMA	iNO × 1 wk	484
NCT00931632	iNO	Placebo	450
NCT01828957	Mesenchymal stem cells	Normal saline	70
NCT01039285	Poractant alfa	Sham	100
NCT02140580	Poractant alfa	Sham	606
NCT02013115	Poractant alfa + budesonide	Poractant alfa	300
NCT01941745	Recombinant human Clara cell 10 protein	Half normal saline	88
NCT01116921	Surfactant via LMA	Nasal CPAP	144
NCT02164734	Surfactant via LMA	Surfactant via ETT	130
NCT01848262	Surfactant via endotracheal vascular catheter	Surfactant via ETT	100
Systemic Therapies			
NCT02282176	Azithromycin	Placebo	810
NCT01778634	Azithromycin	Placebo	180
NCT01751724	Caffeine	Placebo	110
NCT00623740	Hydrocortisone	Placebo	523
NCT01353313	Hydrocortisone	Placebo	800
NCT02128191	Ibuprofen	Placebo	142
NCT01954082	Inositol	Placebo	1760
NCT01717625	Montelukast	No therapy	72
NCT02102711	Vitamin A (oral)	No therapy	30
NCT01600430	Vitamin D	Placebo	100

Abbreviations: CPAP, continuous positive airway pressure; ETT, endotracheal tube; iNO, inhaled nitric oxide; LMA, laryngeal mask airway.

risk of BPD in extremely preterm infants.[78] The observational studies included in this review suggest that vitamin A supplementation in the current era may not prevent BPD, but the evidence from these studies is of lower quality. Tolia and colleagues[81] provides low-quality evidence because of the observational design of the study. Gadhia and colleagues[79] and Uberos and colleagues[82] were further downgraded to *very low* because of a lack of adjustment for potential confounders in the analyses (−1).

Recommendation

The available high-quality evidence indicates that IM supplementation of extremely preterm infants with vitamin A during the first month of life results in a small but statistically significant reduction in BPD. Moreover, there is no evidence that the dosage of vitamin A used in the published RCTs results in significant adverse effects. Although recent observational studies suggest vitamin A may not be effective for the prevention of BPD, these studies do not provide high-quality evidence. Therefore, the authors suggest that IM vitamin A supplementation during the first month of life should be used to prevent BPD in extremely preterm infants (see **Box 2**).

CLINICAL TRIALS REGISTRY SEARCH RESULTS

The authors identified 23 ongoing or completed but not yet published RCTs of therapeutic agents that include BPD as a primary or secondary outcome (**Table 5**). Surfactants and inhaled or systemic corticosteroids are the most common medications under investigation. To the authors' knowledge, montelukast and vitamin D are the only medications under investigation for the prevention of BPD that have not been previously evaluated in an RCT. Intratracheally administered human umbilical cord blood derived mesenchymal stem cells and recombinant human Clara cell 10 protein are 2 novel agents currently under phase 2 investigation. The preliminary studies of both agents suggested safety and feasibility.[85,86]

SUMMARY

Caffeine and vitamin A are the only medications with high-quality evidence to support routine use for the prevention of BPD in extremely preterm infants. Dexamethasone is effective at reducing BPD risk; but the side effects include hypertrophic cardiomyopathy, gastrointestinal complications, and CP. For many infants, the risk of these adverse effects outweighs the potential benefits. Further studies are needed to determine whether low doses of dexamethasone in selected infants at high risk of BPD will prevent BPD without increasing the rates of neurodevelopmental impairment. Azithromycin should not be used to prevent BPD until further safety and efficacy data are available. Although several ongoing trials are evaluating medications for the prevention of BPD, relatively few are investigating novel agents.

REFERENCES

1. American Lung Association. Bronchopulmonary dysplasia. Available at: http://www.lung.org/assets/documents/publications/lung-disease-data/ldd08-chapters/LDD-08-RDS-BPD.pdf. Accessed October 2, 2014.
2. Martin JA, Hamilton BE, Ventura SJ, et al. Births: final data for 2011. Natl Vital Stat Rep 2013;62:1–69.
3. Stoll BJ, Hansen NI, Bell EF, et al. Neonatal outcomes of extremely preterm infants from the NICHD Neonatal Research Network. Pediatrics 2010;126:443–56.

4. Berkelhamer SK, Mestan KK, Steinhorn RH. Pulmonary hypertension in broncho-pulmonary dysplasia. Semin Perinatol 2013;37:124–31.
5. Bott L, Béghin L, Devos P, et al. Nutritional status at 2 years in former infants with bronchopulmonary dysplasia influences nutrition and pulmonary outcomes during childhood. Pediatr Res 2006;60:340–4.
6. Carraro S, Filippone M, Da Dalt L, et al. Bronchopulmonary dysplasia: the earliest and perhaps the longest lasting obstructive lung disease in humans. Early Hum Dev 2013;89:S3–5.
7. Cristea AI, Carroll AE, Davis SD, et al. Outcomes of children with severe broncho-pulmonary dysplasia who were ventilator dependent at home. Pediatrics 2013; 132:e727–34.
8. Doyle LW, Faber B, Callanan C, et al. Bronchopulmonary dysplasia in very low birth weight subjects and lung function in late adolescence. Pediatrics 2006; 118:108–13.
9. Ehrenkranz RA, Walsh MC, Vohr BR, et al. Validation of the National Institutes of Health consensus definition of bronchopulmonary dysplasia. Pediatrics 2005; 116:1353–60.
10. Cotten MC, Oh W, Mcdonald S, et al. Prolonged hospital stay for extremely premature infants: risk factors, center differences, and the impact of mortality on selecting a best-performing center. J Perinatol 2005;25:650–5.
11. Bancalari E, Claure N, Sosenko IR. Bronchopulmonary dysplasia: changes in pathogenesis, epidemiology and definition. Semin Neonatol 2003;8:63–71.
12. Botet F, Figueras-Aloy J, Miracle-Echegoyen X, et al. Trends in survival among extremely-low-birth-weight infants (less than 1000g) without significant broncho-pulmonary dysplasia. BMC Pediatr 2012;12:63–70.
13. Fanaroff A, Stoll B, Wright L, et al. Trends in neonatal morbidity and mortality for very low birthweight infants. Am J Obstet Gynecol 2007;196:147.e1–8.
14. Horbar JD, Carpenter JH, Badger GJ, et al. Mortality and neonatal morbidity among infants 501 to 1500 grams from 2000 to 2009. Pediatrics 2012;129:1019–26.
15. Smith VC, Zupancic JA, Mccormick MC, et al. Trends in severe bronchopulmo-nary dysplasia rates between 1994 and 2002. J Pediatr 2005;146:469–73.
16. Beam K, Aliaga S, Ahlfeld S, et al. A systematic review of randomized controlled trials for the prevention of bronchopulmonary dysplasia in infants. J Perinatol 2014;34:705–10.
17. Guyatt GH, Oxman AD, Vist GE, et al. GRADE: an emerging consensus on rating quality of evidence and strength of recommendations. BMJ 2008;336:924–6.
18. Schünemann HJ, Jaeschke R, Cook DJ, et al. An official ATS statement: grading the quality of evidence and strength of recommendations in ATS guidelines and recommendations. Am J Respir Crit Care Med 2006;174:605–14.
19. Jaffe A, Bush A. Anti-inflammatory effects of macrolides in lung disease. Pediatr Pulmonol 2001;31:464–73.
20. Aghai Z, Kode A, Saslow J, et al. Azithromycin suppresses activation of nuclear factor-kappa b and synthesis of pro-inflammatory cytokines in tracheal aspirate cells from premature infants. Pediatr Res 2007;62:483–8.
21. Southern K, Barker P, Solis-Moya A, et al. Macrolide antibiotics for cystic fibrosis. Cochrane Database Syst Rev 2012;(11):CD002203.
22. Herath S, Poole P. Prophylactic antibiotic therapy for chronic obstructive pulmo-nary disease. Cochrane Database Syst Rev 2013;(11):CD009764.
23. Wang E, Ohlsson A, Kellner J. Association of ureaplasma urealyticum coloniza-tion with chronic lung disease of prematurity: results of a meta-analysis. J Pediatr 1995;127:640–4.

24. Schelonka R, Katz B, Waites K, et al. Critical appraisal of the role of ureaplasma in the development of bronchopulmonary dysplasia with meta-analytic techniques. Pediatr Infect Dis J 2005;24:1033–9.

25. Nair V, Loganathan P, Soraisham AS. Azithromycin and other macrolides for prevention of bronchopulmonary dysplasia: a systematic review and meta-analysis. Neonatology 2014;106:337–47.

26. Ozdemir R, Erdeve O, Dizdar E, et al. Clarithromycin in preventing bronchopulmonary dysplasia in ureaplasma urealyticum-positive preterm infants. Pediatrics 2011;128:e1496–501.

27. Mabanta C, Pryhuber G, Weinberg G, et al. Erythromycin for the prevention of chronic lung disease in intubated preterm infants at risk for, or colonized or infected with ureaplasma urealyticum. Cochrane Database Syst Rev 2003;(4):CD003744.

28. Ballard HO, Shook LA, Bernard P, et al. Use of azithromycin for the prevention of bronchopulmonary dysplasia in preterm infants: a randomized, double-blind, placebo controlled trial. Pediatr Pulmonol 2011;46:111–8.

29. Ballard HO, Anstead MI, Shook LA. Azithromycin in the extremely low birth weight infant for the prevention of bronchopulmonary dysplasia: a pilot study. Respir Res 2007;8:41.

30. Gharehbaghi M, Peirovifar A, Ghojazadeh M, et al. Efficacy of azithromycin for prevention of bronchopulmonary dysplasia. Turk J Med Sci 2012;42:1070–5.

31. Dunwiddie T, Masino S. The role and regulation of adenosine in the central nervous system. Annu Rev Neurosci 2001;24:31–55.

32. Julien C, Joseph V, Bairam A. Caffeine reduces apnea frequency and enhances ventilatory long-term facilitation in rat pups raised in chronic intermittent hypoxia. Pediatr Res 2010;68:105–11.

33. Kassim Z, Greenough A, Rafferty G. Effect of caffeine on respiratory muscle strength and lung function in prematurely born, ventilated infants. Eur J Pediatr 2009;168:1491–5.

34. Schmidt B, Roberts RS, Davis P, et al. Caffeine therapy for apnea of prematurity. N Engl J Med 2006;354:2112–21.

35. Schmidt B, Roberts RS, Davis P, et al. Long-term effects of caffeine therapy for apnea of prematurity. N Engl J Med 2007;357:1893–902.

36. Hsieh EM, Hornik CP, Clark RH, et al. Medication use in the neonatal intensive care unit. Am J Perinatol 2014;31:811–21.

37. Davis PG, Schmidt B, Roberts RS, et al. Caffeine for apnea of prematurity trial: benefits may vary in subgroups. J Pediatr 2010;156:382–7.

38. Dobson NR, Patel RM, Smith PB, et al. Trends in caffeine use and association between clinical outcomes and timing of therapy in very low birth weight infants. J Pediatr 2014;164:992–8.e3.

39. Lodha A, Seshia M, Mcmillan DD, et al. Association of early caffeine administration and neonatal outcomes in very preterm neonates. JAMA Pediatr 2015;169:33–8.

40. Patel R, Leong T, Carlton D, et al. Early caffeine therapy and clinical outcomes in extremely preterm infants. J Perinatol 2013;33:134–40.

41. Taha D, Kirkby S, Nawab U, et al. Early caffeine therapy for prevention of bronchopulmonary dysplasia in preterm infants. J Matern Fetal Neonatal Med 2014; 27:1698–702.

42. Henderson-Smart D, Davis P. Prophylactic methylxanthines for endotracheal extubation in preterm infants. Cochrane Database Syst Rev 2010;(12):CD000139.

43. Henderson-Smart D, De Paoli A. Methylxanthine treatment for apnoea in preterm infants. Cochrane Database Syst Rev 2010;(12):CD000140.

44. Henderson-Smart D, De Paoli A. Prophylactic methylxanthine for prevention of apnoea in preterm infants. Cochrane Database Syst Rev 2010;(12):CD000432.
45. Schoen K, Yu T, Stockmann C, et al. Use of methylxanthine therapies for the treatment and prevention of apnea of prematurity. Paediatr Drugs 2014;16:169–77.
46. Schmidt B, Davis PG, Roberts RS. Timing of caffeine therapy in very low birth weight infants. J Pediatr 2014;164:957–8.
47. Schmidt B, Roberts R, Millar D, et al. Evidence-based neonatal drug therapy for prevention of bronchopulmonary dysplasia in very-low-birth-weight infants. Neonatology 2008;93:284–7.
48. Meikle A, Tyler F. Potency and duration of action of glucocorticoids: effects of hydrocortisone, prednisone and dexamethasone on human pituitary-adrenal function. Am J Med 1977;63:200–7.
49. Cummings J, D'eugenio D, Gross S. A controlled trial of dexamethasone in preterm infants at high risk for bronchopulmonary dysplasia. N Engl J Med 1989;320:1505–10.
50. Mammel M, Green T, Johnson D, et al. Controlled trial of dexamethasone therapy in infants with bronchopulmonary dysplasia. Lancet 1983;8338:1356–8.
51. Avery G, Fletcher A, Kaplan M, et al. Controlled trial of dexamethasone in respirator-dependent infants with bronchopulmonary dysplasia. Pediatrics 1985;75:106–11.
52. Demauro S, Dysart K, Kirpalani H. Stopping the swinging pendulum of postnatal corticosteroid use. J Pediatr 2014;164:9–11.
53. Yeh T, Lin Y, Huang C, et al. Early dexamethasone therapy in preterm infants: a follow-up study. Pediatrics 1998;101:e7.
54. O'shea T, Kothadia J, Klinepeter K, et al. Randomized placebo-controlled trial of a 42-day tapering course of dexamethasone to reduce the duration of ventilator dependency in very low birth weight infants: outcome of study participants at 1-year adjusted age. Pediatrics 1999;104:15–21.
55. Barrington K. The adverse neuro-developmental effects of postnatal steroids in the preterm infant: a systematic review of RCTs. BMC Pediatr 2001;1:1.
56. Yeh T, Lin Y, Lin H, et al. Outcomes at school age after postnatal dexamethasone therapy for lung disease of prematurity. N Engl J Med 2004;350:1304–13.
57. Doyle L, Davis P, Morley C, et al. Low-dose dexamethasone facilitates extubation among chronically ventilator-dependent infants: a multicenter, international, randomized, controlled trial. Pediatrics 2006;117:75–83.
58. Doyle L, Davis P, Morley C, et al. Outcome at 2 years of age of infants from the dart study: a multicenter, international, randomized, controlled trial of low-dose dexamethasone. Pediatrics 2007;119:716–21.
59. Doyle LW, Ehrenkranz RA, Halliday HL. Early (<8 days) postnatal corticosteroids for preventing chronic lung disease in preterm infants. Cochrane Database Syst Rev 2014;(5):CD001146.
60. Doyle LW, Ehrenkranz RA, Halliday HL. Late (>7 days) postnatal corticosteroids for chronic lung disease in preterm infants. Cochrane Database Syst Rev 2014;(5):CD001145.
61. Onland W, De Jaegere AP, Offringa M, et al. Effects of higher versus lower dexamethasone doses on pulmonary and neurodevelopmental sequelae in preterm infants at risk for chronic lung disease: a meta-analysis. Pediatrics 2008;122:92–101.
62. Halliday H, Patterson C, Halahakoon C, et al. A multicenter, randomized open study of early corticosteroid treatment (OSECT) in preterm infants with respiratory illness: comparison of early and late treatment and of dexamethasone and inhaled budesonide. Pediatrics 2001;107:232–40.

63. Merz U, Peschgens T, Kusenbach G, et al. Early versus late dexamethasone treatment in preterm infants at risk for chronic lung disease: a randomized pilot study. Eur J Pediatr 1999;158:318–22.
64. Odd D, Armstrong D, Teele R, et al. A randomized trial of two dexamethasone regimens to reduce side-effects in infants treated for chronic lung disease of prematurity. J Paediatr Child Health 2004;40:282–9.
65. Papile L, Tyson J, Stoll B, et al. A multicenter trial of two dexamethasone regimens in ventilator-dependent premature infants. N Engl J Med 1998;338:1112–8.
66. Yates H, Newell S. Minidex: very low dose dexamethasone (0.05 mg/kg/day) in chronic lung disease. Arch Dis Child Fetal Neonatal Ed 2011;96:F190–4.
67. Onland W, Van Kaam A, De Jaegere A, et al. Open-label glucocorticoids modulate dexamethasone trial results in preterm infants. Pediatrics 2010;2010: e954–64.
68. Onland W, Offringa M, De Jaegere AP, et al. Finding the optimal postnatal dexamethasone regimen for preterm infants at risk of bronchopulmonary dysplasia: a systematic review of placebo-controlled trials. Pediatrics 2009;123:367–77.
69. Doyle LW, Halliday HL, Ehrenkranz RA, et al. Impact of postnatal systemic corticosteroids on mortality and cerebral palsy in preterm infants: effect modification by risk for chronic lung disease. Pediatrics 2005;115:655–61.
70. Doyle LW, Halliday HL, Ehrenkranz RA, et al. An update on the impact of postnatal systemic corticosteroids on mortality and cerebral palsy in preterm infants: effect modification by risk of bronchopulmonary dysplasia. J Pediatr 2014;165: 1258–60.
71. Gregory JF. Vitamins. In: Damodaran S, Parkin K, Fennema O, editors. Fennema's food chemistry. 4th edition. Boca Rato (FL): CRC Press Taylor & Francis Group; 2007. p. 454–5.
72. Niederreither K, Dolle P. Retinoic acid in development: towards an integrated view. Nat Rev Genet 2008;9:541–53.
73. Biesalski H, Nohr I. Importance of vitamin A for lung function and development. Mol Aspects Med 2003;24:431–40.
74. Shenai J, Chytil F, Stahlman M. Vitamin A status of neonates with bronchopulmonary dysplasia. Pediatr Res 1985;19:185–8.
75. Hustead V, Gutcher G, Anderson S, et al. Relationship of vitamin A (retinol) status to lung disease in the preterm infant. J Pediatr 1984;104:610–5.
76. Chytil F. The lungs and vitamin A. Am J Physiol 1992;262:L517–27.
77. Tyson JE, Wright LL, Oh W, et al. Vitamin A supplementation for extremely-low-birth-weight infants. National institute of child health and human development neonatal research network. N Engl J Med 1999;340:1962–8.
78. Darlow BA, Graham PJ. Vitamin A supplementation to prevent mortality and short- and long-term morbidity in very low birthweight infants. Cochrane Database Syst Rev 2011;(10):CD000501.
79. Gadhia MM, Cutter GR, Abman SH, et al. Effects of early inhaled nitric oxide therapy and vitamin A supplementation on the risk for bronchopulmonary dysplasia in premature newborns with respiratory failure. J Pediatr 2014;164:744–8.
80. Ravishankar C, Nafday S, Green RS, et al. A trial of vitamin A therapy to facilitate ductal closure in premature infants. J Pediatr 2003;143:644–8.
81. Tolia VN, Murthy K, Mckinley PS, et al. The effect of the national shortage of vitamin A on death or chronic lung disease in extremely low-birth-weight infants. JAMA Pediatr 2014;168:1039–44.
82. Uberos J, Miras-Baldo M, Jerez-Calero A, et al. Effectiveness of vitamin A in the prevention of complications of prematurity. Pediatr Neonatol 2014;55:358–62.

83. Meyer S, Gortner L, NeoVitaA Trial Investigators. Early postnatal additional high-dose oral vitamin A supplementation versus placebo for 28 days for preventing bronchopulmonary dysplasia or death in extremely low birth weight infants. Neonatology 2014;105:182–8.

84. Pearson E, Bose C, Snidow T, et al. Trial of vitamin A supplementation in very low birth weight infants at risk for bronchopulmonary dysplasia. J Pediatr 1992;121: 420–7.

85. Chang Y, Ahn S, Yoo H, et al. Mesenchymal stem cells for bronchopulmonary dysplasia: phase 1 dose-escalation clinical trial. J Pediatr 2014;164:966–72.e6.

86. Levine C, Gewolb I, Allen K, et al. The safety, pharmacokinetics, and anti-inflammatory effects of intratracheal recombinant human Clara cell protein in premature infants with respiratory distress syndrome. Pediatr Res 2005;58:15–21.

87. Normand SL. Meta-analysis: formulating, evaluating, combining, and reporting. Stat Med 1999;18:321–59.

Mechanical Ventilation and Bronchopulmonary Dysplasia

Martin Keszler, MD[a],*, Guilherme Sant'Anna, MD, PhD, FRCPC[b]

KEYWORDS

- Mechanical ventilation • Bronchopulmonary dysplasia
- Ventilator-associated lung injury • Volume-targeted ventilation
- Lung-protective ventilation

KEY POINTS

- Mechanical ventilation (MV) is an important potentially modifiable risk factor for the development of bronchopulmonary dysplasia (BPD).
- Effective use of noninvasive respiratory support reduces the risk of lung injury.
- Lung volume recruitment and avoidance of excessive tidal volume (V_T) are key elements of lung-protective ventilation strategies.
- Avoidance of oxidative stress, less invasive methods of surfactant administration, and high-frequency ventilation (HFV) are also important factors in lung injury prevention.

INTRODUCTION

MV is undoubtedly one of the key advances in neonatal care. Even in this era of noninvasive respiratory support, MV remains a mainstay of therapy in the extremely preterm population. Data from the Neonatal Research Network show that 89% of extremely low birth weight (ELBW) infants were treated with MV during the first day of life.[1] Among survivors, almost 95% were invasively ventilated at some point during their hospital stay. In the Surfactant, Positive Pressure, and Oxygenation Randomized Trial

Conflict of Interest Statement: Dr M. Keszler has been a consultant to Draeger Medical. He has received honoraria for lectures and research grant support from the company. Dr M. Keszler also chairs the scientific advisory board of Discovery Laboratories and the Data Safety Monitoring Board of a clinical trial supported by Medipost America. None of the companies had any input into the content of this article.

[a] Department of Pediatrics, Women and Infants Hospital of Rhode Island, Alpert Medical School of Brown University, 101 Dudley Street, Providence, RI 02905, USA; [b] Department of Pediatrics, Neonatal Division, Montreal Children's Hospital, McGill University, 1001 Decarie Boulevard, Room B05.2711, Montreal, Quebec H4A 3J1, Canada
* Corresponding author.
E-mail address: mkeszler@wihri.org

Clin Perinatol 42 (2015) 781–796
http://dx.doi.org/10.1016/j.clp.2015.08.006
0095-5108/15/$ – see front matter © 2015 Elsevier Inc. All rights reserved.

(SUPPORT), 83% of the ELBW infants initially assigned to noninvasive support required endotracheal intubation and MV at some point.[2] The CPAP or Intubation trial enrolled infants between 25 and 28 weeks of gestational age only if they had adequate respiratory effort at birth, but even in this group, 46% of the infants assigned to noninvasive support required endotracheal intubation and MV.[3]

Although often lifesaving, MV has many untoward effects. Although this article focuses on the adverse effects of MV on the lungs, protracted MV is also strongly associated with adverse neurologic outcomes.[1] In preterm baboons, 5 days of elective MV resulted in greater degree of brain injury compared with ventilation for 1 day.[4] Cohort data from the Neonatal Research Network show that each week of additional MV is associated with a significant increase in the likelihood of neurodevelopmental impairment.[1] Additionally, the endotracheal tube acts as a foreign body, quickly becoming colonized and acting as a portal of entry for pathogens, increasing the risk of ventilator-associated pneumonia and late-onset sepsis.[5] For these reasons, avoidance of MV in favor of noninvasive respiratory support is seen as perhaps the most important step in preventing neonatal morbidity.

BPD was originally described by Northway and colleagues[6] more than 45 years ago in large moderately and late preterm babies who survived MV. Thus, BPD has always been associated with the use of MV, but many other factors play an important role in the pathogenesis of BPD (**Fig. 1**). The classic, so-called old BPD occurred as a consequence of unsophisticated ventilatory support in infants with surfactant deficiency and was characterized by marked fibrosis, increased interstitium, marked airway alterations, and reactive airway disease.[7] New BPD, characterized mostly by simplified lung architecture as a consequence of an arrest in pulmonary development, occurs in infants who are far more immature, received surfactant replacement therapy, and are likely to have been treated with antenatal steroids.[8] Nevertheless, there is considerable overlap between the 2 forms, and old BPD has by no means disappeared from neonatal ICUs.

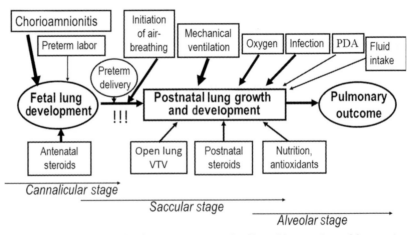

Fig. 1. The ultimate neonatal pulmonary outcome is affected by a variety of factors, beginning in utero. The immediate postnatal period is one of the most critical times, as indicated by the 3 exclamation marks. Adverse influences are listed in the upper part of the panel and mitigating factors in the lower portion. The multifactorial pathogenesis of BPD explains why no single therapeutic intervention is likely to have a large impact on its incidence. PDA, patent ductus arteriousus.

WHAT IS VENTILATOR-ASSOCIATED LUNG INJURY?

The huge number of articles published since the first description of ventilator-associated lung injury (VALI) highlights its importance and the incomplete understanding of this complex subject. The central role of MV and oxygen exposure in VALI and subsequent development of BPD have been recognized since the early days of neonatal medicine. In 1975, Alistair Philip described the etiology of BPD as "oxygen plus pressure plus time."[9] Although fundamentally this concept still holds, it has since been refined by recognizing that excessive volume, rather than pressure, is the most important factor that contributes to VALI, a concept that has been slow to gain complete acceptance, despite strong evidence in its favor.

Many terms have been coined to describe the mechanism of lung injury in VALI. *Barotrauma* refers to damage caused by pressure. The conviction that pressure is the key determinant of lung injury has fostered a deeply ingrained "barophobia," causing clinicians to focus on limiting inflation pressure, sometimes to the point of precluding adequate ventilation. There is convincing evidence, however, that high pressure by itself, without correspondingly high volume, does not result in lung injury. Rather, injury related to high inflation pressure is mediated through the tissue stretch resulting from excessive V_T. Dreyfuss and colleagues[10] demonstrated more than 20 years ago that severe acute lung injury occurred in small animals ventilated with large V_T, regardless of whether that volume was generated by positive or negative inflation pressure. In contrast, animals exposed to the same high inflation pressure but with an elastic bandage over the chest and abdomen to limit V_T delivery experienced much less acute lung damage. Hernandez and colleagues[11] similarly showed that animals exposed to pressure as high as 45 cm H_2O did not show evidence of acute lung injury when their chest and abdomen were enclosed in a plaster cast. *Volutrauma* refers to injury caused by overdistention and excessive stretch of tissues, which leads to disruption of alveolar and small airway epithelium, resulting in acute edema; outpouring of proteinaceous exudate; and release of proteases, cytokines, and chemokines, which in turn leads to activation of macrophages and invasion of activated neutrophils. Collectively, this complex process is referred to as *biotrauma*. Another important concept is that of *atelectrauma*, or lung damage caused by tidal ventilation in the presence of atelectasis.[12] Atelectrauma exerts lung injury via several mechanisms. The portion of the lungs that remains atelectatic has increased surfactant turnover and high critical opening pressure. There are shear forces at the boundary between aerated and atelectatic parts of the lung, leading to structural damage. Ventilation of injured lungs using inadequate end-expiratory pressure results in repeated alveolar collapse and expansion (RACE), which rapidly leads to lung injury. Perhaps most importantly, when a large portion of the lungs is atelectatic, whatever V_T is entering the lungs preferentially enters the aerated portion of the lung, which is more compliant than the atelectatic lung with its high critical opening pressure (Laplace's law). This maldistribution of V_T leads to overdistention of that portion of the lungs and regional volutrauma. Thus, it becomes clear that the risk of lung damage from MV is multifactorial and cannot be linked to any single variable.

The key concept regarding VALI is that the initiating event is biophysical injury from excessive tissue stretch, which in turn leads to biotrauma and initiates the complex cascade of lung injury and repair (**Fig. 2**). It is important to recognize, however, that VALI is only one of several mechanisms that may ultimately lead to BPD. Although infants with severe neonatal lung disease are more likely to develop severe BPD, it is well known that BPD also afflicts infants who require only minimal respiratory support in the first weeks of life.[13] Exposure to intrauterine inflammation is known to result in

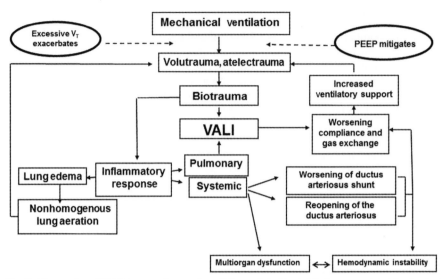

Fig. 2. The cycle of VALI is complex and multifactorial. The initiating event is biophysical injury from excessive tissue stretch, which in turn leads to biotrauma and initiates the complex cascade of lung injury and repair. Both systemic and pulmonary inflammatory responses become operative and lead to secondary adverse effects that in turn worsen pulmonary status, leading to a need for escalating ventilatory settings, which in turn may result in more injury.

accelerated lung maturation in the short term but ultimately triggers biotrauma directly, initiating the cascade of injury and repair that leads to the development of moderate or severe BPD.[14–16]

MITIGATING VENTILATOR-ASSOCIATED LUNG INJURY

Because some degree of impairment of normal pulmonary development is probably inevitable when an extremely preterm fetus is suddenly thrust into a hyperoxic (by fetal standards) environment and must initiate air breathing with lungs that are incompletely developed, it is unlikely that advances in neonatal care, including avoidance of MV, can completely prevent impairment of lung structure and function. Optimal respiratory and general supportive care, however, can minimize the overlay of ventilator-induced lung injury and facilitate lung growth and repair.

IMPORTANCE OF THE GOLDEN FIRST HOUR

The time immediately after birth when air breathing is initiated in a structurally immature surfactant deficient lung has been recognized as a critical time that may rapidly and irrevocably initiate the process of lung injury and repair. To achieve a successful transition to extrauterine life, newborn infants must rapidly aerate their lungs, clear lung fluid from the air spaces, and maintain a functional residual capacity (FRC), ultimately facilitating a dramatic increase in pulmonary blood flow. A healthy full-term infant is able to achieve this remarkable transition quickly and effectively,[17] but this is often not the case in very preterm infants. Preterm infants may be unable to generate the critical opening pressure to achieve adequate lung aeration because of their limited muscle strength, excessively compliant chest wall, limited surfactant pool, and incomplete lung development. Additionally, their excessively compliant chest wall fails to sustain any lung aeration that may have been achieved spontaneously or with positive pressure ventilation. They may also be unable to generate sufficient negative intrathoracic pressure to effectively move lung fluid from the air spaces to the interstitium, lymphatics and veins. Consequently, subsequent tidal breathing, whether spontaneous or generated by positive pressure ventilation, takes place in lungs that are still partially fluid filled and partially atelectatic. This situation leads to maldistribution of the V_T to a fraction of the preterm lung, which leads to volutrauma even when the V_T is in a safe physiologic range.

POSITIVE END-EXPIRATORY PRESSURE IN THE DELIVERY ROOM

The use of positive end-expiratory pressure (PEEP)/continuous positive airway pressure (CPAP) during initial stabilization of preterm infants mitigates the effect of excessively compliant chest wall and surfactant deficiency by stabilizing alveoli during the expiratory phase and has been shown to help establish FRC. Siew and colleagues[18] demonstrated the beneficial effects of PEEP by using phase-contrast radiography in preterm rabbits, showing that virtually no FRC was established after several minutes when PPV was delivered without PEEP. In contrast, FRC was rapidly established when 5 cm H_2O of PEEP was applied.

Both the Neonatal Resuscitation Program and International Liaison Committee on Resuscitation guidelines state, "PEEP is likely to be beneficial during initial stabilization of apneic preterm infants and should be used if suitable equipment is available."[19,20] The physiologic rationale and experimental evidence from preclinical studies is so persuasive that this practice has become the standard of care in much of the developed world. Provision of end-expiratory pressure alone, however, may not entirely address the inadequate muscle strength of the preterm infant or help clear lung fluid sufficiently rapidly to avoid regional volutrauma and atelectrauma, which can occur in minutes.

SUSTAINED INFLATION

Because liquid has much greater viscosity than air, resistance to moving liquid through small airways is orders of magnitude higher than that for air, making the time constants required to clear fluid from the airways much longer. Recognition of these factors supports the concept that a prolonged (sustained) inflation applied soon after birth should be more effective than short inflations in clearing lung fluid in the first minutes of life. Theoretically, ensuring effective lung recruitment with even distribution of V_T immediately after birth should reduce VALI.

Despite a substantial body of evidence that supports the theoretic advantages of sustained inflation in extremely preterm infants,[21] the evidence that this measure can substantially reduce VALI remains inconclusive.[22–24] Additionally, the most appropriate way to deliver an sustained inflation is unclear. Therefore, the procedure cannot currently be recommended outside of well-controlled clinical trials.

HYPEROXIC INJURY

Preterm infants have immature antioxidant defenses, making them more susceptible to oxidative stress from relative or absolute hyperoxia. Several studies of early respiratory management in the delivery room evaluated whether reducing oxygen exposure results in improved respiratory outcomes. A single-center randomized clinical trial (RCT) in infants born at 24 to 28 weeks' gestation demonstrated less oxidative stress, lower proinflammatory cytokine levels, and a lower incidence of BPD (15.4% vs 31.7%; $P<.05$) in infants resuscitated with a fraction of inspired oxygen (FIO_2) of 0.30, compared with 0.90, and then titrated to achieve target oxygen saturation as measured by pulse oximetry (SpO_2) levels.[25] Kapadia and colleagues[26] compared rates of BPD in infants with gestational age of 24 to 34 weeks randomized to receive either 21% or 100% oxygen, which was then titrated to achieve the Neonatal Resuscitation Program recommended SpO_2 target of 85% to 94%. BPD rates were lower in the infants initially resuscitated with room air (7% vs 25%; $P<.04$). In contrast, the Room-Air Versus Oxygen Administration for Resuscitation of Preterm Infants study found no difference in BPD rates between preterm infants treated with room air, despite randomizing greater than 1000 infants.[27] This may be in part because initiating resuscitation with room air in very preterm infants often resulted in inadequate response and a rapid increase to 100% oxygen. Therefore, the best approach probably is to initiate support with FIO_2 of 0.30 and avoid an excessively rapid increase, recognizing that several minutes are needed for SpO_2 to reach 90%.

Although avoidance of oxidative stress is desirable, it has turned out to be a more complicated issue than was initially thought. A series of RCTs that compared lower versus higher SpO_2 targets (SUPPORT, Canadian Oxygen Trial, and Benefits of Oxygen Saturation Targeting II) failed to show a significant reduction in BPD and, unexpectedly showed a higher mortality rate in the low SpO_2 target group.[28–30] A recent meta-analysis of those trials confirmed a significant increase in mortality and necrotizing enterocolitis and a decrease in the rate of severe retinopathy of prematurity in low compared with high oxygen saturation target infants.[31] No differences in physiologic BPD, brain injury, or patent ductus arteriosus were noted between the groups. Based on these results, definitive recommendations regarding saturation targets during continued care of preterm infants are difficult to make. Nevertheless, it seems prudent to target functional SpO_2 at 90% to 95% in infants with gestational age less than 28 weeks until 36 weeks' postmenstrual age. Most NICUs have revised their saturation targets to be close to this higher range, with alarm limits slightly wider, or approximately 88% to 97%. Anecdotally, this change has again increased the risk of significant retinopathy of prematurity.

NONINVASIVE RESPIRATORY SUPPORT

There is little doubt that avoiding MV reduces iatrogenic lung injury superimposed on the inevitable arrest of pulmonary development. Although earlier cohort comparisons of CPAP or MV suggested a large reduction in the risk of BPD,[32] a series of more recent RCTs showed a much more modest benefit of avoiding MV. A meta-analysis of 4 recent RCTs[2,3,33,34] that enrolled nearly 2800 preterm infants showed that BPD rates were not significantly reduced by the use of different types of nasal CPAP (32.4% vs 34.0%).[35] A modest benefit with the use of CPAP, however, was demonstrated for the combined outcome of death or BPD with a reduction of approximately 10% (relative risk [RR] 0.91; 95% CI, 0.84–0.99); with 1 additional infant surviving to 36 weeks without BPD for every 25 babies treated with nasal CPAP in the delivery room rather than being intubated. This latter finding is more important because death and BPD are competing outcomes and, therefore, should be evaluated in combination. There was also a significant decrease in the duration of MV and a nonsignificant trend toward shorter duration of oxygen exposure with early CPAP in the 2 largest trials.[2,3]

Nasal intermittent positive pressure ventilation may be able to augment an immature infant's inadequate respiratory effort without the complications associated with endotracheal intubation.[36] In theory, this approach offers the benefit of avoiding the use of an endotracheal tube, thus reducing the incidence of VALI and ventilator-associated pneumonia and avoiding the contribution of postnatal inflammatory response to the development of BPD.[37] Although a meta-analysis of several small single center studies concluded that nasal intermittent positive pressure ventilation was superior to CPAP,[38] a recent large pragmatic multinational RCT in infants with birth weight less than 1000 g failed to substantiate these benefits, showing no reduction in BPD, mortality, or the combined outcome.[39]

LESS INVASIVE SURFACTANT ADMINISTRATION

Traditionally, the avoidance of intubation and MV and the use of noninvasive respiratory support have meant a trade-off between the presumed benefits of this approach and the well documented benefits of surfactant replacement therapy. Early surfactant trials suggested that prophylactic surfactant administration was superior to rescue use[40]; thus, some clinicians still intubate very premature infants in the delivery room for the sole purpose of administering surfactant. It must be recognized, however, that most surfactant RCTs were done many years ago in a different population of infants and with a less sophisticated approach to delivery room stabilization. A recent meta-analysis comparing prophylactic versus selective surfactant use in the modern era concluded that a prophylactic approach was associated with increased risk of BPD (RR 1.13; 95% CI, 1.00–1.28).[41]

In recent years, a variety of approaches have been proposed to preserve the benefits of avoiding delivery room intubation while still providing surfactant therapy. These include the intubation-surfactant-extubation approach (INSURE) and several methods of administering surfactant through small catheters under direct laryngoscopic visualization.[33,42–45] Although these techniques avoid endotracheal intubation, they still require direct laryngoscopy, typically without sedation and thus are still invasive. Administration of nebulized surfactant during CPAP is a potentially attractive approach that is currently under investigation.[46]

LUNG-PROTECTIVE STRATEGIES OF MECHANICAL VENTILATION

There are numerous modes and modalities of MV and little high-quality evidence to guide clinicians in selecting the optimal method. A detailed discussion of these techniques is beyond the scope of this article; interested readers are referred to several recent reviews of the topic.[47,48] Key principles of lung-protective strategies, however, are outlined.

Volume-targeted Ventilation

Pressure-controlled ventilation (PCV) became the standard mode of ventilation in neonates because early attempts at volume-controlled ventilation proved ineffective in small preterm infants using equipment available at the time. PCV remains the accepted mode of ventilation in neonatal ICUs because of its simplicity, ability to ventilate despite a large endotracheal tube leak, and improved intrapulmonary gas distribution due to the decelerating gas flow pattern.[49,50] Perhaps most importantly, clinicians continue to hold onto the belief that directly controlling peak inflation pressure is important. The danger of using PCV is that V_T varies with changes in lung compliance. Rapid improvement in compliance may occur rapidly in the immediate postnatal period as a result of resorption of lung fluid, recruitment of optimal lung volume, and surfactant replacement therapy, leading to hyperventilation and volutrauma from excessively large V_T. Insufficient V_T may develop because of decreasing lung compliance, increasing airway resistance, airway obstruction, air-trapping, and/or decreased spontaneous respiratory effort. Inadequate V_T leads to hypercapnia, tachypnea, increased work of breathing and oxygen consumption, agitation, fatigue, atelectasis/atelectrauma, and possibly increased risk of intraventricular hemorrhage (IVH) and thus should also be avoided. Low V_T also leads to inefficient gas exchange due to an increased dead space:V_T ratio. These factors suggest that tight control of V_T delivery during MV is highly desirable and are the reason volume-controlled ventilation remains the standard of care in adult and pediatric respiratory support.

There are many ways to regulate V_T delivery during MV. Although there are important differences in how volume targeting is performed, it is likely that the primary benefit of volume-targeted ventilation (VTV) rests in the ability to regulate V_T, regardless of how that goal is achieved. When V_T is the primary control variable, inflation pressure decreases as lung compliance and patient inspiratory effort improve. This process results in real-time weaning of pressure, in contrast to intermittent manual lowering of pressure in response to blood gas measurement, avoiding volutrauma, hypocapnia, and shortening the duration of MV. Volume guarantee, introduced in the 1990s as an option in the Babylog ventilator (Draeger Medical, Telford, Pennsylvania), is the most thoroughly studied form of VTV and the basic control algorithm is increasingly adopted by other ventilator manufacturers.[48] Among the benefits documented in 2 recent meta-analyses that encompassed several different modalities of VTV are significant reduction in the combined outcome of death or BPD, the risk of pneumothorax, shorter duration of MV, and lower rate of severe IVH and periventricular leukomalacia (**Table 1**).[51,52] Although encouraging, these meta-analyses cannot provide definitive evidence of the superiority of VTV, because the clinical trials in these analyses were small and used different devices, and some key outcomes reported in the meta-analysis were not prospectively defined. In some studies, other variables besides volume versus pressure targeting also differed. All the included studies focused on short-term physiologic outcomes rather than BPD. Only 1 study provided some long-term pulmonary and developmental outcomes, but this was based only on a parental questionnaire. Nonetheless, this is more evidence than currently available for any other approach to MV.

Table 1
Summary of major outcomes assessed in the meta-analysis of 11 randomized clinical trials of volume-targeted versus pressure-limited ventilation

Outcome	No. of Studies	No. of Subjects	RR (95% CI) or Mean Difference (95% CI)
Mortality	11	767	0.73 (0.51–1.05)
Any IVH	11	759	0.65 (0.42–0.99)*
Grade 3–4 IVH	11	707	0.55 (0.39–0.79)*
BPD at 36 wk	9	596	0.61 (0.46–0.82)*
Cystic PVL	7	531	0.33 (0.15–0.72)*
Pneumothorax	8	595	0.46 (0.25–0.86)*
Failure of assigned mode	4	405	0.64 (0.43–0.94)*
Any hypocapnia	2	58	0.56 (0.33–0.96)*
Duration of supplemental O_2 (d)	2	133	−1.68 (−2.5 to −0.88)*

* $P<.05$.

Data from Peng WS, Zhu HW, Shi H, et al. Volume-targeted ventilation is more suitable than pressure-limited ventilation for preterm infants: a systematic review and meta-analysis. Arch Dis Child Fetal Neonatal Ed 2014;99:F158–65.

Importance of the Open Lung Strategy

The benefits of VTV cannot be fully realized unless the V_T is evenly distributed into an open lung, avoiding atelectrauma. Adequate PEEP is widely recognized as a means of mitigating lung injury. The admonition of Burkhard Lachman more than 20 years ago to "OPEN THE LUNG AND KEEP IT OPEN!"[53] has been ignored by many during conventional MV despite a sound physiologic basis and strong experimental evidence in its favor. Caruso and colleagues[54] demonstrated that when using PEEP of 0 cm H_2O, lung injury in rats was not reduced by the use of low, compared with high, V_T. Tsuchida and colleagues[55] showed that in the presence of atelectasis, the nondependent (ie, aerated) lung was the most injured area. This is because, as seen in **Fig. 3**, if partially atelectatic lungs are ventilated, the V_T entering only the open alveoli inevitably leads to overexpansion of this relatively healthy portion of the lung with subsequent volutrauma/biotrauma even when the V_T is in the normal range. Additionally, atelectasis leads to exudation of protein-rich fluid with increased surfactant inactivation and release of inflammatory mediators. Shear forces and uneven stress in areas where atelectasis and overinflation coexist add to the damage. Thus, the open lung concept (OLC),[56] which ensures that the V_T is distributed evenly throughout the lungs, is a fundamental component of any lung-protective ventilation strategy.

In practical terms, the open lung is achieved by applying adequate PEEP.[57] One of the most important obstacles to optimizing the way conventional MV is practiced is the persistence of "PEEP-o-phobia", the fear of using adequate levels of end-expiratory pressure. This may be in part because the OLC has not been extensively evaluated in the clinical setting.[58] There is no single optimal PEEP level. The level of end-expiratory pressure must be tailored to the degree of lung injury (ie, lung compliance). For infants with healthy lungs and thus normal lung compliance, PEEP of 3 cm H_2O may be appropriate; PEEP of 6 cm H_2O may well lead to overexpansion of normal lungs with circulatory impairment and elevated cerebral venous pressure. On the other hand, atelectatic, poorly compliant lungs may transiently require PEEP levels as high as 8 to 10 cm H_2O or more to achieve adequate alveolar recruitment and optimize ventilation/perfusion ratio. Because infants with healthy lungs are seldom ventilated, PEEP of less than 5 cm H_2O should be uncommon.

High-frequency Ventilation

In contrast to conventional ventilation, the importance of optimizing lung inflation has been recognized since its early days by users of HFV, where the optimal lung volume strategy has become standard practice and is widely understood to be critical to its success.[59,60] HFV includes several modes of ventilation, including high-frequency oscillatory ventilation (HFOV), high-frequency jet ventilation, and high-frequency percussive ventilation, that have been used in neonatology since the 1980s. The benefit of HFV is believed to be a function of reduced pressure and volume swings transmitted to the periphery of the lungs. For optimal effectiveness, the lungs need to be recruited and then stabilized with the lowest possible mean airway pressure. Several early animal studies demonstrated the short-term benefits of HFOV with an optimal lung volume strategy.[61] More recently, Yoder and colleagues[62] compared the effect of more prolonged HFOV and low V_T positive pressure ventilation using the immature baboon model for BPD, demonstrating that prolonged use of HFOV significantly improved early lung function with sustained improvement in pulmonary mechanics up to 28 days of life and less pulmonary inflammation in the recovery phase of their RDS. Several RCTs of HFOV and high-frequency jet ventilation showed improved outcomes, including reduction in BPD and/or duration of MV,[63–67] whereas

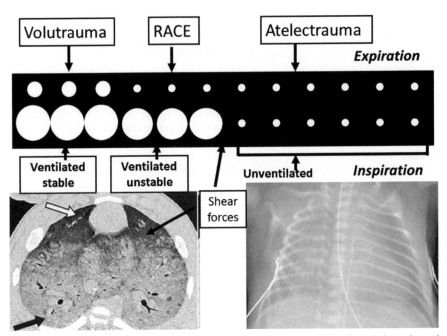

Fig. 3. Tidal ventilation in the presence of extensive atelectasis leads to lung injury via multiple mechanisms. Although lung pathology in an infant with respiratory distress syndrome is commonly thought of as homogeneous, based on an anteroposterior radiograph (*right lower corner*), the lung is heterogeneous due to gravitational effects, as seen on the CT scan (*left lower corner*). This results in 2 populations of alveoli with very different critical opening pressures, illustrated in cartoon form in the upper panel. From Laplace's law, it is known that the already aerated alveoli (*white arrow*) have a lower critical opening pressure; therefore, gas enters the already aerated portion of the lung preferentially, causing overexpansion with each inflation (*black arrow* in lower left corner). This results in volutrauma even with a normal V_T, whereas the atelectatic portion is also damaged by outpouring of protein-rich edema fluid that inactivates surfactant. The ventilated but unstable alveoli undergo repeated alveolar collapse and expansion (RACE) and shear forces at the boundary between aerated and unaerated lung further add to damage. Adequate lung volume recruitment and keeping the lung open throughout the respiratory cycle achieve even distribution of V_T and mitigate all the factors involved in VALI.

other trials showed no improvement.[68–72] Interpretation of RCTs of HFV is made more challenging by the fact that most were done many years ago in patient populations that differ markedly from infants treated today and compared HFV with less sophisticated (more injurious) modes of CMV than those in use today.[58] The only HFV trials that showed benefit were those that used the optimal lung volume strategy. Thus, there were 2 key differences between study and control strategies: higher frequency and use of the OLC in the intervention arm and lower frequency with lower distending pressure. The latter may be the more important difference. HFOV used without the open lung strategy was relatively ineffective in reducing lung injury[73] and several animal studies have indicated that conventional ventilation, when used with the OLC, can achieve similar degrees of lung protection as HFOV, suggesting that optimizing lung volume, rather than frequency, is the key factor.[74–76] Clinical application of the OLC with conventional ventilation, however, may not be an easy task and has not been extensively evaluated in clinical trials.[77]

With the inclusion of more recent clinical trials that reflect advances in conventional ventilation strategies, the protective effect of HFOV is less clear than earlier studies suggested.[78] A recent meta-analysis of individual patient data from several RCTs did not demonstrate any superiority of HFOV over conventional ventilatory strategies.[79] The analysis also did not support the selection of a specific subgroup of preterm infants who might uniquely benefit from HFOV on the basis of gestational age, birth weight for gestation, initial lung disease severity, or exposure to antenatal corticosteroids. The long-term pulmonary follow-up from the United Kingdom Oscillation Study, however, which demonstrated less severe long-term pulmonary abnormalities in the HFOV group, suggests that the dichotomous outcome of BPD versus No BPD is too blunt a tool to assess possible benefits of lung-protective ventilation strategies.[80]

PUTTING IT ALL TOGETHER

Based on the key concepts discussed previously, certain general guidelines for the use of MV can be formulated. The overarching goal is to support adequate gas exchange with the minimum of adverse effects on the infant's lungs, hemodynamics, and brain. Longer duration of ventilation is associated with increased likelihood of chronic lung disease, late-onset sepsis, and neurodevelopmental impairment; therefore, successful extubation at the earliest possible time is desirable. Ventilation strategies should be individualized to address each patient's specific condition, but optimizing lung volume and preventing atelectasis, which improve lung compliance, minimize oxygen requirement, avoid surfactant inactivation and achieve even V_T distribution, remain fundamental imperatives. The second key element of lung-protective strategy is to avoid excessively large V_T, which minimizes volutrauma and hypocapnia, 2 potentially preventable elements of lung and brain injury. This is best accomplished by the use of one of the volume-targeted modes available on most widely used ventilators. When high distending and inflation pressures are needed to achieve these goals, HFV is a reasonable option.

Mild permissive hypercapnia and minimal FiO_2 to achieve adequate oxygen saturation are generally considered appropriate, but Pco_2 greater than 60 mm Hg should be avoided in the first 3 days of life due to increased risk of IVH. There is no evidence to support the routine use of sedation and, therefore, infants should be allowed to breathe spontaneously. Routine suctioning should be avoided, because it leads to derecruitment, transient hypoxemia, and perturbation of cerebral hemodynamics. Only when secretions are detected by auscultation or by perturbation of the flow waveform is gentle rapid suctioning without instillation of normal saline indicated.

In the absence of definitive evidence from RCTs, the choice of synchronized intermittent mandatory ventilation (SIMV) or assist/control (A/C) remains a matter of personal preference and practice style. There is little difference between the two in the acute phase of respiratory failure or in a patient who has little or no respiratory effort but becomes more pronounced during weaning, especially in the smallest infants with narrow endotracheal tubes. Prolonged ventilation with low SIMV rates should be avoided in these infants, because of the mechanical inflations it imposes an undesirably high work of breathing. SIMV also results in larger V_T compared with A/C, because small preterm infants typically do not generate adequate spontaneous V_T resulting in a high dead space:V_T ratio. To a significant degree, this problem may be overcome by adding pressure support ventilation (PS) to the spontaneous breaths during SIMV.[81] Although this approach is effective, it adds complexity and does not seem to have any advantage over A/C or PS used alone as long as atelectasis is avoided by using adequate level of PEEP. Additionally, it is important to recognize that volume targeting is only applied to the SIMV inflations when using SIMV with PS and volume guarantee.

SUMMARY

Although even with optimized respiratory care it is likely that some degree of lung injury is inevitable in ELBW infants, the wide variation in the risk-adjusted incidence of BPD among the academic medical centers that comprise the Neonatal Research Network suggests that MV and other clinical practices are potentially modifiable risk factors.[82,83] Although the evidence to guide respiratory support strategies remains incomplete, the key concepts outlined in this review are based on the best available evidence and physiologic rationale and may provide an opportunity to minimize adverse respiratory outcomes in ELBW infants requiring respiratory support.

REFERENCES

1. Walsh MC, Morris BH, Wrage LA, et al. Extremely low birthweight neonates with protracted ventilation: mortality and 18-month neurodevelopmental outcomes. J Pediatr 2005;146(6):798–804.
2. NICHD Neonatal Research Network, Support Study Group of the Eunice Kennedy Shriver. Early CPAP versus surfactant in extremely preterm infants. N Engl J Med 2010;362:1970–9.
3. Morley CJ, Davis PG, Doyle LW, et al. Nasal CPAP or intubation at birth for very preterm infants. N Engl J Med 2008;358(7):700–8.
4. Loeliger M, Inder T, Cain S, et al. Cerebral outcomes in a preterm baboon model of early versus delayed nasal continuous positive airway pressure. Pediatrics 2006;118(4):1640–53.
5. Garland JS. Strategies to prevent ventilator-associated pneumonia in neonates. Clin Perinatol 2010;37(3):629–43.
6. Northway WH Jr, Rosan RC, Porter DY. Pulmonary disease following respirator therapy of hyaline-membrane disease. Bronchopulmonary dysplasia. N Engl J Med 1967;276(7):357–68.
7. Northway WH Jr, Rosan RC. Radiographic features of pulmonary oxygen toxicity in the newborn: bronchopulmonary dysplasia. Radiology 1968;91(1):49–58.
8. Jobe AH, Bancalari E. Bronchopulmonary dysplasia. Am J Respir Crit Care Med 2001;163(7):1723–9.
9. Philip AG. Oxygen plus pressure plus time: the etiology of bronchopulmonary dysplasia. Pediatrics 1975;55(1):44–50.
10. Dreyfuss D, Soler P, Basset G, et al. High inflation pressure pulmonary edema. Respective effects of high airway pressure, high tidal volume, and positive end-expiratory pressure. Am Rev Respir Dis 1988;137(5):1159–64.
11. Hernandez LA, Peevy KJ, Moise AA, et al. Chest wall restriction limits high airway pressure-induced lung injury in young rabbits. J Appl Physiol (1985) 1989;66(5):2364–8.
12. Mols G, Priebe HJ, Guttmann J. Alveolar recruitment in acute lung injury. Br J Anaesth 2006;96(2):156–66.
13. Laughon M, Bose C, Allred EN, et al. Antecedents of chronic lung disease following three patterns of early respiratory disease in preterm infants. Arch Dis Child Fetal Neonatal Ed 2011;96(2):F114–20.
14. Jobe AH. Effects of chorioamnionitis on the fetal lung. Clin Perinatol 2012;39(3):441–57.

15. Hendson L, Russell L, Robertson CMT, et al. Neonatal and neurodevelopmental outcomes of very low birth weight infants with histologic chorioamnionitis. J Pediatr 2011;158(3):397–402.
16. Speer CP. Chorioamnionitis, postnatal factors and proinflammatory response in the pathogenetic sequence of bronchopulmonary dysplasia. Neonatology 2009;95(4):353–61.
17. Mortola JP, Fisher JT, Smith JB, et al. Onset of respiration in infants delivered by cesarean section. J Appl Physiol Respir Environ Exerc Physiol 1982;52(3):716.
18. Siew ML, Te Pas AB, Wallace MJ, et al. Positive end-expiratory pressure enhances development of a functional residual capacity in preterm rabbits ventilated from birth. J Appl Physiol (1985) 2009;106:1487–93.
19. Kattwinkel J, Perlman JM, Aziz K, et al. Neonatal Resuscitation: 2010 American heart association guidelines for cardiopulmonary resuscitation and emergency cardiovascular care. Pediatrics 2010;126(5):e1400–13.
20. Perlman JM, Wyllie J, Kattwinkel J, et al. Neonatal resuscitation: 2010 international consensus on cardiopulmonary resuscitation and emergency cardiovascular care science with treatment recommendations. Pediatrics 2010;126(5):e1319–44.
21. Keszler M. Sustained inflation during neonatal resuscitation. Curr Opin Pediatr 2015;27(2):145–51.
22. Hillman NH, Kemp MW, Miura Y, et al. Sustained inflation at birth did not alter lung injury from mechanical ventilation in surfactant-treated fetal lambs. PLoS One 2014;9(11):e113473.
23. Hillman NH, Kemp MW, Noble PB, et al. Sustained inflation at birth did not protect preterm fetal sheep from lung injury. Am J Physiol Lung Cell Mol Physiol 2013; 305(6):L446–53.
24. Schmölzer GM, Kumar M, Aziz K, et al. Sustained inflation versus positive pressure ventilation at birth - a systematic review and meta-analysis. Arch Dis Child Fetal Neonatal Ed 2015;100(4):F361–8.
25. Vento M, Moro M, Escrig R, et al. Preterm resuscitation with low oxygen causes less oxidative stress, inflammation, and chronic lung disease. Pediatrics 2009; 124(3):e439–49.
26. Kapadia VS, Chalak LF, Sparks JE, et al. Resuscitation of preterm neonates with limited versus high oxygen strategy. Pediatrics 2013;132(6):e1488–96.
27. Rabi Y, Singhal N, Nettel-Aguirre A. Room-air versus oxygen administration for resuscitation of preterm infants: the ROAR study. Pediatrics 2011;128(2): e374–81.
28. SUPPORT Study Group of the Eunice Kennedy Shriver NICHD Neonatal Research Network. Target ranges of oxygen saturation in extremely preterm infants. N Engl J Med 2010;362(21):1970–9.
29. Stenson BJ, Tarnow-Mordi WO, Darlow BA, et al. Oxygen saturation and outcomes in preterm infants. N Engl J Med 2013;368(22):2094–104.
30. Schmidt B, Whyte RK, Asztalos EV, et al. Effects of targeting higher vs lower arterial oxygen saturations on death or disability in extremely preterm infants: a randomized clinical trial. JAMA 2013;309(20):2111–20.
31. Saugstad OD, Aune D. Optimal oxygenation of extremely low birth weight infants: a meta-analysis and systematic review of the oxygen saturation target studies. Neonatology 2014;105(1):55–63.
32. Van Marter LJ, Allred EN, Pagano M, et al. Do clinical markers of barotrauma and oxygen toxicity explain interhospital variation in rates of chronic lung disease? The Neonatology Committee for the Developmental Network. Pediatrics 2000; 105:1194–201.

33. Sandri F, Plavka R, Ancora G, et al. Prophylactic or early selective surfactant combined with nCPAP in very preterm infants. Pediatrics 2010;125(6):e1402–9.
34. Dunn MS, Kaempf J, de Klerk A, et al. Randomized trial comparing 3 approaches to the initial respiratory management of preterm neonates. Pediatrics 2011; 128(5):e1069–76.
35. Schmolzer GM, Kumar M, Pichler G, et al. Non-invasive versus invasive respiratory support in preterm infants at birth: systematic review and meta-analysis. BMJ 2013;347:f5980.
36. Moretti C, Gizzi C, Papoff P, et al. Comparing the effects of nasal synchronized intermittent positive pressure ventilation (nSIPPV) and nasal continuous positive airway pressure (nCPAP) after extubation in very low birth weight infants. Early Hum Dev 1999;56(2–3):167–77.
37. Davis PG, Morley CJ, Owen LS. Non-invasive respiratory support of preterm neonates with respiratory distress: continuous positive airway pressure and nasal intermittent positive pressure ventilation. Semin Fetal Neonatal Med 2009;14(1):14–20.
38. Meneses J, Bhandari V, Alves JG. Nasal intermittent positive-pressure ventilation vs nasal continuous positive airway pressure for preterm infants with respiratory distress syndrome: a systematic review and meta-analysis. Arch Pediatr Adolesc Med 2012;166(4):372–6.
39. Kirpalani H, Millar D, Lemyre B, et al. A trial comparing noninvasive ventilation strategies in preterm infants. N Engl J Med 2013;369(7):611–20.
40. Bahadue FL, Soll R. Early versus delayed selective surfactant treatment for neonatal respiratory distress syndrome. Cochrane Database Syst Rev 2012;(11):CD001456.
41. Rojas-Reyes MX, Morley CJ, Soll R. Prophylactic versus selective use of surfactant in preventing morbidity and mortality in preterm infants. Cochrane Database Syst Rev 2012;(3):CD000510.
42. Dargaville PA, Aiyappan A, Cornelius A, et al. Preliminary evaluation of a new technique of minimally invasive surfactant therapy. Arch Dis Child Fetal Neonatal Ed 2011;96(4):F243–8.
43. Kribs A, Härtel C, Kattner E, et al. Surfactant without intubation in preterm infants with respiratory distress: first multicenter data. Klin Padiatr 2010;222(1):13–7.
44. Dargaville PA, Aiyappan A, De Paoli AG, et al. Minimally-invasive surfactant therapy in preterm infants on continuous positive airway pressure. Arch Dis Child Fetal Neonatal Ed 2013;98(2):F122–6.
45. More K, Sakhuja P, Shah PS. Minimally invasive surfactant administration in preterm infants: a meta-narrative review. JAMA Pediatr 2014;168(10):901–8.
46. Finer N, Merritt T, Bernstein G, et al. A multicenter pilot study of Aerosurf delivered via nasal continuous positive airway pressure (nCPAP) to prevent respiratory distress syndrome in preterm neonates. J Aerosol Med Pulm Drug Deliv 2010; 23(5):303–9.
47. Keszler M. State of the art in conventional mechanical ventilation. J Perinatol 2009;29(4):262–75.
48. Morley CJ. Volume-limited and volume-targeted ventilation. Clin Perinatol 2012; 39(3):513–23.
49. Dani C, Bresci C, Lista G, et al. Neonatal respiratory support strategies in the intensive care unit: an Italian survey. Eur J Pediatr 2013;172(3):331–6.
50. van Kaam AH, Rimensberger PC, Borensztajn D, et al. Ventilation practices in the neonatal intensive care unit: a cross-sectional study. J Pediatr 2010;157(5):767–71.
51. Wheeler K, Klingenberg C, McCallion N, et al. Volume-targeted versus pressure-limited ventilation in the neonate. Cochrane Database Syst Rev 2010;(11):CD003666.

52. Peng WS, Zhu HW, Shi H, et al. Volume-targeted ventilation is more suitable than pressure-limited ventilation for preterm infants: a systematic review and meta-analysis. Arch Dis Child Fetal Neonatal Ed 2014;99:F158–65.
53. Lachmann B. Open up the lung and keep the lung open. Intensive Care Med 1992;18(6):319–21.
54. Caruso P, Meireles SI, Reis LFL, et al. Low tidal volume ventilation induces proinflammatory and profibrogenic response in lungs of rats. Intensive Care Med 2003;29:1808–11.
55. Tsuchida S, Engelberts D, Peltekova V, et al. Atelectasis causes alveolar injury in nonatelectatic lung regions. Am J Respir Crit Care Med 2006;174(3):279–89.
56. Rimensberger PC, Cox PN, Frndova H, et al. The open lung during small tidal volume ventilation: concepts of recruitment and "optimal" positive end-expiratory pressure. Crit Care Med 1999;27:1946–52.
57. Castoldi F, Daniele I, Fontana P, et al. Lung recruitment maneuver during volume guarantee ventilation of preterm infants with acute respiratory distress syndrome. Am J Perinatol 2011;28:521–8.
58. van Kaam AH, Rimensberger PC. Lung-protective ventilation strategies in neonatology: what do we know - what do we need to know? Crit Care Med 2007;35:925–31.
59. Bryan AC. The oscillations of HFO. Am J Respir Crit Care Med 2001;163(4):816–7.
60. Froese AB. Role of lung volume in lung injury: HFO in the atelectasis-prone lung. Acta Anaesthesiol Scand 1989;90:126.
61. Keszler M, Durand D. High-frequency ventilation. Clin Perinatol 2001;28(3):579–607.
62. Yoder BA, Siler-Khodr T, Winter VT, et al. High-frequency oscillatory ventilation: effects on lung function, mechanics, and airway cytokines in the immature baboon model for neonatal chronic lung disease. Am J Respir Crit Care Med 2000;162:1867–76.
63. Clark RH, Gertsmann DR, Null DM, et al. Prospective randomized comparison of high-frequency oscillatory and conventional ventilation in respiratory distress syndrome. Pediatrics 1992;89:5–12.
64. Gerstmann DR, Minton SD, Stoddard RA, et al. The Provo multicenter early high frequency oscillatory ventilation trial: improved pulmonary and clinical outcome in respiratory distress syndrome. Pediatrics 1996;98:1044–57.
65. Keszler M, Modanlou HD, Brudno DS, et al. Multi-center controlled clinical trial of high-frequency jet ventilation in preterm infants with uncomplicated respiratory distress syndrome. Pediatrics 1997;100:593–9.
66. Plavka R, Kopecky P, Sebron V, et al. A prospective randomized comparison of conventional mechanical ventilation and very early high-frequency oscillatory ventilation in extremely premature newborns with respiratory distress syndrome. Intensive Care Med 1999;25:68–75.
67. Courtney SE, Durand DJ, Asselin JM, et al, The Neonatal Ventilation Study Group. High-frequency oscillatory ventilation versus conventional mechanical ventilation for very-low-birth-weight infants. N Engl J Med 2002;347:643–52.
68. Wiswell TE, Graziani LJ, Kornhauser MS, et al. High-frequency jet ventilation in the early management of respiratory distress syndrome is associated with a greater risk for adverse outcomes. Pediatrics 1996;98:1035–43.
69. Rettwitz-Volk W, Veldman A, Roth B, et al. A prospective, randomized, multicenter trial of high-frequency oscillatory ventilation compared with conventional ventilation

in preterm infants with respiratory distress syndrome receiving surfactant. J Pediatr 1998;132:249–54.

70. Moriette G, Paris-Llado J, Walti H, et al. Prospective randomized multicenter comparison of high-frequency oscillatory ventilation and conventional ventilation in preterm infants of less than 30 weeks with respiratory distress syndrome. Pediatrics 2001;107:363–72.

71. Johnson AH, Peacock JL, Greenough A, et al. High-frequency oscillatory ventilation for the prevention of chronic lung disease of prematurity. N Engl J Med 2002; 347:633–42.

72. Van Reempts P, Borstlap C, Laroche S, et al. Early use of high frequency ventilation in the premature neonate. Eur J Pediatr 2003;162:219–26.

73. McCulloch PR, Forkert PG, Froese AB. Lung volume maintenance prevents lung injury during high-frequency oscillatory ventilation in surfactant deficient rabbits. Am Rev Respir Dis 1988;137:1185–92.

74. Gommers D, Hartog A, Schnabel R, et al. High-frequency oscillatory ventilation is not superior to conventional mechanical ventilation in surfactant-treated rabbits with lung injury. Eur Respir J 1999;14:738–44.

75. Vazquez de Anda GF, Hartog A, Verbrugge SJ, et al. The open lung concept: pressure-controlled ventilation is as effective as high-frequency oscillatory ventilation in improving gas exchange and lung mechanics in surfactant-deficient animals. Intensive Care Med 1999;25:990–6.

76. Vazquez de Anda GF, Gommers D, Verbrugge SJ, et al. Mechanical ventilation with high positive end-expiratory pressure and small driving pressure amplitude is as effective as high-frequency oscillatory ventilation to preserve the function of exogenous surfactant in lung-lavaged rats. Crit Care Med 2000;28:2921–5.

77. Jobe AH. Lung recruitment for ventilation: does it work, and is it safe? J Pediatr 2009;154(5):635–6.

78. Cools F, Henderson-Smart DJ, Offringa M, et al. Elective high frequency oscillatory ventilation versus conventional ventilation for acute pulmonary dysfunction in preterm infants. Cochrane Database Syst Rev 2009;(3):CD000104.

79. Cools F, Askie LM, Offringa M, et al, PreVILIG Collaboration. Elective high-frequency oscillatory versus conventional ventilation in preterm infants: a systematic review and meta-analysis of individual patients' data. Lancet 2010; 375(9731):2082–91.

80. Zivanovic S, Peacock J, Alcazar-Paris M, et al. Late outcomes of a randomized trial of high-frequency oscillation in neonates. N Engl J Med 2014;370(12): 1121–30.

81. Osorio W, Claure N, D'Ugard C, et al. Effects of pressure support during an acute reduction of synchronized intermittent mandatory ventilation in preterm infants. J Perinatol 2005;25(6):412–6.

82. Laughon MM, Langer JC, Bose CL, et al. Prediction of bronchopulmonary dysplasia by postnatal age in extremely premature infants. Am J Respir Crit Care Med 2011;183(12):1715–22.

83. Ambalavanan N, Walsh M, Bobashev G, et al. Intercenter differences in bronchopulmonary dysplasia or death among very low birth weight infants. Pediatrics 2011;127(1):e106–16.

Impact of Nutrition on Bronchopulmonary Dysplasia

Brenda B. Poindexter, MD, MS[a],*, Camilia R. Martin, MD, MS[b]

KEYWORDS

- Nutrition • Bronchopulmonary dysplasia • Growth • Premature infants

KEY POINTS

- Suboptimal intrauterine and postnatal growth is associated with an increased risk of bronchopulmonary dysplasia (BPD).
- Premature infants with BPD are at high risk for poor growth attainment after discharge from the neonatal intensive care unit.
- A multidisciplinary approach to postdischarge management is critical to optimize nutrition, growth, and medical outcomes.
- Pilot human data and animal data support the critical role of specific immunonutrients in lung development and in the protection from lung injury. Additional research and bedside translation are needed to optimize nutritional strategies in the neonatal intensive care unit and following hospital discharge.

INTRODUCTION

Bronchopulmonary dysplasia (BPD) remains a common morbidity of prematurity. Although the pathogenesis of BPD is recognized to be both multifactorial and complex, much of the focus is traditionally on injurious factors, such as oxygen toxicity, volutrauma, and inflammation. Discussion of the role of nutrition in the pathophysiology of BPD is typically limited to management after a diagnosis has been made. In this article, the association between growth and pulmonary outcomes is reviewed, including the role of nutrition in lung development and function, the consequences of various treatments for lung disease on nutritional status, and the nutritional strategies to optimize growth of infants at risk for or diagnosed with BPD, including management

[a] Perinatal Institute, Cincinnati Children's Hospital Medical Center, 3333 Burnet Avenue, MLC 7009, Cincinnati, OH 45229, USA; [b] Beth Israel Deaconess Medical Center, Harvard Medical School, Rose Building, 330 Brookline Avenue, 3rd Floor, Boston, MA 02215, USA
* Corresponding author.
E-mail address: brenda.poindexter@cchmc.org

Clin Perinatol 42 (2015) 797–806
http://dx.doi.org/10.1016/j.clp.2015.08.007   **perinatology.theclinics.com**
0095-5108/15/$ – see front matter © 2015 Elsevier Inc. All rights reserved.

following hospital discharge. Finally, research opportunities on the role of nutrition and lung disease are considered.

INTRAUTERINE GROWTH AND PULMONARY OUTCOMES

Although infants with BPD are more likely to experience postnatal growth failure, it is important to recognize that suboptimal intrauterine growth is also associated with an increased risk of adverse pulmonary outcomes. Although the incidence of small for gestational age (weight less than the 10th percentile) among very low birth weight infants is approximately 20%,[1] large cohort and observational studies have demonstrated significantly higher neonatal mortality and rates of BPD in small-for-gestational-age neonates compared with preterm infants born appropriate for gestational age.[2,3]

Indeed, fetal growth restriction based on birth weight z scores was found to be independently associated with the risk of chronic lung disease in the (ELGAN) Extremely Low Gestational Age Newborn study cohort.[4] Although not completely understood, decreased lung growth is hypothesized to be the mechanism. Using a well-established animal model of placental insufficiency, Rozance and colleagues[5] found decreased alveolar and vascular growth in fetal lambs with intrauterine growth restriction. These investigators hypothesize that a similar mechanism may contribute to the increased risk of BPD in infants with suboptimal intrauterine growth. A review of clinical and animal data discussed later in greater detail suggests that these changes in lung growth may be amenable to nutritional interventions.

POSTNATAL GROWTH AND CLINICAL OUTCOMES

Postnatal growth failure, typically defined as weight less than the tenth percentile for gestational age at 36 weeks postmenstrual age (PMA), is an all too common byproduct of several months in the neonatal intensive care unit (NICU). Although the incidence of postnatal growth failure in extremely premature infants has steadily declined over the past 2 decades,[1,6,7] further efforts to decrease growth faltering are urgently needed. In a recent cohort of more than 2000 infants less than 27 weeks' gestation reported by the Eunice Kennedy Shriver National Institute of Child Health and Human Development (NICHD) Neonatal Research Network, 55% were found to have weight less than the tenth percentile at 36 weeks PMA based on the Olsen postnatal growth curves.[6,8] Infants who have experienced one or more major morbidity, such as BPD, necrotizing enterocolitis, severe intracranial hemorrhage, or late-onset sepsis, have a higher incidence of postnatal growth failure than infants who survive without a major morbidity. Factors commonly associated with postnatal growth failure include male gender, need for assisted ventilation on the first day of life, necrotizing enterocolitis, need for respiratory support at 28 days of age, and treatment with postnatal corticosteroids.[9]

Ehrenkranz and colleagues[10] evaluated the relationship between in-hospital weight gain and neonatal morbidities in a cohort of extremely low birth weight (501–1000 g) infants cared for in centers participating in the Eunice Kennedy Shriver NICHD Neonatal Research Network. Infants were divided into quartiles of weight gain, with those in the lowest quartile gaining an average of 12 g/kg/d, whereas those in the highest quartile gaining an average of 21 g/kg/d. Not surprisingly, the incidence of BPD and receipt of postnatal corticosteroids were higher in the infants in the lowest quartile of in-hospital weight gain (BPD: 56% vs 31%; postnatal steroids: 64% vs 30% for lowest weight gain quartile and highest weight gain quartile, respectively). In-hospital weight gain was also found to have a significant and independent effect on neurodevelopmental outcomes in this cohort, with infants in the lowest quartile of in-hospital weight gain having a greater odd of cerebral palsy, Bayley Mental Developmental Index less than 70, and neurodevelopmental impairment at 18 months corrected age. A more recent cohort of infants has confirmed these findings.[6,10,11]

Although weight gain is the primary assessment of postnatal growth, linear growth is also an important parameter to monitor, particularly in infants with significant lung disease. Linear growth may be more closely linked to organ growth and development. The association between linear growth and improved cognitive outcomes at 2 years of age was recently demonstrated by Ramel and colleagues.[12] In order to optimize outcomes not only of infants with BPD but also of all premature infants, proportional growth of weight, length, and head circumference is needed.

GROWTH OUTCOMES OF INFANTS WITH BRONCHOPULMONARY DYSPLASIA

Numerous observational studies have demonstrated slower rates of postnatal growth in infants diagnosed with BPD compared with preterm infants without lung disease.[13–15] The reasons for suboptimal growth are varied and include failure to meet nutrient requirements and also to the adverse effects related to some of the therapeutic interventions used for treatment of lung disease, such as diuretics and systemic corticosteroids.

Whatever the cause, the suboptimal postnatal growth observed in infants with BPD does not resolve quickly. Investigators from the Netherlands evaluated growth and body composition of preterm infants (mean gestational age 27 weeks and birth weight 850 g) with BPD and found deficits in fat-free mass and total body fat that persisted through the first year of life.[16] Future studies are needed to determine whether specific nutritional interventions can improve growth and body composition in these infants.

CAUSE OF POOR GROWTH IN INFANTS WITH BRONCHOPULMONARY DYSPLASIA

Severity of illness can impact provider decisions regarding provision of nutritional support. Ehrenkranz and colleagues[17] found that infants receiving mechanical ventilation for the first 7 days after birth received significantly less nutritional support (both parenteral and enteral) during each of the first 3 weeks compared with less critically ill infants who did not require ventilation. These findings are intriguing, if not paradoxic, because the infants arguably needing early nutritional support the most were receiving less. Given the association between suboptimal nutrition, growth failure, and impaired neurodevelopment, these findings also support the utility of standardized feeding guidelines to ensure that the sickest infants receive optimal nutritional support.

NUTRITIONAL INTERVENTIONS TO PREVENT BRONCHOPULMONARY DYSPLASIA

All too often, attempts to prevent postnatal growth failure are not made soon enough, resulting in nutrient deficits that can be difficult to recoup and long-term consequences. As BPD is not typically diagnosed until 36 weeks PMA, it is important to prevent growth failure in all extremely premature infants at risk for BPD. A combined approach of early parenteral and enteral nutrition is a key factor and has been reviewed previously.[18] It is important to point out that there is no contraindication to either parenteral or enteral nutrition in critically ill infants receiving mechanical ventilation.

Very few randomized trials have demonstrated efficacy of drugs or nutritional interventions for the prevention or treatment of BPD.[19] One intervention shown to be efficacious is vitamin A. Two randomized clinical trials have evaluated the use of vitamin A for the prevention of BPD in 856 extremely premature infants,[20,21] although some have questioned whether a higher dose of vitamin A supplementation is necessary to reduce the risk of BPD.[22] There is no evidence that vitamin A supplementation reduces hospitalizations or pulmonary morbidity after hospital discharge.[23]

In a secondary analysis of data from a cohort of nearly 1400 extremely low birth weight infants, Oh and colleagues[24] found an association between fluid intake and weight loss and the risk of BPD. The risk of death or BPD was associated with higher fluid intake and less weight loss in the first 10 days of life. However, physiologic contraction of the extracellular fluid compartment must be balanced with the risk of accumulating significant nutrient deficits if adequate nutrition is not provided.

IMPACT OF TREATMENT FOR BRONCHOPULMONARY DYSPLASIA ON NUTRITIONAL STATUS

Although the evidence (or lack thereof) for various treatments for bronchopulmonary dysplasia is discussed elsewhere in this issue, many commonly used therapies can have a significant impact on nutritional status and growth.

Fluid restriction is sometimes used in the management of pulmonary edema that can accompany evolving BPD. Fluid restriction can interfere with delivery of recommended nutrient intake.

Although the efficacy of diuretic therapy may be viewed as controversial, there is no disputing the increased risk of hyponatremia and hypokalemia in infants who receive diuretics. In animal models, sodium restriction, even with relatively normal serum sodium levels, is associated with poor weight gain and linear growth and may also impact lung growth.[25] If diuretics are given, sodium supplementation may be required to maintain sodium stores necessary for optimal growth.

The mechanism of decreased weight gain velocity during administration of systemic corticosteroids does not seem to be related to increased energy expenditure,[26] although some studies evaluating changes in body composition in infants receiving dexamethasone were conducted before early parenteral nutrition. Increased rates of protein breakdown may be a direct effect of steroids or could reflect suboptimal protein intake in these infants.

NUTRITIONAL STRATEGIES TO OPTIMIZE GROWTH

Provision of nutritional support for infants with evolving lung disease is not fundamentally different from that provided to premature infants without lung disease. Prevention of growth faltering requires focused attention to adequate protein and energy intake in the first few weeks after birth. In a prospective cohort study, Senterre and Rigo[27] found that providing recommended intake of 3.8 g/kg/d of protein and 120 kcal/kg/d to extremely premature infants in the first week of life reduced the incidence of postnatal growth failure. In this cohort, postnatal weight loss was limited to the first 3 days after birth, but pulmonary outcomes were not reported for this cohort. Martin and colleagues[28] also demonstrated the association between nutritional intake at 7 days with growth velocity over the first month of life, reinforcing the concept that early nutritional support is a key determinant to subsequent growth outcomes.

A minimum of 2 g/kg/d of intravenous amino acids should be provided as soon as possible following birth in extremely low gestational age neonates. Within 48 to 72 hours, a target of 3.5 to 4.0 g/kg/d of amino acids is recommended. In order to meet recommended energy intake, intravenous lipids should also be provided. There is no evidence to support the need for a stepwise increase in lipid intake; a minimum of 2 g/kg/d is recommended with a target of 3.0 to 4.0 g/kg/d shortly thereafter.[29]

In infants who are fluid restricted, it is critical to maintain total energy and macronutrient provision; this can be achieved using fortifiers to increase caloric density as well as protein and fat delivery. Optimization of protein is essential for adequate utilization of total calories for energy. After ensuring optimal protein delivery, further increases in carbohydrate and fats may be necessary to maintain total energy delivery. In reviewing these options, it is important to consider that fats provide the highest concentrated energy source relative to carbohydrates and have a lower respiratory quotient and thus lower production of carbon dioxide.[30]

POSTDISCHARGE MANAGEMENT OF INFANTS WITH BRONCHOPULMONARY DYSPLASIA

A coordinated medical home should be created that consists of a multidisciplinary team that meets the complex medical needs of a former preterm infant with bronchopulmonary disease. The full complement of this team will vary based on the infant's precise needs, but at a minimum the team should include, in addition to the infant's pediatrician, a pulmonologist and a nutritionist, given the high prevalence of residual pulmonary concerns and the high rate of postdischarge growth failure.[31,32] Frequent assessments should be made to track growth on appropriate growth charts, allowing for timely intervention when needed.

Decreased weight, length, head circumference, fat mass, and fat-free mass seen during the NICU hospitalization often continue after discharge.[33] Medical management that interfered with optimal nutritional delivery during the NICU hospitalization may persist, such as fluid restriction, salt and mineral wasting due to chronic diuretics, increased energy expenditure from medications (caffeine, theophylline, other bronchodilators),[33] and poor protein accretion with steroid use. In addition, other medical issues may persist or evolve that interfere with nutritional delivery and desirable growth, such as gastrointestinal reflux, oral aversion, unrecognized hypoxia, repeated intercurrent illnesses, and neurocognitive impairment.[31–33]

Energy needs for an infant with BPD have been estimated to be 15% to 25% greater than for an infant without BPD, and thus, in the range of 140 to 150 kcal/kg/d.[33] Often, increased calorie and protein delivery is required to meet the increased energy expenditures and metabolic needs of these vulnerable infants.[31] Studies on the use of a fortified discharge formula have demonstrated improved length, lean mass, and bone mass.[33–35] Oxygen may improve weight gain; however, it should be noted that the criteria for home oxygen remain controversial.[31]

Nutritional status at 2 years of age is a positive predictor of pulmonary outcomes later in childhood.[36] Thus, multidisciplinary oversight and frequent assessments are critical to maintain nutrition and growth in infants diagnosed with BPD.[31] **Box 1** outlines the general predischarge and postdischarge clinical principles to optimize growth and nutritional status in infants with BPD.

Close monitoring of nutritional status and growth is important not only to ensure an adequate growth trajectory but also to monitor for excess in weight gain due to intensive nutritional support. Excess weight gain in early infancy may increase the risk of insulin resistance and adult onset metabolic disease.[37,38]

RESEARCH OPPORTUNITIES IN THE ROLE OF NUTRITION AND LUNG DISEASE

As discussed earlier, the only nutrient to date that has been shown to have a positive effect in reducing BPD in a large clinical trial is vitamin A.[20] Prior rationale for this clinical trial and continued subsequent validation of the role of vitamin A in lung development include data from animal models of neonatal lung injury. Supplementation of

---

Box 1
Predischarge and postdischarge nutritional management of the preterm infant with bronchopulmonary dysplasia

Predischarge nutritional management

1. Determine discharge diet that optimizes total energy delivery and provision of macronutrients

2. If unable to meet total requirements orally alone, nasogastric or gastric tube feedings

3. Teach family how to prepare discharge diet

4. Copy growth chart and send to pediatrician, infant follow-up program, outpatient nutritionist, and subspecialists

5. Obtain recent biochemical parameters (electrolytes, trace minerals) before discharge if infant is on diuretics

Postdischarge nutritional management

1. Regular outpatient follow-up with pediatrician and subspecialists

2. Track weight, length, and head circumference on a regular basis

3. Modify diet to meet growth goals as needed

4. Regular monitoring of serum electrolytes and trace minerals if infant remains on diuretics

5. If infant is on chronic diuretics, obtain renal ultrasound for nephrocalcinosis

6. If poor growth
   a. Consider increasing caloric density of diet
   b. Rule out significant gastrointestinal reflux disease, oral aversion, or aspiration as a cause for poor growth due to limited intakes
   c. Rule out unrecognized hypoxia

---

vitamin A or retinoic acid attenuates lung injury and alveolar simplification in models of neonatal lung injury, including rescuing alveolar hypoplasia induced by caloric restriction.[39,40] In the NICHD-supported clinical trial, 5000 IU of vitamin A administered intramuscularly 3 times a week resulted in a reduction in death or BPD by 7% versus controls.[20] Despite this modest effect, bedside translation has not been universal with varying beliefs in the overall effectiveness, concerns about ease of implementation, and the perception of a large number of injections for a small benefit.[41] The clinical experience with vitamin A illustrates the challenges in implementing a potential therapeutic and that additional research in maximizing dosing effectiveness in addition to exploring other routes of delivery may be warranted. This finding is true of all potential nutrient interventions.

In addition to the immunomodulatory effects of vitamin D in T-cell differentiation, vitamin D has also been shown in animal studies to play a critical role in lung development, improving alveolarization and alveolar type II cell maturation.[42] In a recent rodent model of antenatal endotoxin-mediated neonatal lung injury, maternal treatment with vitamin D attenuated the morphologic features of lung injury in the pups.[43] Further analysis revealed that vitamin D mediated its effects through proangiogenesis, upregulation of VEGF (vascular endothelial growth factor) and KDR (kinase domain receptor), and increasing alveolar epithelial type II cell proliferation. Clinical trials of vitamin D supplementation in infants at high risk for BPD are lacking. The animal data suggest this may be worth pursuing.

Inositol is a carbohydrate that is an important component of phosphatidylinositol, and thus, the phospholipid bilayer of a cell that determines cell membrane structure, function, and signaling. Likely through the previously described function of increasing surfactant production, small early clinical trials demonstrated reduced respiratory distress syndrome and subsequent survival without BPD in preterm infants who received inositol supplementation compared with control infants.[44–46] There is currently no intravenous preparation of inositol available clinically. However, a large multicenter randomized clinical trial evaluating the efficacy of myo-inositol to reduce severe retinopathy of prematurity is underway (NCT01954082); BPD will be assessed as a secondary outcome measure in this trial conducted by the NICHD Neonatal Research Network.

Also integral to cell membrane function and signaling is the long-chain polyunsaturated fatty acid (LCPUFA) composition of the phospholipid bilayer. In addition, LCPUFAs possess anti-inflammatory, proangiogenic, and pro-organogenesis properties. Animal data suggest potential effectiveness of LCPUFAs in the prevention of BPD. In multiple studies using the murine model of neonatal hyperoxia-induced lung injury, increased exposure to docosahexaenoic acid (DHA), either through increased maternal content in dam milk or directly through oral administration to the mouse pups, or the provision of the terminal bioactive metabolites of DHA and arachidonic acid (Resolvin D1 and Lipoxin A4, respectively), attenuated the morphologic features of lung injury.[47–49] In each of these studies, optimizing exposure to LCPUFAs or to their derivatives resulted in a reduction of inflammation and improved alveolarization. Observation and clinical trial data of improved DHA delivery in preterm infants support these observations. In a cohort study of preterm infants less than 30 weeks of gestation, for every 1 mol% decline in DHA, there was a 2.5-fold increase in the odds of developing BPD.[50] In breast milk-fed preterm infants less than 1250 g, infants of mothers who were supplemented with a high-DHA diet had a 12% decrease in the incidence of BPD compared with infants whose mothers were not supplemented.[51] Finally, in a small clinical trial comparing 2 different lipid emulsions (soy-based vs an emulsion containing 15% fish oil) in preterm infants less than 1500 g, the infants who received the fish oil-based lipid emulsion were less likely to develop BPD compared with the infants receiving the soybean oil-based lipid emulsion.[52] A large study specifically evaluating the reduction in BPD with LCPUFA supplementation has not been reported to date.

The potential for nutrition to modulate the risk of BPD is not limited to the above-mentioned nutrients. Additional elements worth pursuing also include trace elements and amino acids. Nutrition plays a critical role in susceptibility to chronic lung disease, not only through energy delivery and promoting somatic growth but also through specific nutrient immunomodulation in the developmental pathways of lung development. Increased research efforts in nutrient-gene interaction in lung development as well as optimizing nutritional management strategies to ensure adequate provision of essential immunonutrients are needed to pave the way for further reduction in the development of BPD. For each nutrient, the dose, timing, duration, and route of administration will need to be defined through thoughtful and iterative study designs.

REFERENCES

1. Fanaroff AA, Stoll BJ, Wright LL, et al. Trends in neonatal morbidity and mortality for very low birthweight infants. Am J Obstet Gynecol 2007;196(2): 147.e1–8.
2. Reiss I, Landmann E, Heckmann M, et al. Increased risk of bronchopulmonary dysplasia and increased mortality in very preterm infants being small for gestational age. Arch Gynecol Obstet 2003;269(1):40–4.

3. Eriksson L, Haglund B, Odlind V, et al. Perinatal conditions related to growth restriction and inflammation are associated with an increased risk of bronchopulmonary dysplasia. Acta Paediatr 2015;104(3):259–63.

4. Bose C, Van Marter LJ, Laughon M, et al. Fetal growth restriction and chronic lung disease among infants born before the 28th week of gestation. Pediatrics 2009; 124(3):e450–8.

5. Rozance PJ, Seedorf GJ, Brown A, et al. Intrauterine growth restriction decreases pulmonary alveolar and vessel growth and causes pulmonary artery endothelial cell dysfunction in vitro in fetal sheep. Am J Physiol Lung Cell Mol Physiol 2011;301(6):L860–71.

6. Poindexter B, Langer J, Hintz S, et al. Have we caught up? Growth and neurodevelopmental outcomes in extremely premature infants. Pediatric Academic Societies annual meeting. 2013. 1395.2.

7. Stoll BJ, Hansen NI, Bell EF, et al. Neonatal outcomes of extremely preterm infants from the NICHD Neonatal Research Network. Pediatrics 2010;126(3):443–56.

8. Olsen IE, Groveman SA, Lawson ML, et al. New intrauterine growth curves based on United States data. Pediatrics 2010;125(2):e214–24.

9. Clark RH, Thomas P, Peabody J. Extrauterine growth restriction remains a serious problem in prematurely born neonates. Pediatrics 2003;111(5 Pt 1):986–90.

10. Ehrenkranz RA, Dusick AM, Vohr BR, et al. Growth in the neonatal intensive care unit influences neurodevelopmental and growth outcomes of extremely low birth weight infants. Pediatrics 2006;117(4):1253–61.

11. Ehrenkranz RA. Nutrition, growth and clinical outcomes. World Rev Nutr Diet 2014;110:11–26.

12. Ramel SE, Demerath EW, Gray HL, et al. The relationship of poor linear growth velocity with neonatal illness and two-year neurodevelopment in preterm infants. Neonatology 2012;102(1):19–24.

13. Vohr BR, Bell EF, Oh W. Infants with bronchopulmonary dysplasia. Growth pattern and neurologic and developmental outcome. Am J Dis Child 1982; 136(5):443–7.

14. Markestad T, Fitzhardinge PM. Growth and development in children recovering from bronchopulmonary dysplasia. J Pediatr 1981;98(4):597–602.

15. Davidson S, Schrayer A, Wielunsky E, et al. Energy intake, growth, and development in ventilated very-low-birth-weight infants with and without bronchopulmonary dysplasia. Am J Dis Child 1990;144(5):553–9.

16. Huysman WA, de Ridder M, de Bruin NC, et al. Growth and body composition in preterm infants with bronchopulmonary dysplasia. Arch Dis Child Fetal Neonatal Ed 2003;88(1):F46–51.

17. Ehrenkranz RA, Das A, Wrage LA, et al. Early nutrition mediates the influence of severity of illness on extremely LBW infants. Pediatr Res 2011;69(6):522–9.

18. Poindexter B. Approaches to growth faltering. World Rev Nutr Diet 2014;110: 228–38.

19. Beam KS, Aliaga S, Ahlfeld SK, et al. A systematic review of randomized controlled trials for the prevention of bronchopulmonary dysplasia in infants. J Perinatol 2014;34(9):705–10.

20. Tyson JE, Wright LL, Oh W, et al. Vitamin A supplementation for extremely-low-birth-weight infants. National Institute of Child Health and Human Development Neonatal Research Network. N Engl J Med 1999;340(25):1962–8.

21. Pearson E, Bose C, Snidow T, et al. Trial of vitamin A supplementation in very low birth weight infants at risk for bronchopulmonary dysplasia. J Pediatr 1992; 121(3):420–7.

22. Kennedy KA, Stoll BJ, Ehrenkranz RA, et al. Vitamin A to prevent bronchopulmonary dysplasia in very-low-birth-weight infants: has the dose been too low? The NICHD Neonatal Research Network. Early Hum Dev 1997;49(1):19–31.
23. Ambalavanan N, Tyson JE, Kennedy KA, et al. Vitamin A supplementation for extremely low birth weight infants: outcome at 18 to 22 months. Pediatrics 2005;115(3):e249–54.
24. Oh W, Poindexter BB, Perritt R, et al. Association between fluid intake and weight loss during the first ten days of life and risk of bronchopulmonary dysplasia in extremely low birth weight infants. J Pediatr 2005;147(6):786–90.
25. Wassner SJ. Altered growth and protein turnover in rats fed sodium-deficient diets. Pediatr Res 1989;26(6):608–13.
26. Leitch CA, Ahlrichs J, Karn C, et al. Energy expenditure and energy intake during dexamethasone therapy for chronic lung disease. Pediatr Res 1999;46(1): 109–13.
27. Senterre T, Rigo J. Optimizing early nutritional support based on recent recommendations in VLBW infants and postnatal growth restriction. J Pediatr Gastroenterol Nutr 2011;53(5):536–42.
28. Martin CR, Brown YF, Ehrenkranz RA, et al. Nutritional practices and growth velocity in the first month of life in extremely premature infants. Pediatrics 2009; 124(2):649–57.
29. Koletzko B, Poindexter B, Uauy R. Recommended nutrient intake levels for stable, fully enterally fed very low birth weight infants. World Rev Nutr Diet 2014;110: 297–9.
30. Forsyth JS, Crighton A. Low birthweight infants and total parenteral nutrition immediately after birth. I. Energy expenditure and respiratory quotient of ventilated and non-ventilated infants. Arch Dis Child Fetal Neonatal Ed 1995;73(1):F4–7.
31. Groothuis JR, Makari D. Definition and outpatient management of the very low-birth-weight infant with bronchopulmonary dysplasia. Adv Ther 2012;29(4): 297–311.
32. Bancalari E, Wilson-Costello D, Iben SC. Management of infants with bronchopulmonary dysplasia in North America. Early Hum Dev 2005;81(2):171–9.
33. Carlson SJ. Current nutrition management of infants with chronic lung disease. Nutr Clin Pract 2004;19(6):581–6.
34. Carver JD. Nutrition for preterm infants after hospital discharge. Adv Pediatr 2005;52:23–47.
35. Brunton JA, Saigal S, Atkinson SA. Growth and body composition in infants with bronchopulmonary dysplasia up to 3 months corrected age: a randomized trial of a high-energy nutrient-enriched formula fed after hospital discharge. J Pediatr 1998;133(3):340–5.
36. Bott L, Béghin L, Devos P, et al. Nutritional status at 2 years in former infants with bronchopulmonary dysplasia influences nutrition and pulmonary outcomes during childhood. Pediatr Res 2006;60(3):340–4.
37. Brands B, Demmelmair H, Koletzko B, et al. How growth due to infant nutrition influences obesity and later disease risk. Acta Paediatr 2014;103(6):578–85.
38. Lapillonne A, Griffin IJ. Feeding preterm infants today for later metabolic and cardiovascular outcomes. J Pediatr 2013;162(3 Suppl):S7–16.
39. Maden M, Hind M. Retinoic acid in alveolar development, maintenance and regeneration. Philos Trans R Soc Lond B Biol Sci 2004;359(1445):799–808.
40. Londhe VA, Maisonet TM, Lopez B, et al. Retinoic acid rescues alveolar hypoplasia in the calorie-restricted developing rat lung. Am J Respir Cell Mol Biol 2013; 48(2):179–87.

41. Kaplan HC, Tabangin ME, McClendon D, et al. Understanding variation in vitamin A supplementation among NICUs. Pediatrics 2010;126(2):e367–73.

42. Lykkedegn S, Sorensen GL, Beck-Nielsen SS, et al. The impact of vitamin D on fetal and neonatal lung maturation. A systematic review. Am J Physiol Lung Cell Mol Physiol 2015;308(7):L587–602.

43. Mandell E, Seedorf G, Gien J, et al. Vitamin D treatment improves survival and infant lung structure after intra-amniotic endotoxin exposure in rats: potential role for the prevention of bronchopulmonary dysplasia. Am J Physiol Lung Cell Mol Physiol 2014;306(5):L420–8.

44. Hallman M, Jarvenpaa AL, Pohjavuori M. Respiratory distress syndrome and inositol supplementation in preterm infants. Arch Dis Child 1986;61(11):1076–83.

45. Hallman M, Bry K, Hoppu K, et al. Inositol supplementation in premature infants with respiratory distress syndrome. N Engl J Med 1992;326(19):1233–9.

46. Hallman M, Pohjavuori M, Bry K. Inositol supplementation in respiratory distress syndrome. Lung 1990;168(Suppl):877–82.

47. Martin CR, Zaman MM, Gilkey C, et al. Resolvin D1 and lipoxin A4 improve alveolarization and normalize septal wall thickness in a neonatal murine model of hyperoxia-induced lung injury. PLoS One 2014;9(6):e98773.

48. Ma L, Li N, Liu X, et al. Arginyl-glutamine dipeptide or docosahexaenoic acid attenuate hyperoxia-induced lung injury in neonatal mice. Nutrition 2012; 28(11–12):1186–91.

49. Rogers LK, Valentine CJ, Pennell M, et al. Maternal docosahexaenoic acid supplementation decreases lung inflammation in hyperoxia-exposed newborn mice. J Nutr 2011;141(2):214–22.

50. Martin CR, Dasilva DA, Cluette-Brown JE, et al. Decreased postnatal docosahexaenoic and arachidonic acid blood levels in premature infants are associated with neonatal morbidities. J Pediatr 2011;159(5):743–9.e2.

51. Manley BJ, Makrides M, Collins CT, et al. High-dose docosahexaenoic acid supplementation of preterm infants: respiratory and allergy outcomes. Pediatrics 2011;128(1):e71–7.

52. Skouroliakou M, Konstantinou D, Agakidis C, et al. Cholestasis, bronchopulmonary dysplasia, and lipid profile in preterm infants receiving MCT/omega-3-PUFA-containing or soybean-based lipid emulsions. Nutr Clin Pract 2012;27(6): 817–24.

Oxygen Saturation Targeting and Bronchopulmonary Dysplasia

Brian A. Darlow, MD, FRCP, FRACP, FRCPCH[a],*,
Colin J. Morley, MD, FRCPCH[b]

KEYWORDS

- Oxygen saturation • Bronchopulmonary dysplasia • Retinopathy of prematurity
- Neonatal free radical disease • Randomized controlled trial • Very preterm infant

KEY POINTS

- Four out of 5 trials of higher and lower oxygen saturation targeting in very preterm infants have shown increased mortality in the lower target group, significantly so in meta-analysis of all trials.
- The trend to use lower oxygen saturation targets in very preterm infants, principally to avoid retinopathy of prematurity, should cease and a target higher than 85% to 89% chosen.
- There is little impact of higher or lower oxygen saturation targeting on bronchopulmonary dysplasia when the latter is defined by physiologic criteria.
- It is reassuring that longer-term neurodevelopmental outcomes, including severe visual impairment with reported rates around 1%, show no differences between oxygen saturation target groups.

INTRODUCTION

Oxygen saturation (Sp_{O_2}) monitors, although convenient, provide an indirect measure of oxygenation, and technological innovations are needed to better guide clinical care.

The 2005 workshop on oxygen in neonatal therapies, sponsored by the National Institute of Child Health and Human Development and dubbed "one of the most complex areas in perinatal/neonatal medicine," explored gaps in knowledge and opportunities for research.[1] For more than 10 years an international effort has been addressing one key research question: "How low can oxygen saturations be set before causing

The authors have no financial or other conflicts of interest.
[a] Department of Paediatrics, University of Otago at Christchurch, PO Box 4345, Christchurch 8140, New Zealand; [b] Department of Obstetrics and Gynaecology, University of Cambridge, 223, Level 2, The Rosie Hospital, Robinson Way, Cambridge CB2 2SW, UK
* Corresponding author.
E-mail address: brian.darlow@otago.ac.nz

Clin Perinatol 42 (2015) 807–823
http://dx.doi.org/10.1016/j.clp.2015.08.008   **perinatology.theclinics.com**
0095-5108/15/$ – see front matter © 2015 Elsevier Inc. All rights reserved.

harm?"[1,2] Although there are still unanswered questions about the optimal target ranges for very preterm infants, the emerging evidence from this effort is beginning to affect practice.

This review focuses on oxygen targeting in acute and continuing care of very preterm infants and its relationship to bronchopulmonary dysplasia (BPD). The technology of oxygen monitoring and the role of oxygen toxicity are briefly reviewed.

OXYGEN MONITORING

The principles of pulse oximetry monitoring in neonates were well described in *Clinics in Perinatology* more than 20 years ago[3] and in more recent publications including another *Clinics* review.[4]

Oximeters in clinical use have 2 light-emitting diodes (LEDs) with wavelengths of 660 nm (red) and 940 nm (infrared), respectively. The light is passed through a translucent part of the body (the hand or foot of a newborn) and measured by a facing photodiode. Oxyhemoglobin (Hbo_2) and deoxyhemoglobin or reduced hemoglobin (RHb) have different light absorption spectra; in the red region Hbo_2 absorbs less light than RHb, whereas the opposite occurs in the infrared region (**Fig. 1**).

The device measures the absorption of these wavelengths in the pulsatile portion of blood flow, which varies with each heartbeat, eliminating absorption by nonpulsatile venous and capillary blood, myoglobulin, and other tissue.[5] Readings taken multiple times per second are averaged (every 2–16 seconds: "averaging time") and the value of the red-to-infrared ratio compared with a stored calibration algorithm to give Spo_2. The calibration algorithm is generated from direct in vitro measurement of arterial blood saturation (Sao_2) from adult volunteers by CO-oximetry, which measures absorption at several wavelengths. Accuracy of oximeters is limited below an Sao_2 level of 75% to 80% because of difficulties achieving such values in healthy volunteers, and

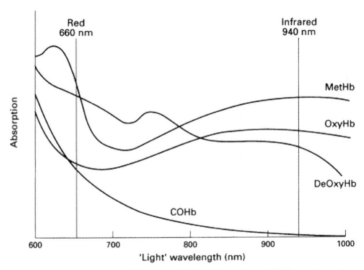

Fig. 1. Light absorption curves of hemoglobin derivatives. COHb, carboxyhemoglobin; DeOxyHb, deoxyhemoglobin or reduced hemoglobin; MetHb, methemoglobin; OxyHb, oxyhemoglobin. The vertical lines indicate red and infrared wavelengths used in most pulse oximeters. (*From* Moyle JT. Uses and abuses of pulse oximetry. Arch Dis Child 1996;74:77; with permission.)

values lower than this are extrapolated from the measured data. Pulse oximeters usually display the plethysmographic waveform (pulsatile signal) to detect whether the signal is affected by low perfusion, noise, or motion artifact.[6] The displayed SpO_2 is affected by the averaging time, longer times reducing signal artifact but also limiting the ability to detect brief hypoxemic episodes.[7] Inaccurate readings may occur when there is an optical shunt, that is, the photodiode receives ambient light, or when partially detached and only one of the transmitted wavelengths is received.

Although the accuracy of commercially available oximeters varies, they must all meet international standards.[8,9] Oximeter performance is reported as bias, being the mean difference between the reference SaO_2 and displayed SpO_2; precision, which is the standard deviation of the differences between SaO_2 and SpO_2[6]; and most recently as the root mean squared, which combines bias and precision.[10] Most manufacturers state an "accuracy" (how far a value is from a reference standard) of $\pm2\%$ to 3% at least two-thirds of the time.[8,9,11]

Traditionally clinical oximeters measure functional oxygen saturation, which is a measure of the amount of oxygen bound to each hemoglobin molecule as a percentage of its maximal capacity [$HbO_2/(HbO_2 + RHb)] \times 100$. Fractional saturation represents the fraction of oxyhemoglobin in relation to the total hemoglobin present, including non–oxygen-binding hemoglobins [$HbO_2/(HbO_2 + RHb + MetHb + COHb)] \times 100$. Clinical instruments that display "fractional" hemoglobin measure functional hemoglobin, and 1.5% to 2% is then subtracted from this in the displayed value.[12] Newer-generation oximeters, including the Masimo Radical-7 (Masimo Corp, Irving, CA, USA) used in recent trials of oxygen saturation monitoring in very preterm infants (vide infra), use LEDs with more than 7 wavelengths, but still display functional saturation.[13]

Oxygen is transported in the blood in 2 forms: free oxygen molecules dissolved in the plasma or combined with hemoglobin. Although the former comprises only around 2% of the total oxygen content, oxygen delivery to tissues depends on the oxygen tension (PaO_2) or partial pressure of dissolved oxygen in the blood, together with pulmonary function, cardiac output, and tissue perfusion. The amount of dissolved oxygen determines the amount combined with hemoglobin as depicted in the oxyhemoglobin dissociation curve (**Fig. 2**). However, the relationship between SaO_2 and PaO_2 depends on various factors including the proportion of fetal hemoglobin (HbF; which shifts the curve to the left) and pH (with a lower pH shifting the curve to the right), thus complicating the interpretation of SpO_2.

A large international survey highlighted the wide variation in transfusion practices in very preterm infants and, hence, in the proportion of HbF.[14] Some data suggest that HbF may result in a 4% overestimation of oxygen saturation,[15] but not all investigators agree.[16] A recommendation that CO-oximetry, which can correct for HbF, be performed intermittently to set safety limits for pulse oximetry[17] is not routinely practiced. Poets and Southall[12] noted that a change in pH can have a similarly large effect; at a PaO_2 of 45 mm Hg, SaO_2 increases from 80% to 88% if arterial pH is raised from 7.25 to 7.4.

OXYGEN TOXICITY

Oxygen is necessary for our existence, but excess oxygen can be harmful. Healthy adults who breathe higher inspired oxygen (up to 100%) at normal barometric pressure become unwell with retrosternal discomfort and breathing difficulties within a few hours.[18,19] Experimental animal data tell a similar story,[20,21] although there are species differences and, intriguingly, newborn animals of some species are more tolerant of high oxygen concentrations than are adults.[22]

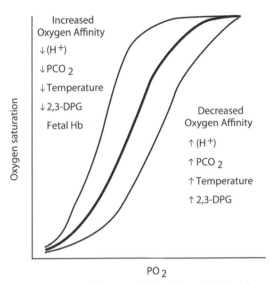

Fig. 2. Oxygen dissociation curve of hemoglobin. 2,3-DPG, 2,3-diphosphoglycerate; Fetal Hb, fetal hemoglobin. The thick line represents the oxygen dissociation curve of normal adult hemoglobin. Fetal hemoglobin has high oxygen affinity and shifts the curve to the left. (*From* Hay WW. Physiology of oxygenation and its relation to pulse oximetry in neonates. J Perinatol 1987;7:310; with permission.)

At the cellular level, oxygen is normally fully reduced by the cytochrome oxidase pathway. However, even in health small amounts of highly reactive oxygen species are produced, being sequentially the superoxide radical, hydrogen peroxide, and the hydroxyl radical (**Fig. 3**).[23]

Although small amounts of such oxygen radicals are required for normal physiologic functioning,[24] all have the potential to cause damage by reacting with adjacent molecules. Organisms that depend on oxygen have antioxidant defenses, comprising both enzymatic (eg, superoxide dismutase, catalase, glutathione peroxidase) and nonenzymatic free radical scavengers (eg, β-carotene, vitamin E, vitamin C, glutathione, bilirubin).

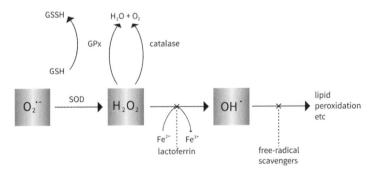

Fig. 3. Oxygen-derived reactive species and antioxidant protectants. Fe^{2+}, ferrous iron; Fe^{3+}, ferric iron; GPx, glutathione peroxide; GSH, reduced glutathione; GSSH, oxidized glutathione; H_2O_2, hydrogen peroxide; $O_2^{\bullet-}$, superoxide radical; $OH^{\bullet}$, hydroxyl radical; SOD, superoxide dismutase. Pathway of increasingly reactive oxygen species, role of prooxidants (transition metals such as iron), and enzymatic and nonenzymatic defenses (see text).

There are other sources of free radicals, such as those produced by ionizing radiation. One important source in the newborn is through the action of xanthine oxidase. Following a hypoxemic-ischemic episode, hypoxanthine, the breakdown product of adenine nucleotides, accumulates and is converted by xanthine oxidase to uric acid with the generation of superoxide and hydrogen peroxide.[23]

The premise that very preterm infants are especially vulnerable to oxidative damage is based on several factors. In utero the fetus develops normally in a low oxygen environment (Sao_2 and Pao_2) and so has low concentrations of antioxidant defenses; these mature during the last trimester. For preterm infants even air is relatively hyperoxic, yet they often require high inspired oxygen for many days because of lung immaturity. The evidence for the first 2 elements largely comes from animal data, but is less certain in human infants.[25]

Exposure to increased inspired oxygen (Fio_2) for several days is a key insult resulting in changes that mimic BPD in both large and small animal models.[26] Biomarkers of oxidative damage, including lipid peroxidation products in exhaled breath[27] and protein carbonyls in endotracheal aspirates,[28] have been reported to be elevated in preterm infants who later develop BPD, but these are nonspecific products and do not indicate the processes involved.[24] The current evidence indicates that BPD has a multifactorial etiology, and that much of the damage is the result of inflammation and free radicals generated from neutrophils and macrophages.[21,29–32] Preventing initiation of the inflammatory cascade by minimizing barotrauma, volutrauma, and infection might have as great an impact on decreasing rates of BPD as a focus purely on oxygen exposure.

HISTORY OF OXYGEN MONITORING IN PRETERM INFANTS

The history of oxygen use in neonates has been described in numerous reviews, including the well-known monograph by Silverman.[33] Ten years after the first description of retinopathy of prematurity (ROP) in 1942, 3 randomized controlled trials (RCTs) showed convincingly that severe ROP can be caused by unrestricted oxygen.[34] Mortality was reported in 2 trials, and was nonsignificantly increased with restricted compared with unrestricted oxygen (25.9% vs 17.7%; risk ratio 1.23; 95% confidence interval [CI] 0.80–1.90).[34]

In the years of frequent oxygen restriction which followed these trials, it has been estimated that for every infant whose sight was saved there may have been 16 additional deaths.[35] In the 1960s and 1970s oxygen therapy was monitored by Pao_2 measurement on intermittent arterial blood samples, but a large cohort study was unable to establish a relationship between Pao_2 and ROP.[36] The American Academy of Pediatrics (1976, 1988) recommendation of target ranges for Pao_2 in preterm infants of 50 to 80 mm Hg was based on consensus.

Following the development of continuous transcutaneous oxygen tension monitoring ($TcPo_2$), a Miami study investigated whether this would reduce ROP compared with intermittent monitoring, in the first month of life, with the aim of keeping $TcPo_2$ or Pao_2 less than 70 mm Hg.[37] Overall there was no reduction in any or severe ROP with $TcPo_2$ monitoring. However, a post hoc analysis in a subset of infants weighing 900 to 1300 g showed that the longer the time with $TcPo_2$ greater than 80 mm Hg, the greater was the risk of ROP.[38] Intriguingly, in all infants of 1300 g or smaller, mortality was nonsignificantly higher in the $TcPo_2$ monitoring group (32% vs 24%)[37] $TcPo_2$ monitoring requires frequent calibration through arterial blood sampling, and may cause skin burns in fragile preterm infants. By the 1990s, therefore, continuous Spo_2 monitoring was being widely used because it is simple to undertake and noninvasive.

Despite variation between units, many adopted Spo_2 targets in the range of 85% to 95%, and this was endorsed as "pragmatic" by the American Academy of Pediatrics in 2007, while also noting that the optimal range was unknown.[39]

TRIALS OF OXYGEN SATURATION TARGETING AND BRONCHOPULMONARY DYSPLASIA

Changing practices at birth aimed at decreasing barotrauma and volutrauma and exposure to hyperoxia have coincided with the emergence of a less severe form of neonatal chronic lung disease dubbed "the new BPD."[40] In a meta-analysis of 9 randomized trials of commencing resuscitation with higher or lower Fio_2 in infants of gestational age 32 weeks or less (BPD being the primary outcome in only 2 trials[41,42]), Saugstad and colleagues[43] reported no significant association with BPD (relative risk [RR] 1.11; 95% CI 0.73–1.68). As other aspects of resuscitation could not be controlled for, these results are somewhat hard to interpret.

In the 1990s there was speculation that higher O_2 may prevent progression of ROP. There was also concern that too low an O_2 level would increase pulmonary hypertension and impair growth and neurodevelopment, especially in infants with chronic lung disease.[44] Two RCTs in convalescing infants, both of which hypothesized that a higher Spo_2 target would be beneficial, investigated these issues.

The Supplemental Therapeutic Oxygen for Prethreshold Retinopathy of Prematurity (STOP-ROP) trial randomized infants with prethreshold ROP to an Spo_2 target of 89% to 94% or 96% to 99% for at least 2 weeks.[45] The mean postmenstrual age (PMA) at enrollment was 35.4 ± 2.5 weeks. The higher target was associated with a nonsignificant increase in episodes of pneumonia/chronic lung disease, but this was confined to infants with a worse lung disease at trial entry. The Benefits of Oxygen Saturation Targeting (BOOST) trial randomized infants who were born at less than 30 weeks' gestation and still requiring supplementary oxygen at 32 weeks PMA to a Spo_2 target of 91% to 94% or 95% to 98%, with caregivers masked to the intervention through the use of oximeters that were offset at $\pm2\%$ in this range, and staff targeting a displayed value of 93% to 96%.[46] There were no differences between the groups in growth or development at 1 year of age, but the higher target was associated with significantly increased rates of supplementary oxygen at 36 weeks PMA and requirement for home oxygen. Of note, the lower target in both the STOP-ROP and BOOST I trials is close to the higher target in the NeOProM trials (see later discussion). "Lower" and "higher" are relative terms.

Two influential observational studies also suggested that lower Spo_2 targets might be beneficial. A North-East England study reported the 1-year outcome for infants of less than 28 weeks' gestation cared for in neonatal units, which set Spo_2 alarms at 70% and 90% compared with 88% and 98% (staff were said to "aim to keep saturation in the upper half of the range," ie, 80%–90% and 94%–98%, respectively).[47] The lower target range was associated with a reduced likelihood of ROP treatment (6.2% vs 27.2%) and a reduced need for oxygen at 36 weeks (17% vs 45%). At 1 year there were no differences in either survival or incidence of cerebral palsy. These differing targets were mostly applied in different units; hence, other aspects of care could have contributed to the differences. A single-unit study from California reported that lowering the Spo_2 target to 85% to 93% for infants of less than 32 weeks' gestation, and to 83% to 93% for the smallest and sickest infants, was associated with a decrease in severe ROP and a trend toward increased survival in infants with birth weights less than 1250 g compared with historical controls when a Spo_2 of 90% to 98% was targeted.[48] Respiratory outcomes were not reported.

THE NEONATAL OXYGENATION PROSPECTIVE META-ANALYSIS TRIALS OF OXYGEN SATURATION TARGETING

As other reports demonstrate, much of the practice in this period was driven by the desire to avoid severe ROP, and many units adopted lower SpO_2 targets in very preterm infants.[49] Surveys from North America[50] and the United Kingdom[51] both reported a wide range of SpO_2 targets and alarms with little consensus. As stated by both Tin and Wariyar[51] and Silverman,[52] the more precise problem was that it was unclear where the balance should lie to avoid the competing outcomes of ROP, BPD, death, and neurodevelopmental impairment.

In 2002-2003 an international group of investigators met to plan an RCT of SpO_2 targeting in very preterm infants in an attempt to resolve this issue.[53] Recognizing the difficulties of funding a single study with sufficient power, the collaborators agreed early on to submit separate studies but, as far as possible, to use a common protocol so that data could be combined in a prospective individual patient data (IPD) meta-analysis known as the Neonatal Oxygenation Prospective Meta-analysis (NeOProM) collaboration.[2] Six studies were planned and 5 were funded to give a total of more than 5000 infants (**Table 1**).

All NeOProM studies used a Masimo oximeter with the display offset by $\pm3\%$ in the range 85% to 95%, with nurses targeting 88% to 92%. The objective of these studies was to assess in infants of less than 28 weeks' gestation whether targeting SpO_2 85% to 89% compared with 91% to 95% from within 24 hours of birth until the infant was in air (or until 36 weeks) reduces or increases the risk of death or neurodevelopmental disability at 2 years of age. A total NeOProM sample size of 5230 infants would have 80% power to detect an absolute 4% increase or decrease in this outcome from a baseline rate of 42%. Halfway through 3 of the trials (COT, BOOST II Australia, BOOST UK) the pulse oximeter software was upgraded to eliminate a small (2%) overestimation of SpO_2 in the 87% to 90% range.[11,54]

Three studies (SUPPORT, COT, BOOST-NZ) have reported the primary outcome at 18 to 24 months, with no significant differences between the groups (see **Table 1**; **Table 2**).[55–57]

In 2010 the SUPPORT study, which also randomized infants to early continuous positive airway pressure (CPAP) or intubation and surfactant using a 2-by-2 factorial design, published outcomes at hospital discharge.[58] There was no significant difference between the lower and higher target groups in the primary outcome of death or severe ROP (28.3% vs 32.1%; RR 0.90; 95% CI 0.76–1.06). However, severe ROP was significantly less frequent in the lower target group (8.6% vs 17.9%; RR 0.52; 95% CI 0.37–0.73) ($P<.001$) and, unexpectedly, mortality was increased (19.9% vs 16.2%; RR 1.27; 95% CI 1.01–1.60) ($P = .04$).[58]

The consequences of this finding for the remaining 4 trials have been detailed elsewhere.[56,59,60] Review by the data-monitoring committees of combined data from the 3 BOOST studies, together with data from SUPPORT, confirmed higher mortality in the lower target group and led to recruitment to the BOOST UK and BOOST II Australia trials being stopped on December 24, 2010. Recruitment to the BOOST-NZ trial had already been completed. A research letter on 36-week outcomes was published[54] followed by outcomes at hospital discharge for the combined BOOST studies.[61]

An interim meta-analysis has been published, combining these hospital discharge data with 18- to 22-month data from SUPPORT and COT.[62] This analysis confirms increased mortality in the lower target group (RR 1.18; 95% CI 1.04–1.34) (**Fig. 4**). It is noteworthy that all studies except the smaller BOOST-NZ had higher mortality in

Table 1
Oxygen saturation targeting studies: the NeOProM collaboration

Study	Countries	Enrollment Planned	Actual	Timeline	18–24 mo Primary Outcome Measures
SUPPORT[55,58]	USA	1200	1316	February 2005 to February 2009	18–22 mo corrected. Death or major disability (severe visual impairment, deafness requiring aids, CP with GMFCS level ≥2, a CCS on BSID-III of <70)
COT[56]	Canada, USA, Argentina, Finland, Germany	1200	1201	December 2006 to August 2010	18–22 mo corrected. Death or major disability (severe visual impairment, deafness requiring aids, CP with GMFCS level ≥2, a CCS or CLS on BSID-III of <85)
BOOST-NZ[57,61]	New Zealand	320	340	September 2006 to December 2009	24 mo corrected. Death or major disability (severe visual impairment, deafness requiring aids, CP with GMFCS level ≥2, a CCS or CLS on BSID-III of <85)
BOOST II Australia[61]	Australia	1200	1135	March 2006 to December 2010	24 mo corrected. Death or major disability (severe visual impairment, deafness requiring aids, CP with GMFCS level ≥2, a CCS or CLS on BSID-III of <85)
BOOST UK[61]	UK	1200	973	October 2007 to December 2010	24 mo corrected. Death or major disability (severe visual impairment, deafness requiring aids, CP with GMFCS level ≥2, a CCS or CLS on BSID-III of <85)

Abbreviations: BSID-III, Bayley scales of infant and toddler development, third edition; CCS, composite cognitive score; CLS, composite language score; CP, cerebral palsy; GMFCS, Gross Motor Function Classification System.

Table 2
Death or major neurodevelopmental disability at 18–24 months corrected age in infants randomized to a lower or higher oxygen saturation target

Study	N	SpO_2 Target (%) 85%–89%	91%–95%	RR (95% CI)
SUPPORT[55]	1234	30.2	27.5	1.12 (0.94–1.32)
COT[56]	1147	51.6	49.7	1.10 (0.9–1.4)[a]
BOOST-NZ[57]	335	38.9	45.2	0.87 (0.68–1.11)

Abbreviations: CI, confidence interval; RR, relative risk.
[a] Odds ratio: See **Table 1** for definitions of major neurodevelopmental disability.

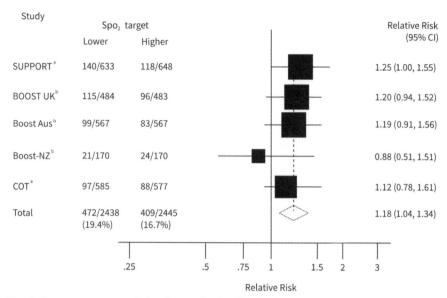

Fig. 4. Summary meta-analysis of mortality in all infants randomized to a lower or higher Spo₂ target. RR >1 favors higher oxygen saturation target. [a] Mortality before 18 months. [b] Mortality at hospital discharge. (*Adapted from* Saugstad OD, Aune D. Optimal oxygenation of extremely low birth weight infants: a meta-analysis and systematic review of the oxygen saturation target studies. Neonatology 2014;105(Suppl):S10; with permission.)

this group. Since then the 2-year outcomes from the BOOST-NZ trial have been published,[57] and most recently partial 2-year results from BOOST UK have appeared in an abstract.[63] Little would be gained from another interim meta-analysis with these additional data. The complete Cochrane review will be undertaken following publication of the Australian and United Kingdom trials,[64] to be followed by the IPD meta-analysis.[2] Given that there were very few additional deaths from hospital discharge to follow-up at 18 to 24 months in the 3 published studies, it seems unlikely that the major conclusion, namely that the lower target is associated with increased mortality, will change materially.

THE NEONATAL OXYGENATION PROSPECTIVE META-ANALYSIS TRIALS AND BRONCHOPULMONARY DYSPLASIA

The definitions of BPD have varied among the 5 trials (**Tables 3** and **4**). Oxygen treatment at 36 weeks' gestation has been reported from the SUPPORT trial and for pooled data from the 3 BOOST II trials.[58,61] A meta-analysis of these data shows that the lower target was significantly associated with a lower incidence of BPD as defined (RR 0.86; 95% CI 0.77–0.96).[62] However, meta-analysis of data from the 3 trials using physiologic criteria (SUPPORT, COT, BOOST UK) showed no significant difference between the Spo₂ target groups (RR 0.95; 95% CI 0.86–1.04).[62] In addition, the pooled data from the 3 BOOST trials has been reported according to the whether the infant was treated with the original or revised oximeter algorithm, as has the BOOST UK physiologic data.[61] In both cases this separation made little difference to the RRs and, although oxygen at 36 weeks was significantly less in the pooled BOOST data overall, this was not the case when grouped by algorithm.

Table 3
Duration of intervention, alarm settings for nursing Spo2 target of 88%–92%, and definitions of bronchopulmonary dysplasia

Study	Intervention Timing	Alarm Settings	Definition of BPD	BPD Additional Criteria
SUPPORT[55]	From within first 2 h of age to 36 wk PMA or in air with no CPAP for >72 h	Suggested: 85% and 95%	O2 requirement at 36 wk PMA	Physiologic definition: Walsh and colleagues[88] Either: positive pressure or supplemental O2 of ≥30% at 36 wk PMA Or: if <30%, the need for any oxygen after an attempt at O2 withdrawal
COT[56]	From 24 h until 36 wk PMA even if in air. If on any respiratory support at 35 wk continued until 40 wk PMA, unless discharged home	Mandated: 86% and 94%	O2 requirement at 36 wk PMA (not reported to date)	Severe BPD: positive pressure or supplemental O2 of ≥30% at 36 wk PMA after at least 28 d of oxygen therapy for more than 12 h per day[89]
BOOST-NZ[57]	From 24 h until 36 wk PMA; after first 2 wk could be discontinued if in air and Spo2 >96% for >95% of the time for 3 d	Recommended: 87% and 93%	Respiratory support or O2 requirement at 36 wk PMA (in combined BOOST report,[61] O2 at 36 wk)	—
BOOST II Australia[61]	From 24 h until 36 wk PMA; after first 2 wk could be discontinued if in air and Spo2 >96% for >95% of the time for 3 d	Recommended: 86% (or between 80% and 85%) and 95%	O2 requirement at 36 wk PMA	—
BOOST UK[61]	From 24 h until 36 wk PMA, except in exceptional circumstances, until the baby is discharged home	Recommended: lower as per local protocol, upper at 94%	O2 requirement at 36 wk PMA	Physiologic definition: Jones criteria (derived from Ref.[90]) effectively, requiring supplemental O2 to maintain an actual Spo2 of 90% or more

Abbreviations: BPD, bronchopulmonary dysplasia; CPAP, continuous positive airway pressure; O2, oxygen; PMA, postmenstrual age.

Table 4
Bronchopulmonary dysplasia (BPD) outcomes by Spo_2 target groups in NeOProM trials

Study (BPD Definition)	85%–89%	90%–95%	RR (95% CI)
SUPPORT (standard)	203/540 (37.6%)	265/568 (46.7%)	0.82 (0.72–0.93)[a]
SUPPORT (physiologic)	205/540 (38.0%)	237/568 (41.7%)	0.92 (0.81–1.05)[a]
COT (physiologic/severe)	164/515 (31.8%)	171/517 (33.1%)	0.94 (0.71–1.23)[b]
BOOST-NZ (standard)	58/153 (37.9%)	70/148 (47.3%)	0.80 (0.62–1.04)[c]
BOOST II Australia (standard)	161/473 (34.0%)	191/492 (38.8%)	0.88 (0.74–1.04)
BOOST UK (standard)	193/372 (51.9%)	212/392 (54.1%)	0.96 (0.84–1.10)
BOOST II Pooled (standard)	394/998 (39.5%)	461/1031 (44.7%)	0.90 (0.81–0.99)[d]
BOOST UK (physiologic/Jones)	160/353 (45.3%)	172/376 (45.7%)	0.99 (0.85–1.16)

For explanation of BPD definitions, see **Table 3**.
[a] Adjusted for stratification (study center, GA groups) and familial clustering.
[b] Odds ratio, adjusted for center.
[c] Unadjusted because of small sample size. This comparison from correction to original publication.
[d] Data from hospital discharge report from BOOST II Australia, BOOST UK, BOOST-NZ.[61] Unadjusted.

WHAT CAN BE CONCLUDED FROM THE EVIDENCE PUBLISHED TO DATE?

- Collectively these studies confirm that too little oxygen increases mortality.
- The drift to using lower and lower Spo_2 targets, principally to avoid ROP, should cease.
- In very preterm infants the Spo_2 target range should be higher than 85% to 89%.
- Measures should be used to minimize the number and duration of hypoxemic episodes.
- Vigilance is needed to minimize the time very preterm infants treated with oxygen have an Spo_2 greater than 95% (to avoid a further epidemic of oxygen toxicity).
- It is reassuring that longer-term neurodevelopmental outcomes show no differences between Spo_2 target groups.
- Spo_2 monitors, although convenient, provide an indirect measure of oxygenation; therefore, improved technology is needed.

It was already known that too little oxygen is harmful and may increase mortality. We now know that in infants of less than 28 weeks' gestation "too little" is when the Spo_2 target is 85% to 89%. However, it should be recognized that infants who were eligible but not enrolled in SUPPORT had a hospital mortality of 24%, which is higher than the 19.9% in that trial's lower target group, although nonenrolled infants were slightly more immature and less likely to have been exposed to antenatal steroids.[65] Infants in the SUPPORT, and other NeOProM studies, had comparatively good outcomes, but this does not alter the conclusion that an Spo_2 target of 85% to 89% should not be used.

Deaths in all studies were spread throughout the ages and occurred from a range of causes in both groups. In a subcohort of 115 infants enrolled in the SUPPORT trial, the lower target was associated with a greater risk of significant hypoxemia.[66] Spo_2 may overestimate Pao_2, particularly at lower saturations.[67] Changing from Pao_2 to Spo_2 targets has likely led to a shift downward in the Pao_2 ranges very preterm infants are exposed to, with values below 50 and even 40 mm Hg being frequent in both NeOProM target groups.[68] It seems plausible, as suggested by others,[62] that hypoxemic episodes might underlie increased vulnerability to later death from a range of causes, for instance, necrotizing enterocolitis, pulmonary hypertension and BPD, or sepsis.

Less secure is which alternative Spo_2 target to adopt. Most commentators suggest targeting 90% to 95% pending further results,[62,69–71] although wider targets have been suggested.[16,72] Given that it is important to avoid hyperoxemia (Spo_2 >95%) and a further epidemic of oxygen toxicity, there seems merit in a high target of 94%, which allows the high alarm to be set at 95%.[57] Observational evidence suggests that tighter alarm limits (1% above the upper target limit and 1%–2% below the lower limit) are associated with improved compliance.[73]

Other targets, including the middle ground of 88% to 92% frequently adopted before the trials, have not been and may never be studied, given the number of infants required. Exploration of the relationship between achieved saturations for infants in both groups compared with outcomes, both for individual studies and combined data, may well provide more insight. In the meantime it is reassuring that long-term neurodevelopmental outcomes among surviving infants in the published trials showed no difference between the groups.

It may be an illusion that there is a precise target that is optimal (just as there is no exact bilirubin concentration at which kernicterus occurs, or blood glucose concentration that is consistently harmful). Moreover, nurses know it is not possible to consistently stay "on target." A prospective multicenter observational study of very preterm infants with modifiable oxygenation found the Spo_2 target to be achieved less than 50% of the time (range 16%–64%).[73] Another study of infants on CPAP and supplementary oxygen reported compliance with Spo_2 targets only 31% of the time.[74] Compliance with Spo_2 targets was improved, mostly by a reduction in hyperoxemia, by a more optimal nurse/patient ratio.[75] Nurse opinion is a factor in achieving target compliance,[76] and may be modifiable by education and clear-cut protocols.[77] Infants in the SUPPORT study collectively experienced a lower mortality than similar infants not in the trial, suggesting that the extra effort to maintain compliance with the Spo_2 target in the trial was valuable. Claims are made that what is possible within the context of a trial may be more difficult to achieve in "general care." However, it is unclear why general care should not demand similar standards, as, for instance, is the case with measures to prevent nosocomial infection.[78]

Among other morbidities, the lower target was associated with an increased rate of serious necrotizing enterocolitis (NEC) in the interim meta-analysis,[62] but the definitions of NEC varied between the studies, and the planned IPD meta-analysis should be more informative. Not surprisingly, the requirement for oxygen at 36 weeks was increased for infants randomized to the higher Spo_2 target, but there was no increased risk of BPD when data were analyzed using a physiologic definition. Furthermore, in SUPPORT both those with and without BPD had ongoing respiratory morbidity at 2 years, although less respiratory morbidity in those randomized to initial CPAP versus intubation.[79] In addition, although rates of severe ROP were increased in the higher target group, severe visual impairment at 2 years was very low (for the lower and higher targets in SUPPORT 1.0% and 1.2%; in COT 1.0% and 0.6%; in BOOST-NZ 0% and 0.7%),[55–57] indicating that current detection and treatment of ROP in these infants was largely successful.

OTHER ISSUES THAT ARISE

Given the problems with Spo_2 target compliance, there is increasing interest in automated control of Fio_2 using feedback systems.[80,81] Two recent studies in preterm infants both demonstrated better Spo_2 target compliance and, respectively, fewer prolonged hypoxemic episodes[82] and fewer manual changes.[83] The latter study included both ventilated infants and others on CPAP.[83]

One issue throughout this review concerns the limitations of Spo_2 monitoring. The pulse oximeter is used in neonates because it is simple to operate, noninvasive, and gives a continuous readout. However, Spo_2 monitoring only provides an indirect measurement of what is desired, namely oxygen tension and tissue oxygenation.[16] The problem lies in the fact that no other method of monitoring is ideal either. A 2005 survey of neonatal intensive care units in Germany, Austria, and Switzerland showed that $TcPo_2$ monitoring continued to be widely used.[84] Quine and Stenson[85] reported that preterm infants on respiratory support and $TcPo_2$ monitoring had significantly less variable oxygenation than those on Spo_2 monitoring. However, this might be because the slow response time of $TcPo_2$ monitors dampens variability.[86] Near-infrared spectroscopic technology has been developed to measure continuous regional tissue oxygenation, and trials are under way to assess whether both cerebral hypoxia and hyperoxia can be reduced using this technique.[87] Only time will tell whether such methods will become part of routine monitoring in very preterm infants.

REFERENCES

1. Higgins RD, Bancalari E, Willinger M, et al. Executive summary of the workshop on oxygen in neonatal therapies: controversies and opportunities for research. Pediatrics 2006;119:790–6.
2. Askie LM, Brocklehurst P, Darlow BA, et al. NeOProM: neonatal oxygen prospective meta-analysis collaboration study protocol. BMC Pediatr 2011;11:6. Available at: http://www.biomedcentral.com/1471-2431/11/6.
3. Hay WW, Thilo E, Culander JB. Pulse oximetry in neonatal medicine. Clin Perinatol 1991;18:441–72.
4. Polin RA, Bateman DA, Sahni R. Pulse oximetry in very low birth weight infants. Clin Perinatol 2014;41:1017–32.
5. Salyer JW. Neonatal and pediatric pulse oximetry. Respir Care 2003;48:386–96.
6. Juban A. Pulse oximetry. Intensive Care Med 2004;30:2017–20.
7. Vagedes J, Poets CF, Dietz K. Averaging time, desaturation level, duration and extent. Arch Dis Child Fetal Neonatal Ed 2012;98:F265–6.
8. Milner QJW, Mathews GR. An assessment of the accuracy of pulse oximeters. Anaesthesia 2012;67:396–401.
9. Moyle JTB. Uses and abuses of pulse oximetry. Arch Dis Child 1996;74:77–80.
10. Ross PA, Newth CJL, Khemani RG. Accuracy of pulse oximetry in children. Pediatrics 2014;133:22–9.
11. Johnston ED, Boyle B, Juszczak E, et al. Oxygen targeting in preterm infants using the Masimo Set Radical pulse oximeter. Arch Dis Child Fetal Neonatal Ed 2011;96:F429–33.
12. Poets CF, Southall DP. Noninvasive monitoring of oxygenation in infants and children: practical considerations and areas of concern. Pediatrics 1994;93:737–46.
13. Masimo Corporation. Radical-7 signal extraction pulse co-oximeter operator's manual. Irving (CA): Masimo Corporation; 2007.
14. Guillén U, Cummings JJ, Bell EF, et al. International survey of transfusion practices for extremely premature infants. Semin Perinatol 2012;36:244–7.
15. Nitzan M, Romem A, Koppel R. Pulse oximetry: fundamentals and technology update. Med Devices 2014;7:231–9.
16. Lakshminrusimha S, Manja V, Mathew B, et al. Oxygen targeting in preterm infants: a physiological interpretation. J Perinatol 2015;35:8–15.

17. Whyte RK, Jangaard KA, Dooley KC. From oxygen content to pulse oximetry: completing the picture in the newborn. Acta Anaesthesiol Scand 1995; 39(Suppl 107):95–100.
18. Jackson RM. Pulmonary oxygen toxicity. Chest 1985;88:900–5.
19. Bitterman H. Bench-to-bedside review: oxygen as a drug. Crit Care 2009;13:205.
20. Bhandari V. Hyperoxia-derived lung damage in preterm infants. Semin Fetal Neonatal Med 2010;15:223–9.
21. Chess PR, D'Angio CT, Pryhuber GS, et al. Pathogenesis of bronchopulmonary dysplasia. Semin Perinatol 2006;30:171–8.
22. Buczynski BW, Maduekwe ET, O'Reilly MA. The role of hyperoxia in the pathogenesis of experimental BPD. Semin Perinatol 2013;37:69–78.
23. Winterbourn CC. Free radicals, oxidants and antioxidants. In: Gluckman PD, Heymann MA, editors. Pediatrics and Perinatology: the scientific basis. 2nd edition. London: Arnold Publisher; 1996. p. 168–75.
24. Murphy MP, Holmgren A, Larsson NG, et al. Unraveling the biological roles of reactive oxygen species. Cell Metab 2011;13:361–6.
25. Jankov RP, Negus A, Tanswell AK. Antioxidants as therapy in the newborn: some words of caution. Pediatr Res 2001;50:681–7.
26. Jobe AH, Kallapur SG. Long term consequences of oxygen therapy in the neonatal period. Semin Fetal Neonatal Med 2010;15:230–5.
27. Pitkänen OM, Hallman M, Andersson SM. Correlation of free oxygen radical-induced lipid peroxidation with outcome in very low birth weight infants. J Pediatr 1990;116:760–4.
28. Gladstone IM Jr, Levine RL. Oxidation of proteins in neonatal lungs. Pediatrics 1994;93:764–8.
29. Saugstad OD. Chronic lung disease: oxygen dogma revisited. Acta Paediatr 2001;90:113–5.
30. Speer CP. Inflammation and bronchopulmonary dysplasia: a continuing story. Semin Fetal Neonatal Med 2006;11:354–62.
31. Harwood T, Darlow BA, Cheah F-C, et al. Biomarkers of neutrophil-mediated glutathione and protein oxidation in tracheal aspirates from preterm infants: association with bacterial infection. Pediatr Res 2011;69:28–33.
32. Wright CJ, Kirpalani H. Targeting inflammation to prevent bronchopulmonary dysplasia: can new insights be translated into therapies? Pediatrics 2011;128: 111–26.
33. Silverman WA. Retrolental fibroplasia: a modern parable. New York: Grune and Stratton; 1980.
34. Askie LM, Henderson-Smart DH. Restricted versus liberal oxygen exposure for preventing morbidity and mortality in preterm or low birth weight infants. Cochrane Database Syst Rev 2001;(4):CD001077.
35. Cross KW. Cost of preventing retrolental fibroplasia. Lancet 1973;2:954–6.
36. Kinsey VE, Arnold HJ, Kalina RE, et al. PaO$_2$ levels and retrolental fibroplasia: a report of the cooperative study. Pediatrics 1977;60:655–68.
37. Bancalari E, Flynn J, Goldberg RN, et al. Influence of transcutaneous oxygen monitoring on the incidence of retinopathy of prematurity. Pediatrics 1987;79:663–9.
38. Flynn JT, Bancalari E, Snyder ES, et al. A cohort study of transcutaneous oxygen tension and the incidence and severity of retinopathy of prematurity. N Engl J Med 1992;326:1050–4.
39. American Academy of Pediatrics. American College of Obstetricians and Gynecologists. Guidelines for perinatal care. 6th edition. Elk Grove Village (IL): American Academy of Pediatrics; 2007.

40. Jobe AJ. The new BPD: an arrest of lung development. Pediatr Res 1999;46: 641–3.
41. Vento M, Moro M, Escrig R, et al. Preterm resuscitation with low oxygen causes less oxidative stress, inflammation, and chronic lung disease. Pediatrics 2009; 124:e439–49.
42. Rook D, Schierbeek H, Vento M, et al. Resuscitation of preterm infants with different inspired oxygen fractions. J Pediatr 2012;164:1322–6.
43. Saugstad OD, Aune D, Aguar M, et al. Systematic review and meta-analysis of optimal initial fraction of oxygen levels in the delivery room at ≤32 weeks. Acta Paediatr 2014;103:744–51.
44. Kotecha S, Allen J. Oxygen therapy for infants with chronic lung disease. Arch Dis Child Fetal Neonatal Ed 2002;87:F11–4.
45. The STOP-ROP Multicenter Study Group. Supplemental therapeutic oxygen for prethreshold retinopathy of prematurity (STOP-ROP), a randomized, controlled trial. I: primary outcomes. Pediatrics 2000;105:295–310.
46. Askie LM, Henderson-Smart DJ, Irwig L, et al. Oxygen-saturation targets and outcomes in extremely preterm infants. N Engl J Med 2003;349:959–67.
47. Tin W, Milligan DW, Pennefather P, et al. Pulse oximetry, severe retinopathy, and outcome at one year in babies of less than 28 weeks gestation. Arch Dis Child Fetal Neonatal Ed 2001;84:F106–10.
48. Chow LC, Wright KW, Sola A, et al. Can changes in clinical practice decrease the incidence of severe retinopathy of prematurity in very low birth weight infants? Pediatrics 2003;111:339–45.
49. VanderVeen DK, Mansfield TA, Eichenwald EC. Lower oxygen saturation alarm limits decrease the severity of retinopathy of prematurity. J AAPOS 2006;10:445–8.
50. Anderson CG, Benitz WE, Madan A. Retinopathy of prematurity and pulse oximetry: a national survey of recent practices. J Perinatol 2004;24:164–8.
51. Tin W, Wariyar U. Giving small babies oxygen: 50 years of uncertainty. Semin Neonatol 2002;7:361–7.
52. Silverman WA. A cautionary tale about supplemental oxygen: the albatross of neonatal medicine. Pediatrics 2004;113:394–6.
53. Cole CH, Wright KW, Tarnow-Mordi W, et al. Resolving our uncertainty about oxygen therapy. Pediatrics 2003;112:1415–9.
54. Stenson B, Brocklehurst P, Tarnow-Mordi W. Increased 36-week survival with high oxygen saturation target in extremely preterm infants. N Engl J Med 2011;364: 1680–2.
55. Vaucher YE, Peralta-Carcelen M, Finer NN, et al. Neurodevelopmental outcomes in the early CPAP and pulse oximetry trial. N Engl J Med 2012;367:2495–504.
56. Schmidt B, Whyte RK, Asztalos EV, et al. Effects of targeting higher vs lower arterial oxygen saturations on death or disability in extremely preterm infants: a randomized clinical trial. JAMA 2013;309:2111–20.
57. Darlow BA, Marschner S, Donoghoe M, et al. Randomized controlled trial of oxygen saturation targets in very preterm infants: two year outcomes. J Pediatr 2014;165:30–5.
58. SUPPORT Study Group of the Eunice Kennedy Shriver NICHD Neonatal Research Network, Carlo WA, Finer NN, et al. Target ranges of oxygen saturation in extremely preterm infants. N Engl J Med 2010;362:1959–69.
59. Fleck BW, Stenson BJ. Retinopathy of prematurity and the oxygen conundrum: lessons learned from recent randomized trials. Clin Perinatol 2013;40:229–40.
60. Modi N. Ethical pitfalls in neonatal comparative effectiveness trials. Neonatology 2014;105:350–1.

61. The BOOST II UK, Australia and New Zealand Collaborative Groups, Stenson BJ, Tarnow-Mordi WO, et al. Oxygen saturation and outcomes in preterm infants. N Engl J Med 2013;368:2094–104.

62. Saugstad OD, Aune D. Optimal oxygenation of extremely low birth weight infants: a meta-analysis and systematic review of the oxygen saturation target studies. Neonatology 2014;105:55–63.

63. Stenson B, Brocklehurst P, Cairns P, et al. Follow-up outcomes from the BOOST-II UK trial of oxygen saturation targeting in preterm infants. Arch Dis Child 2014; 99(Suppl 2):A23.

64. Askie L, Darlow BA, Davis PG, et al. Effects of targeting higher versus lower arterial oxygen saturations on death or disability in preterm infants (Protocol). Cochrane Database Syst Rev 2014;(7):CD011190.

65. Rich W, Finer NN, Gantz MG, et al. Enrolment of extremely low birth weight infants in a clinical research study may not be representative. Pediatrics 2012;129: 480–4.

66. Di Fiore JM, Walsh M, Wrage L, et al. Low oxygen saturation target range is associated with increased incidence of intermittent hypoxemia. J Pediatr 2012;161: 1047–52.

67. Rosychuk RJ, Hudson-Mason A, Eklund D, et al. Discrepancies between arterial oxygen saturation and functional oxygen saturation measured with pulse oximetry in very preterm infants. Neonatology 2012;101:14–9.

68. Quine D, Stenson BJ. Arterial oxygen tension (Pao_2) values in infants <29 weeks of gestation at currently targeted saturations. Arch Dis Child Fetal Neonatal Ed 2009;94:F51–3.

69. Bancalari E, Claure N. Oxygen targets and outcomes in premature infants. JAMA 2013;309:2161–2.

70. Polin RA, Bateman D. Oxygen-saturation targets in preterm infants. N Engl J Med 2013;368:2141–2.

71. Sweet DG, Carnielli V, Greisen G, et al. European consensus guidelines on the management of neonatal respiratory distress syndrome in preterm infants— 2013 update. Neonatology 2013;103:353–68.

72. Sola A, Golombek SG, Montes Bueno MT, et al. Safe oxygen saturation targeting and monitoring in preterm infants: can we avoid hypoxia and hyperoxia? Acta Paediatr 2014;103:1009–18.

73. Hagadorn JI, Furey AM, Nghiem T-H, et al. Achieved versus intended pulse oxygen saturation in infants less than 28 weeks gestation: the AVIOx study. Pediatrics 2006;118:1574–82.

74. Lim K, Wheeler KI, Gale TJ, et al. Oxygen saturation targeting in preterm infants receiving continuous positive airway pressure. J Pediatr 2014;164:730–6.

75. Sink DK, Hope SA, Hagadorn JL. Nurse: patient ratio and achievement of oxygen saturation goals in premature infants. Arch Dis Child Fetal Neonatal Ed 2011;96: F93–8.

76. Nghiem TH, Hagadorn JI, Terrin N, et al. Nurse opinions and pulse oximeter saturation target limits for preterm infants. Pediatrics 2008;121:e1039–46.

77. Armbruster J, Schmidt B, Poets CF, et al. Nurses' compliance with alarm limits for pulse oximetry: qualitative study. J Perinatol 2010;30:531–4.

78. Billett AL, Colletti RB, Mandel KE, et al. Exemplar pediatric collaborative improvement networks: achieving results. Pediatrics 2013;131(Suppl 4):S196–203.

79. Stevens TP, Finer NN, Carlo WA, et al. Respiratory outcomes of the surfactant positive pressure and oximetry randomized trial (SUPPORT). J Pediatr 2014; 165:240–9.

80. Bancalari E, Claure N. Control of oxygenation during mechanical ventilation in the premature infant. Clin Perinatol 2012;39:563–72.
81. Hummler H, Fuchs H, Schmid M. Automated adjustments of inspired fraction of oxygen to avoid hypoxemia and hyperoxemia in neonates - a systematic review on clinical studies. Klin Padiatr 2014;226:204–10.
82. Waitz M, Schmid MB, Fuchs H, et al. Effects of automated adjustment of the inspired oxygen on fluctuations of arterial and regional cerebral tissue oxygenation in preterm infants with frequent desaturations. J Pediatr 2015;166:401–6.e1.
83. Hallenberger A, Poets CF, Horn W, et al. Closed-loop automatic oxygen control (CLAC) in preterm infants: a randomized controlled trial. Paediatrics 2014;133: e379–85.
84. Rüdiger M, Töpfer K, Hammer H, et al. A survey of transcutaneous blood gas monitoring among European neonatal intensive care units. BMC Pediatr 2005; 5:30.
85. Quine D, Stenson B. Does the monitoring method influence stability of oxygenation in preterm infants?. A randomised crossover study of saturation versus transcutaneous monitoring. Arch Dis Child Fetal Neonatal Ed 2008;93:F347–50.
86. Poets CF, Bassler D. Providing stability in oxygenation for preterm infants: is transcutaneous oxygen monitoring really better than pulse oximetry? Arch Dis Child Fetal Neonatal Ed 2008;93:F330–1.
87. Pellicer A, Bravo Mdel C. Near-infrared spectroscopy: a methodology-focused review. Semin Fetal Neonatal Med 2011;16:42–9.
88. Walsh MC, Wilson-Costello D, Zadell A, et al. Safety, reliability, and validity of a physiologic definition of a bronchopulmonary dysplasia. J Perinatol 2003;23: 451–6.
89. Jobe A, Bancalari E. NICHD/NHLBI/ORD workshop summary—bronchopulmonary dysplasia. Am J Respir Crit Care Med 2001;163:1723–9.
90. Quine D, Wong CM, Boyle EM, et al. Non-invasive measurement of reduced ventilation: perfusion ratio and shunt in infants with bronchopulmonary dysplasia: a physiological definition of the disease. Arch Dis Child Fetal Neonatal Ed 2006; 91:F409–14.

Hypoxic Episodes in Bronchopulmonary Dysplasia

Richard J. Martin, MD[a],*, Juliann M. Di Fiore, BSEE[b],
Michele C. Walsh, MD, MSEpi[a]

KEYWORDS

- Neonatal respiratory control • Apnea of prematurity
- Desaturation episodes in preterm infants

KEY POINTS

- Intermittent hypoxic episodes frequently accompany bronchopulmonary dysplasia (BPD).
- Immature respiratory control superimposed on abnormal pulmonary function is a major contributor to intermittent hypoxia in BPD.
- Pulmonary hypertension may aggravate predisposition to intermittent hypoxia.

INTRODUCTION

Hypoxic episodes remain a major source of frustration for care providers of preterm infants in the neonatal intensive care unit. Although optimizing oxygen saturation remains a challenge, the newest generation of pulse oximeters has enabled us to document the incidence of episodic desaturation in this population. These episodes persist beyond the first weeks and even months of postnatal life and, therefore, are temporally related to the development of bronchopulmonary dysplasia (BPD) in a high proportion of extremely low birth weight infants. Unfortunately, there are limited data on how development of BPD modifies respiratory control, airway function, and the pulmonary vascular contribution to hypoxic episodes during postnatal maturation. Although the primary etiology of intermittent hypoxic episodes in preterm infants is immature respiratory control,[1] abnormal lung function present in developing BPD clearly aggravates vulnerability to desaturation.

Disclosure Statement: The authors have nothing to disclose.
R.J. Martin is supported by NIH [NHLBI] 56470 and NIH [NICHD] 78528.
[a] Division of Neonatology, Department of Pediatrics, Rainbow Babies & Children's Hospital, Case Western Reserve University School of Medicine, 11100 Euclid Avenue, Suite RBC 3100, Cleveland, OH 44106-6010, USA; [b] Division of Neonatology, Department of Pediatrics, Rainbow Babies & Children's Hospital, Case Western Reserve University, 11100 Euclid Avenue, Suite RBC 3100, Cleveland, OH 44106-6010, USA
* Corresponding author.
E-mail address: rxm6@case.edu

ROLE OF IMMATURE RESPIRATORY CONTROL IN BRONCHOPULMONARY DYSPLASIA

The multiple contributors to apnea of prematurity and resultant desaturation are summarized in **Fig. 1**. They comprise upregulation of brainstem-mediated inhibitory pathways, altered peripheral chemosensitivity, decreased central chemosensitivity, enhanced inhibition from upper airway afferents, and an unstable upper airway.[2] Apnea is clearly more likely to elicit desaturation with the low functional residual capacity (and other abnormalities of lung function) that characterizes BPD (see **Fig. 1**).

Data from Animal Models

Large animal models of BPD have proven to be a challenge and very expensive owing to the need for longer term survival. Studies have, therefore, focused primarily on hyperoxia-exposed neonatal rodents who exhibit lung injury somewhat analogous to the BPD seen in preterm infants. Unfortunately, few studies have focused on vulnerability of respiratory control in the face of neonatal lung injury in such a model. Ratner and associates[3,4] have demonstrated that intermittent hypoxia (IH; to which infants with BPD are clearly predisposed) superimposed open hyperoxic lung injury aggravates both alveolar arrest and neurologic handicap in neonatal mice. More recent studies in neonatal rats have documented that an early period of sustained postnatal hypoxia followed by subsequent chronic IH causes a markedly attenuated ventilator response to acute hypoxic exposure.[5] The conditions precipitating this vulnerability of respiratory control may be analogous to the oxygenation status of preterm infants exposed to low baseline levels of oxygen, as described elsewhere in this article.

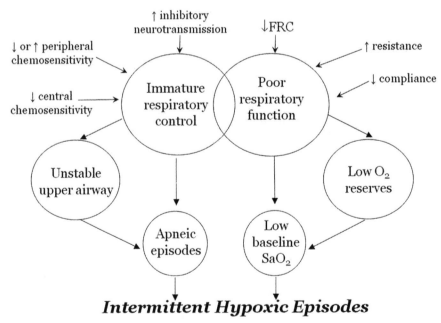

Fig. 1. Multiple factors contribute to both immature respiratory control and poor respiratory function, are potentially aggravated by bronchopulmonary dysplasia, and enhance vulnerability for development of intermittent hypoxic episodes. ↑, increased; ↓, decreased; FRC, functional residual capacity; SaO_2, oxygen saturation.

Inflammation and oxidant stress are both interrelated components of the pulmonary and central nervous system morbidities to which preterm infants are predisposed, especially those with BPD. Available data support the concept that inflammatory mechanisms contribute to instability of neonatal respiratory control. Clinically, apnea increases in frequency and severity during acute infections in premature infants. Although inflammatory cytokines probably do not readily cross the blood–brain barrier, systemic infection does upregulate inflammatory cytokines at the blood–brain barrier, resulting in activation of prostaglandin signaling and consequent inhibition of respiratory neural output.[6] Chorioamnionitis is a major precipitant of preterm birth definitively associated with neonatal brain injury in the form of periventricular leukomalacia and probably BPD. It is possible that antenatal or postnatal exposure of the lung to a proinflammatory stimulus may activate brain circuits via vagally mediated processes. Lipopolysaccharide (LPS; 0.1 mg/kg) instilled into the trachea of newborn rat pups at day of life 10 to 12 increases inflammatory cytokine gene expression in the medulla oblongata and attenuates both the immediate and late hypoxic ventilator response when animals were tested within 3 hours of LPS treatment[7] (**Fig. 2**). This brainstem response to intrapulmonary LPS was diminished after vagotomy, suggesting a lung-to-brainstem communication via vagal afferents. It is, therefore, tempting to speculate that the intrapulmonary inflammation that is an integral part of BPD contributes to impaired respiratory control. It is of interest that caffeine, which is used to prevent BPD, seems to be associated with improved lung function and decreased proinflammatory cytokine expression in rat pups exposed to LPS-induced amnionitis.[8]

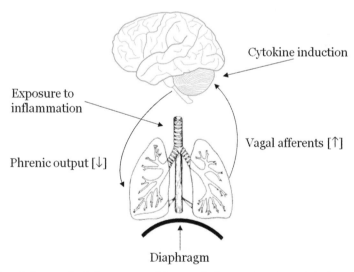

Fig. 2. Prenatal or postnatal exposure of the respiratory system to endotoxin may elicit a proinflammatory cytokine response in the brainstem via stimulation of vagal afferents. This, in turn, may inhibit respiratory neural output. Such vulnerability of respiratory control is likely aggravated by the inflammatory processes that are associated with bronchopulmonary dysplasia. ↑, increased; ↓, decreased. (*Adapted from* Balan KV, KC P, Mayer CA, et al. Intrapulmonary lipopolysaccharide exposure upregulates cytokine expression in the neonatal brainstem. Acta Paediatr 2012;101:467.)

Data from Human Infants

The transition from fetal to neonatal life is accompanied by a dramatic increase in Pao_2 from around 25 to at least 80 torr within 5 to 10 minutes of birth. This postnatal onset of continuous breathing is probably primarily the result of arousal and thermal, rather than chemical, stimuli. The abrupt increase in Pao_2 is widely believed to inhibit O_2-sensitive peripheral chemoreceptors in the early postnatal period. Although CO_2 is the major chemical driver of breathing, ventilatory responses to hypoxia have been extensively studied and well-characterized in human infants and newborn animal models.[9] A transient increase in ventilation in response to hypoxia of 1 to 2 minutes' duration, and mediated via oxygen-sensitive peripheral chemoreceptors, is followed by a decline in ventilation that may even decrease below baseline ventilation, and is presumably centrally mediated. This pattern persists in preterm infants into the second postnatal month.[10]

Although absent peripheral chemosensitivity may inhibit breathing, upregulated peripheral chemoreceptors may also destabilize breathing (**Fig. 3**). Two studies of human preterm infants have shown a direct relationship between apnea frequency and increased peripheral chemosensitivity to hypoxia.[11,12] The mechanisms underlying this relationship are unclear, although if baseline $Paco_2$ and the CO_2 threshold for apnea are close, fluctuations in ventilation associated with increased oxygen-sensitive peripheral chemosensitivity may readily decrease $Paco_2$ to below the apnea threshold.[13]

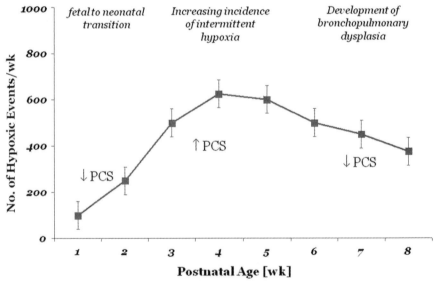

Fig. 3. Proposed relationship between O_2-sensitive peripheral chemosensitivity (PCS) and the natural history of intermittent hypoxia (IH) in a cohort of preterm infants studied over the first 8 weeks of life. The fetal to neonatal transition is associated with decreased PCS and a low incidence of IH. Subsequently, there is an increased incidence of IH associated with increased PCS, and later maturation is accompanied by a declining incidence of IH and decreased PCS in the presence of bronchopulmonary dysplasia. (*Data from* Di Fiore JM, Bloom JN, Orge F, et al. A higher incidence of intermittent hypoxemic episodes is associated with severe retinopathy of prematurity. J Pediatr 2010;157:69–73; and *Adapted from* Nurse CA, Gonzalez C, Peers C, et al, editors. Advances in experimental medicine and biology. Netherlands: Springer; 2012. p. 351–8; with permission.)

Two groups of investigators have studied peripheral chemosensitivity in preterm infants of advanced postnatal age who have developed BPD or chronic neonatal lung disease.[14,15] Such infants with BPD may be exposed to a combination of acute or more chronic hypoxia, although these may coexist. In both studies, BPD was associated with decreased peripheral chemosensitivity, possibly associated with a declining rate of IH episodes (see **Fig. 3**). From these studies it would seem that increased peripheral chemosensitivity may predispose to respiratory pauses and decreased peripheral chemosensitivity may delay recovery from apnea-induced hypoxia episodes. The latter observation in infants with BPD, that is, delayed recovery from hypoxia, may contribute to the reported association between BPD and sudden infant death syndrome.[16]

CONSEQUENCES OF INTERMITTENT HYPOXIC EPISODES

Many diseases of the neonatal period, including BPD, retinopathy of prematurity (ROP), necrotizing enterocolitis, and periventricular leukomalacia, are related to free radical damage, although the specific contribution of oxidative stress has yet to be elucidated. In rodents, intermittent hypoxemia has been shown to elicit an oxidative stress response that occurs during the reoxygenation period.[17] This may, in turn, serve as a proinflammatory stimulus creating a vicious cycle as proposed in **Fig. 4**. In the preterm infant, the incidence of IH during the first few months of life changes dramatically with increasing postnatal age. During the first week of life, there are relatively few IH events, followed by an increase over weeks 2 to 4 with a subsequent plateau or decrease thereafter[18] (see **Fig. 3**). As a result of these alterations in oxygenation, the preterm infant may be exposed to increasing levels of reactive oxygen species during early postnatal life. Consequently, the effect of oxidative stress on morbidity and how to reduce this exposure continues to be of great interest to neonatal care.

Neonatal intermittent hypoxemic exposure may disrupt maturation of the central nervous system at a critical time of development, resulting in neurodevelopmental sequelae. In rodents, IH exposure during the first weeks of life inhibits myelin formation in the corpus callosum[19] and evokes hyperlocomotive behavior and impaired working

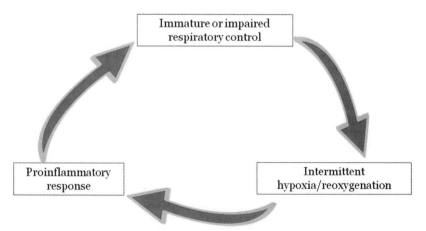

Fig. 4. Proposed vicious cycle whereby immature respiratory control precipitates recurrent intermittent hypoxia/reoxygenation that, in turn, serves as a proinflammatory stimulus and further depresses respiratory neural output.

memory.[20] Although direct effects of IH on neurodevelopmental impairment have yet to be determined in infants, related evidence, including prematurity, caffeine exposure, and apnea reporting, suggest a relationship. Former preterm infants exhibit increased deficits in cognitive ability and academic achievement at 8 to 10 years of age.[21] The risk factor of prematurity may be a marker of the high incidence of cardiorespiratory events during early postnatal maturation. Caffeine therapy for apnea of prematurity decreased the rate of cerebral palsy and cognitive delay at 18 months of age,[22] although the effect of caffeine was no longer significant at the 5-year assessment.[23] There was, however, a decrease in developmental coordination disorder in the caffeine-treated group.[24] Although apnea was not documented in the Schmidt trials, caffeine has been shown to be effective for reducing both apnea[25] and intermittent hypoxemia.[26] Apnea of prematurity during hospitalization, as recorded by nursing staff, has been associated with both abnormal neurodevelopment at 3 years of age[27] and early school age outcomes.[28] However, it is well-known that nursing documentation grossly underestimates the number of cardiorespiratory events. More extensive documentation by home memory monitoring in the Collaborative Home Infant Monitoring Evaluation (CHIME) study demonstrate an association between 5 or more cardiorespiratory events during the first few months of life and poor motor outcome at 7 years of age.[29] Because intermittent hypoxemia and bradycardia are considered the detrimental components of apnea of prematurity, these studies suggest a relationship between oxygenation and brain injury.

Pediatric sleep-disordered breathing is an increasingly recognized disorder associated with behavioral morbidity. Former preterm infants have a higher prevalence of sleep disordered breathing[30] at 8 to 10 years of age, which may be a manifestation of respiratory remodeling during early maturation. In rodents, early postnatal IH exposure is associated with a higher spontaneous apnea frequency during recovery in room air, enhanced acute ventilatory response to hypoxia,[31] and increased carotid body excitation.[32] Similarly, in preterm infants apnea frequency is correlated positively with the ventilatory response to acute hypoxic exposure.[11] These findings suggest that IH exposure may increase markedly carotid body excitation resulting in destabilization of respiration.

Although the optimal oxygen saturation target remains unknown, oxygen saturation levels of greater than 95% are generally avoided in infants requiring supplemental oxygen. To assess whether oxygen supplementation can be further decreased without detrimental consequences, recent collaborative multicenter trials randomized more than 5000 extremely preterm infants to a low (85%–89%) versus high (91%–95%) oxygen saturation target to compare the effect of oxygen saturation targeting on the rate of death or ROP. The outcomes varied among the multinational trials with the Surfactant, Positive Pressure, and Pulse Oximetry Randomization Trial (SUPPORT)[33] and Benefits of Oxygen Saturation Targeting (BOOST II) Trial[34] finding a lower incidence of severe ROP but an unexpected increase in mortality in the low target group. In a subcohort of infants enrolled in SUPPORT, the low target was also associated with an increase in IH events.[35] During the trials, the investigators were met with the underappreciated challenge of keeping the infants within the randomized target range, resulting in numerous fluctuations in oxygen saturation and the actual achieved median oxygen saturation quite often outside of the expected target range. Therefore, both actual achieved baseline oxygen saturation levels and intermittent hypoxemia may have played a role on the increase in mortality, but their potential contribution has yet to be determined.

Trials in both animal and infant models indicate that the development of ROP may be based on the pattern and timing of intermittent hypoxemia events. ROP is triggered by multiple factors, including levels of oxygenation encompassing two phases of development. The first phase includes hyperoxia-induced suppression of normal retinal vascularization predominantly by inhibition of vascular endothelial growth factor. The second phase comprises retinal vascular overproliferation via hypoxia-induced increases in vascular endothelial growth factor and other growth factors.[36] Rodent models have shown that various derivations of IH/hyperoxia cycling can also cause neovascularization[37,38] with clustered, compared with equally dispersed, IH over the same period, yielding increased abnormal vascular morphology.[38] Similar findings have been seen in neonates with distinct patterns and timing of IH associated with severe ROP requiring laser therapy, including a higher incidence of IH, longer duration and short time period (1–20 minutes) between IH events.[39] Interestingly, the time period between IH events reported by Di Fiore and colleagues[39] corresponds with the reactive oxygen species response during the reoxygenation period described in rodents.[17]

Intermittent hypoxemia events have implications on growth trajectory and cardiovascular control. In rodent models, IH exposure during early postnatal life restricts both body[40] and brain growth[19]; however, these effects were reversed after a few weeks of recovery. IH effects on cardiovascular control are more complex and longer lasting. Changes in arterial blood pressure depend on the timing of the IH events with a clustered pattern associated with lower blood pressure than equaling dispersed events[40] with no recovery in either IH paradigm after 7 weeks of exposure. Interestingly, there is an association between extreme prematurity, increased blood pressure in adolescence, and functional vascular changes, although it is speculative whether intermittent hypoxic episodes in early life might be contributory.[41]

ROLE OF THE IMMATURE AIRWAY

Hypoxic episodes in infants with BPD are often attributed to airway closure either during assisted ventilation or spontaneous breathing. The exact pathophysiologic etiology of such events and the underlying biologic mechanisms may be difficult to elucidate. The 2 likely candidates are airway collapse or bronchospasm (**Fig. 5**).

The high compliance and resultant deformability of the trachea in the preterm period seems to be a consequence of decreased airway smooth muscle contractility and diminished cartilaginous support.[42] The obvious result is that lower airways are vulnerable to the injurious effects of positive pressure ventilation. A greater understanding of the detrimental effects of positive pressure ventilation at high inflating pressures has decreased the risk of deformation injury in the immature airway. Lung parenchymal injury is a well-recognized complication of neonatal intensive care and is characterized by the development of enlarged, simplified alveolar structures in infants with BPD. This may result in decreased tethering of intraparenchymal airways and the accompanying decrease in airway lumen would increase baseline airway resistance.[43] A related observation is that lung parenchymal injury elicited by hyperoxic exposure is associated with fewer bronchiolar–alveolar attachments in a rodent model of neonatal lung injury.[44] A resultant increase in baseline lung resistance would likely enhance vulnerability to hypoxic episodes.

Data in rat pups indicate that enhancement of airway reactivity occurs even after short-term mechanical ventilation.[45] In newborn animal models, hyperoxic exposure has also been associated with development of airway hyperreactivity.[46] Although hyperoxic exposure may increase smooth muscle area, this effect is variable and does not, in itself, explain the development of hyperoxia-induced airway hyperresponsiveness, suggesting a functional component for increased airway reactivity.[47]

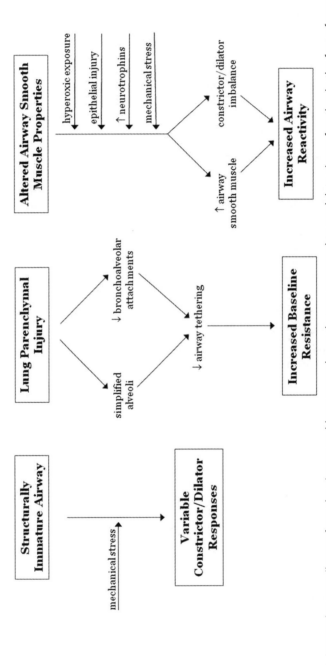

Fig. 5. Interacting contributors from the airways and lung parenchyma that are proposed to modulate airway function in the face of neonatal lung injury, and contribute to airway-related hypoxic episodes. ↑, increased; ↓, decreased. (*Adapted from* Martin RJ. Regulation of lower airway function. Chapter 67. In: Polin, Abman, Bentiz, et al, editors. Fetal and neonatal physiology. 5th edition. Philadelphia: Elsevier (Saunders), in press.)

Many factors may contribute to the increased airway reactivity that is seen after neonatal hyperoxic exposure. Studies have focused on neonatal rodent models exposed to only moderate (eg, 40%–60%) hyperoxic exposure because this more closely simulates the clinical condition. Recent data demonstrate that 40% oxygen exposure elicited a greater increase in airway reactivity than 70% oxygen exposure, associated with greater airway smooth muscle thickness.[48] This might be attributed to a dominant proliferative effect of 40% oxygen on airway smooth muscle versus a predominantly apoptotic effect at the high oxygen level.[49,50] Epithelial injury with loss of airway relaxant factors may also contribute to the hyperoxia-induced increase in airway contractile responses.

It is often difficult to identify specific precipitants of apparent bronchospasm with resultant hypoxia in infants with BPD. Afferent fibers from the upper or lower airway, which precipitate apnea as a protective reflex, may also induce bronchospasm. Earlier studies in infants with BPD have documented a significant increase in lung resistance induced by an abrupt decrease in inspired oxygen.[51] Conversely, exposure to supplemental oxygen in infants with BPD and increased baseline resistance caused relief of bronchoconstriction.[52] Studies in newborn dogs have demonstrated that hypercapnia is more likely than hypoxia to elicit bronchoconstriction.[53] They, therefore, speculated that central chemoreceptors are more effective than peripheral chemoreceptors in altering contractile airway smooth muscle responses. These data support the concept that respiratory depression with superimposed chronic lung disease and resultant hypoxia/hyperoxia may contribute to bronchospasm and establish a vicious cycle of impaired gas exchange. Susceptibility to airway closure may be further aggravated by the increased work of breathing and resultant asynchrony of chest wall movements in infants with BPD.[54,55] Such asynchrony of chest wall motion is aggravated in the supine position. McEvoy and colleagues have[56] documented that prone positioning decreases hypoxic episodes in infants with BPD, although this must be weighed against avoidance of that position before discharge.

ROLE OF PULMONARY VASOCONSTRICTION

The contribution of pulmonary vasoconstriction to hypoxic spells in BPD has been recognized from the earliest descriptions of the disease. Vascular remodeling with intimal hyperplasia leads to abnormal vasoreactivity, as evidenced by the marked vasoconstrictor response seen in even modest episodes of hypoxia.[57,58] Infants with BPD who were assessed at cardiac catheterization were found to have marked increases in pulmonary arterial pressure in response to mild hypoxia, regardless of the severity of BPD.[59] Thus, maintaining normoxic conditions, as measured by oxygen saturation of 92% to 94%, is the mainstay of therapy. However, Lakshminrusimha and associates[60] found that exposure to both brief (30 minutes) or prolonged (24 hours) of 100% oxygen increased pulmonary artery reactivity. Subsequent work demonstrated that this effect was mediated by depletion of antioxidant enzymes.[61] Thus, neonatologists must guard against hyperoxia while avoiding hypoxia.

A second mechanism of vascular impairment has been recognized more recently. Very preterm infants with BPD may have decreased angiogenesis, and this may be a contributing factor to the development of pulmonary hypertension. Reduced vascular growth limits the vascular surface area, and further increases pulmonary vascular resistance, especially when cardiac output is increased, such as with exercise or stress. In animal models, Abman's group has demonstrated in a series of elegant experiments that impaired angiogenesis can lead to impaired alveolarization.[62–66] Thus, a primary contributor to the development of BPD is abnormal vascular

Table 1
Approach to intermittent hypoxic episodes

Clinical Presentation/Etiology	Diagnostic Approach and Therapy
Apneic/bradycardic episodes (spontaneous breathing)	CPAP ± caffeine
Bradycardic episodes (intubated)	Consider extubation Caffeine and CPAP
Pulmonary hypertension	Confirm via echocardiogram Consider iNO
Bronchospasm	Poor air entry Consider bronchodilator

Abbreviations: CPAP, continuous positive airway pressure; iNO, inducible nitrous oxide.

development. Mourani and colleagues[67] prospectively studied 277 preterm infants with echocardiograms at 7 days of age and correlated evidence of pulmonary hypertension with the severity of BPD at 36 weeks postmenstrual age. Infants who ultimately had severe BPD were more likely to have early pulmonary hypertension on the 7-day echo. These findings suggest that early pulmonary vascular disease contributes to the susceptibility for BPD.

Hypoxic episodes are significant challenges in the shorter and longer term management of former preterm infants. Because the etiology may be multifactorial, including immature respiratory control and both airway and vascular related etiologies, an integrated approach to understanding the Pathobiology of these events is essential in this high risk population.

SUMMARY

There is currently no "quick fix" for eliminating the recurrent hypoxic episodes that occur so frequently in infants who are developing, or have established, BPD. **Table 1** summarizes potential etiologies and approaches that may prove effective, although it is important to recognize that recurrent hypoxic episodes may have multifactorial overlapping etiologies in this high-risk population.

REFERENCES

1. Martin RJ, Di Fiore JM, MacFarlane PM, et al. Physiologic basis for intermittent hypoxic episodes in preterm infants. In: Nurse CA, Gonzalez C, Peers C, et al, editors. Arterial chemoreception: from molecules to systems. Dordrecht (The Netherlands): Springer-Science+Business Media; 2012. p. 351–8.
2. Di Fiore JM, Martin RJ, Gauda EB. Apnea of prematurity - perfect storm. Respir Physiol Neurobiol 2013;189:213–22.
3. Ratner V, Kishkurno SV, Slinko SK, et al. The contribution of intermittent hypoxemia to late neurological handicap in mice with hyperoxia-induced lung injury. Neonatology 2007;92:50–8.
4. Ratner V, Slinko S, Sosunova IU, et al. Hypoxic stress exacerbates hyperoxia-induced lung injury in a neonatal mouse model of bronchopulmonary dysplasia. Neonatology 2009;95:299–305.
5. Mayer CA, Ao J, Di Fiore JM, et al. Impaired hypoxic ventilator response following neonatal sustained and subsequent chronic intermittent hypoxia in rats. Respir Physiol Neurobiol 2013;187:167–75.

6. Hofstetter AO, Saha S, Siljehav V, et al. The induced prostaglandin E2 pathway is a key regulator of the respiratory response to infection and hypoxia in neonates. Proc Natl Acad Sci U S A 2007;104:9894–9.
7. Balan KV, Kc P, Hoxha Z, et al. Vagal afferents modulate cytokine-mediated respiratory control at the neonatal medulla oblongata. Respir Physiol Neurobiol 2011;178:458–64.
8. Köroğlu OA, MacFarlane PM, Balan KV, et al. Anti-inflammatory effect of caffeine is associated with improved lung function after lipopolysaccharide-induced amnionitis. Neonatology 2014;106:235–40.
9. Rigatto H, Brady JP. Periodic breathing and apnea in preterm infants I. Evidence for hypoventilation possibly due to central respiratory depression. Pediatrics 1972;50:202–18.
10. Martin RJ, Di Fiore JM, Jana L, et al. Persistence of the biphasic ventilator response to hypoxia in preterm infants. J Pediatr 1998;132:960–4.
11. Nock ML, Di Fiore JM, Arko MK, et al. Relationship of the ventilatory response to hypoxia with neonatal apnea in preterm infants. J Pediatr 2004;144:291–5.
12. Cardot V, Chardon K, Tourneux P, et al. Ventilatory response to a hyperoxic test is related to the frequency of short apneic episodes in late preterm neonates. Pediatr Res 2007;62:591–6.
13. Al-Matary A, Kutbi I, Qurashi M, et al. Increased peripheral chemoreceptor activity may be critical in destabilizing breathing in neonates. Semin Perinatol 2004; 28:264–72.
14. Katz-Salamon M, Jonsson B, Lagercrantz H. Blunted peripheral chemoreceptor response to hyperoxia in a group of infants with bronchopulmonary dysplasia. Pediatr Pulmonol 1995;20:101–6.
15. Calder NA, Williams BA, Smyth J, et al. Absence of ventilator responses to alternating breaths of mild hypoxia and air in neonates who have had bronchopulmonary dysplasia: implications for the risk of sudden infant death. Pediatr Res 1994; 35:677–81.
16. Werthammer J, Brown ER, Neff RK, et al. Sudden infant death syndrome in infants with bronchopulmonary dysplasia. Pediatrics 1982;69:301–4.
17. Fabian RH, Perez-Polo JR, Kent TA. Extracellular superoxide concentration increases following cerebral hypoxia but does not affect cerebral blood flow. Int J Dev Neurosci 2004;22:225–30.
18. Di Fiore JM, Bloom JN, Orge F, et al. A higher incidence of intermittent hypoxemic episodes is associated with severe retinopathy of prematurity. J Pediatr 2010; 157:69–73.
19. Kanaan A, Farahani R, Douglas RM, et al. Effect of chronic continuous or intermittent hypoxia and reoxygenation on cerebral capillary density and myelination. Am J Physiol Regul Integr Comp Physiol 2006;290:R1105–14.
20. Decker MJ, Hue GE, Caudle WM, et al. Episodic neonatal hypoxia evokes executive dysfunction and regionally specific alterations in markers of dopamine signaling. Neuroscience 2003;117:417–25.
21. Emancipator JL, Storfer-Isser A, Taylor HG, et al. Variation of cognition and achievement with sleep-disordered breathing in full-term and preterm children. Arch Pediatr Adolesc Med 2006;160:203–10.
22. Schmidt B, Roberts RS, Davis P, et al. Long-term effects of caffeine therapy for apnea of prematurity. N Engl J Med 2007;357:1893–902.
23. Schmidt B, Anderson PJ, Doyle LW, et al. Survival without disability to age 5 years after neonatal caffeine therapy for apnea of prematurity. JAMA 2012;307: 275–82.

24. Doyle LW, Schmidt B, Anderson PJ, et al. Reduction in developmental coordination disorder with neonatal caffeine therapy. J Pediatr 2014;165:356–9.
25. Erenberg A, Leff RD, Haack DG, et al. Caffeine citrate for the treatment of apnea of prematurity: a double-blind, placebo-controlled study. Pharmacotherapy 2000; 20:644–52.
26. Rhein LM, Dobson NR, Darnall RA, et al. Effects of caffeine on intermittent hypoxia in infants born prematurely: a randomized clinical trial. JAMA Pediatr 2014;168:250–7.
27. Janvier A, Khairy M, Kokkotis A, et al. Apnea is associated with neurodevelopmental impairment in very low birth weight infants. J Perinatol 2004;24:763–8.
28. Taylor HG, Klein N, Schatschneider C, et al. Predictors of early school age outcomes in very low birth weight children. J Dev Behav Pediatr 1998;19:235–43.
29. Hunt CE, Corwin MJ, Baird T, et al. Cardiorespiratory events detected by home memory monitoring and one-year neurodevelopmental outcome. J Pediatr 2004;145:465–71.
30. Rosen CL, Larkin EK, Kirchner HL, et al. Prevalence and risk factors for sleep-disordered breathing in 8- to 11-year-old children: association with race and prematurity. J Pediatr 2003;142:383–9.
31. Julien C, Bairam A, Joseph V. Chronic intermittent hypoxia reduces ventilatory long-term facilitation and enhances apnea frequency in newborn rats. Am J Physiol Regul Integr Comp Physiol 2008;294:R1356–66.
32. Pawar A, Peng YJ, Jacono FJ, et al. Comparative analysis of neonatal and adult rat carotid body responses to chronic intermittent hypoxia. J Appl Physiol (1985) 2008;104:1287–94.
33. Carlo WA, Finer NN, Walsh MC, et al. Target ranges of oxygen saturation in extremely preterm infants. N Engl J Med 2010;362:1959–69.
34. Stenson B, Brocklehurst P, Tarnow-Mordi W. Increased 36-week survival with high oxygen saturation target in extremely preterm infants. N Engl J Med 2011;364: 1680–2.
35. Di Fiore JM, Walsh M, Wrage L, et al. Low oxygen saturation target range is associated with increased incidence of intermittent hypoxemia. J Pediatr 2012;161: 1047–52.
36. Chen J, Smith LE. Retinopathy of prematurity. Angiogenesis 2007;10:133–40.
37. Barnett JM, Yanni SE, Penn JS. The development of the rat model of retinopathy of prematurity. Doc Ophthalmol 2010;120:3–12.
38. Coleman RJ, Beharry KD, Brock RS, et al. Effects of brief, clustered versus dispersed hypoxic episodes on systemic and ocular growth factors in a rat model of oxygen-induced retinopathy. Pediatr Res 2008;64:50–5.
39. Di Fiore JM, Kaffashi F, Loparo K, et al. The relationship between patterns of intermittent hypoxia and retinopathy of prematurity in preterm infants. Pediatr Res 2012;72:606–12.
40. Pozo ME, Cave A, Köroğlu OA, et al. Effect of postnatal intermittent hypoxia on growth and cardiovascular regulation of rat pups. Neonatology 2012;102: 107–13.
41. Lee H, Dichtl S, Mormanova Z, et al. In adolescence, extreme prematurity is associated with significant changes in the microvasculature, elevated blood pressure and increased carotid intima-media thickness. Arch Dis Child 2014;99:907–11.
42. Panitch HB, Deoras KS, Wolfson MR, et al. Maturational changes in airway smooth muscle structure-function relationships. Pediatr Res 1992;31:151–6.
43. Colin AA, McEvoy C, Castile RG. Respiratory morbidity and lung function in preterm infants of 32 to 36 weeks' gestational age. Pediatrics 2010;126:115–28.

44. O'Reilly M, Harding R, Sozo F. Altered airways in aged mice following neonatal exposure to hyperoxic gas. Neonatology 2014;105:39–45.

45. Iben SC, Haxhiu MA, Farver CF, et al. Short-term mechanical ventilation increases airway reactivity in rat pups. Pediatr Res 2006;60:136–40.

46. Belik J, Jankov RP, Pan J, et al. Chronic O_2 exposure enhances vascular and airway smooth muscle contraction in the newborn but not adult rat. J Appl Physiol (1985) 2003;94:2303–12.

47. Hershenson MB, Wylam ME, Punjabi N, et al. Exposure of immature rats to hyperoxia increases tracheal smooth muscle stress generation in vitro. J Appl Physiol (1985) 1994;76:743–9.

48. Wang H, Jafri A, Martin RJ, et al. Severity of neonatal hyperoxia determines structural and functional changes in developing mouse airway. Am J Physiol Lung Cell Mol Physiol 2014;307:L295–301.

49. Yi M, Masood A, Ziimo A, et al. Inhibition of apoptosis by 60% oxygen: a novel pathway contributing to lung injury in neonatal rats. Am J Physiol Lung Cell Mol Physiol 2011;300:L319–29.

50. Hartman WR, Smelter DF, Sathish V, et al. Oxygen dose responsiveness of human fetal airway smooth muscle cells. Am J Physiol Lung Cell Mol Physiol 2012;303: L711–9.

51. Teague G, Pian MS, Heldt GP, et al. An acute reduction in the fraction of inspired oxygen increases airway constriction in infants with chronic lung disease. Am Rev Respir Dis 1988;137:861–5.

52. Tay-Uyboco JS, Kwiatkowski K, Cates DB, et al. Hypoxic airway constriction in infants of very low birth weight recovering from moderate to severe bronchopulmonary dysplasia. J Pediatr 1989;115:456–9.

53. Waldron MA, Fisher JT. Differential effects of CO_2 and hypoxia on bronchomotor tone in the newborn dog. Respir Physiol 1988;72:271–82.

54. Rome ES, Miller MJ, Goldthwait DA, et al. Effect of sleep state on chest wall movements and gas exchange in infants with resolving bronchopulmonary dysplasia. Pediatr Pulmonol 1987;3:259–63.

55. Allen JL, Greenspan JS, Deoras KS, et al. Interaction between chest wall motion and lung mechanics in normal infants and infants with bronchopulmonary dysplasia. Pediatr Pulmonol 1991;11:37–43.

56. McEvoy C, Mendoza ME, Bowling S, et al. Prone positioning decreases episodes of hypoxemia in extremely low birth weight infants [1000 grams or less] with chronic lung disease. J Pediatr 1997;130:305–9.

57. Halliday HL, Dumpit FM, Brady JP. Effects of inspired oxygen on echocardiographic assessment of pulmonary vascular resistance and myocardial contractility in bronchopulmonary dysplasia. Pediatrics 1980;65:536–40.

58. Abman SH, Wolfe RR, Accurso FJ, et al. Pulmonary vascular response to oxygen in infants with severe bronchopulmonary dysplasia. Pediatrics 1985;75: 80–4.

59. Mourani PM, Ivy DD, Gao D, et al. Pulmonary vascular effects of inhaled nitric oxide and oxygen tension in bronchopulmonary dysplasia. Am J Respir Crit Care Med 2004;170:1006–13.

60. Lakshminrusimha S, Russell JA, Steinhorn RH, et al. Pulmonary arterial contractility in neonatal lambs increases with 100% oxygen resuscitation. Pediatr Res 2006;59:137–41.

61. Patel A, Lakshminrusimha S, Ryan RM, et al. Exposure to supplemental oxygen downregulates antioxidant enzymes and increases pulmonary arterial contractility in premature lambs. Neonatology 2009;96:182–92.

62. Mourani PM, Abman SH. Pulmonary vascular disease in bronchopulmonary dysplasia: physiology, diagnosis, and treatment. In: Bronchopulmonary dysplasia. New York: Informa Healthcare; 2010. p. 347–63.

63. Jakkula M, LeCras TD, Gebb S, et al. Inhibition of angiogenesis decreases alveolarization in the developing rat lung. Am J Physiol Lung Cell Mol Physiol 2000;279: L600–7.

64. Abman SH. Bronchopulmonary dysplasia: "a vascular hypothesis". Am J Respir Crit Care Med 2001;164:1755–6.

65. Bhatt AJ, Pryhuber GS, Huyck H, et al. Disrupted pulmonary vasculature and decreased vascular endothelial growth factor, flt-1, and tie-2 in human infants dying with bronchopulmonary dysplasia. Am J Respir Crit Care Med 2001;164: 1971–80.

66. De Paepe ME, Greco D, Mao Q. Angiogenesis-related gene expression profiling in ventilated preterm human lungs. Exp Lung Res 2010;36:399–410.

67. Mourani PM, Sontag MK, Younoszai A, et al. Early pulmonary vascular disease in preterm infants at risk for bronchopulmonary dysplasia. Am J Respir Crit Care Med 2015;191(1):87–95.

Pulmonary Hypertension and Vascular Abnormalities in Bronchopulmonary Dysplasia

Peter M. Mourani, MD[a],*, Steven H. Abman, MD[b]

KEYWORDS

- Bronchopulmonary dysplasia • Pulmonary vascular disease
- Pulmonary hypertension • Echocardiogram • Inhaled nitric oxide

KEY POINTS

- Pulmonary vascular disease (PVD) and cardiovascular abnormalities are increasingly recognized components of bronchopulmonary dysplasia (BPD) and contribute significantly to morbidity and mortality.
- Complex interactions between antenatal and postnatal factors contribute to impair normal pulmonary vascular signaling pathways, leading to altered growth, structure, and function of the developing pulmonary circulation after preterm birth.
- The impairments of the developing pulmonary vasculature may result in prolonged oxygen requirements, exacerbated effects of anatomic shunt lesions, exercise intolerance, altered pulmonary blood flow distribution in response to acute respiratory infections, and ultimately pulmonary hypertension (PH).
- Several studies using echocardiograms to screen preterm infants have determined the incidence of PH in BPD to be 16% to 25%, but some cardiovascular abnormalities may be missed with echocardiograms and require cardiac catheterization.
- Further studies are needed to determine the risk factors, mechanisms of disease, and long-term outcomes, and to better define the clinical approach and treatment of PVD in BPD.

Funding sources: This work was supported in part by grants from the NHLBI HL085703 (P.M. Mourani and S.H. Abman), HL068702 (S.H. Abman), and U01 HL102235 (S.H. Abman).
Conflicts of interest: The authors have no significant conflicts of interest.
Disclosures: The authors do not have any relationships to disclose.
[a] Section of Pediatric Critical Care, Pediatric Heart Lung Center, Department of Pediatrics, University of Colorado, School of Medicine, 13121 East 17th Avenue, MS8414, Aurora, CO 80045, USA; [b] Section of Pulmonary Medicine, Pediatric Heart Lung Center, Department of Pediatrics, University of Colorado, School of Medicine, Mail Stop B395, 13123 East 16th Avenue, Aurora, CO 80045, USA
* Corresponding author.
E-mail address: peter.mourani@childrenscolorado.org

Clin Perinatol 42 (2015) 839–855
http://dx.doi.org/10.1016/j.clp.2015.08.010
0095-5108/15/$ – see front matter

INTRODUCTION

Bronchopulmonary dysplasia (BPD) is a chronic lung disease that occurs in preterm infants who require mechanical ventilation and oxygen therapy for postnatal respiratory distress.[1] BPD is characterized by persistent pulmonary disease with a prolonged need for supplemental oxygen, recurrent respiratory exacerbations with frequent emergency department visits and hospitalizations,[2,3] exercise intolerance, and associated respiratory problems that can extend into adulthood.[4] Improved respiratory support strategies, antenatal steroids, surfactant therapy, and other advances in clinical care have decreased the risk for death and the development of BPD in larger preterm infants. These strategies have also increased the survival of infants born earlier in gestation who then have high risk to develop BPD. Thus, the incidence of BPD has remained fairly stable over the past decade.[5,6] BPD in this new era most often occurs in infants born at 24 to 28 weeks' postmenstrual age (PMA), weighing less than or equal to 1000 g, who have less severe acute respiratory symptoms and require less respiratory support than patients with BPD in the era when the disease was first described.[7,8]

Maternal, genetic, and environmental factors can lead to early injury of the developing lung that impairs angiogenesis and alveolarization, resulting in simplification of the distal lung airspace and clinical manifestations of BPD. The impairments of the developing pulmonary vasculature may result in significant pulmonary vascular disease (PVD) (**Fig. 1**). In its most severe form, PVD results in pulmonary hypertension (PH).[9–12] The impact of clinically apparent PH in the new BPD era suggests that morbidity[13–17] and late mortality are high, with up to 48% mortality 2 years after diagnosis of PH.[18]

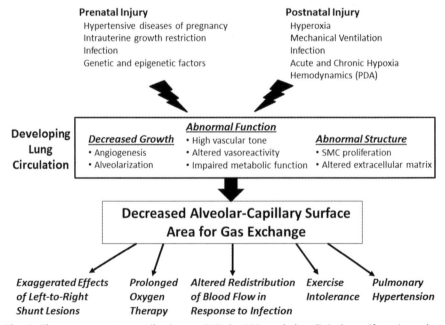

Fig. 1. The components contributing to PVD in BPD and the clinical manifestations that result. PDA, patent ductus arteriosus; SMC, smooth muscle cells.

Prospective studies have shown that PH is common in BPD, affecting 16% to 25% of infants.[15–17] Greater recognition of PH and its impact in this population has led to widespread treatment with pulmonary vasodilator medications. However, there are limited prospective data examining the impact of these medications on pulmonary vascular development as well as the clinical effectiveness of such medications. Thus, there is a need for greater insights into basic mechanisms of BPD and standardized clinical criteria for identifying at-risk infants in order to develop better strategies for the prevention, monitoring, and treatment of preterm newborns. This article discusses recent studies examining the role of the pulmonary circulation in the pathogenesis of BPD and PVD, the epidemiologic studies of PH in BPD, and the rationale for the clinical approach to diagnosis and treatment of PH in BPD.

PATHOGENESIS OF PULMONARY VASCULAR DISEASE IN BRONCHOPULMONARY DYSPLASIA

Pulmonary vascular growth is a dynamic process, beginning in the embryonic period and continuing throughout gestation and during postnatal life. Premature birth exposes the developing lung to an environment that can impair the normal developmental process. On histology, the lungs of preterm infants have revealed reduced numbers of both alveoli and intra-acinar arteries, leading to the description of BPD as an arrest of lung development. The pathogenesis of PVD in BPD is multifactorial, resulting from complex interactions between maternal, genetic, and epigenetic susceptibility, and environmental factors (both prenatal and postnatal), including hyperoxia, hypoxia, hemodynamic stress, infection, and inflammation. Clinical studies strongly suggest that these complex interactions contribute to alterations in normal growth factor expression and signaling pathways, leading to impaired growth, structure, and function of the developing pulmonary circulation after premature birth (see **Fig. 1**).[10,19–27]

Disruption of vascular growth and signaling may contribute to impaired lung structure,[28–32] leading to a marked reduction in alveolar-capillary surface area.[33–35] Abnormal growth of the pulmonary circulation in BPD is characterized by decreased vascular branching, an altered pattern of vascular distribution within the lung interstitium, and persistent intrapulmonary venous anastomoses,[31,36–39] which collectively contribute to the symptoms of BPD.[40] Several recent studies have shown that preeclampsia is a risk factor for BPD and PVD,[41] possibly through disruption of these vascular signaling pathways.[42–45] Intrauterine growth restriction is another condition that has been associated with disruption of vascular signaling[46] and an increased risk for BPD and PH in preterm infants.[47]

The reduction in vessel number resulting from impaired vascular growth coupled with alveolar hypoxia, hyperoxia, or hemodynamic stress may worsen pulmonary arterial structural remodeling in preterm infants. Endothelial injury caused by these environmental stressors[27,48,49] induces the media of small pulmonary arteries to undergo smooth muscle cell proliferation, precocious maturation of immature mesenchymal cells into mature smooth muscle cells, and the incorporation of fibroblasts/myofibroblasts into the vessel wall.[50] Smooth muscle proliferation also extends abnormally into the smaller peripheral arteries.[9] Such pulmonary artery remodeling and disruption of angiogenic factor expression as has been shown in autopsy data from infants dying with BPD[35,51,52] could lead to high pulmonary vascular resistance (PVR) caused by narrowing of the vessel diameter and decreased vascular compliance, especially in response to respiratory infections. Persistent abnormalities of pulmonary vascular growth and/or failure of the lung vasculature to catch up to infants born at term may contribute to PVD that becomes increasing symptomatic later in life.[53,54]

DIAGNOSIS AND EPIDEMIOLOGY OF PULMONARY VASCULAR DISEASE IN PRETERM INFANTS

PH and cor pulmonale, resulting from extreme forms of PVD, are recognized factors associated with high mortality in preterm infants with BPD.[18,55,56] In the past decade, patients with BPD and PH had reported survival rates of 52% 2 years after the diagnosis of PH.[18] The increasing recognition of PVD and its association with poor outcomes in preterm infants born at earlier gestational ages led to renewed interest in determining the incidence of PH in new-era BPD and identifying high-risk infants as early as possible. However, the lack of a data-derived definition of PH in this population and reliable diagnostic assessment measures to diagnose PH has limited study in this area.

Cardiac catheterization remains the gold standard for diagnosis of PH, but its invasive nature has restricted its application to those infants at highest risk. Noninvasive assessment via echocardiography, despite its significant limitations,[14] has become the most often used tool for screening and diagnosis of PH in preterm infants. The most objective measure of PH by echocardiogram is the estimated right ventricular systolic pressure (RVSP) derived from the tricuspid regurgitant jet velocity (TRJV).[57–60] Applied from adult criteria, a threshold of RVSP greater than 35 mm Hg (TRJV >3 m/s) to define PH has been used. Because of low blood pressures in preterm infants, estimated pulmonary pressures greater than 50% of the systemic pressure have also been used to define PH and seem to correlate better with measurements performed during cardiac catheterization.[14,61] Earlier studies of infants with BPD with known or suspected PH revealed a measureable TRJV in only 31% to 61% of these infants.[14–16,62] More recent studies that have screened large groups of preterm infants have found that a measureable TRJV is more rare (6%–10%)[16,17] and was the determining factor to diagnose PH in a very small proportion of infants. Further, the standards for determining the quality of the TRJV used to estimate RVSP and diagnose PH have not been thoroughly reported in some recent studies.[15,16,61,63]

However, the lack of a measureable TRJV does not preclude the presence of PVD or PH. Qualitative echocardiogram findings to diagnose PH, including right atrial enlargement, right ventricular hypertrophy, right ventricular dilatation, pulmonary artery dilatation, and interventricular septal flattening, have correlated with diagnosis of PH by cardiac catheterization. Septal flattening seems to be among the most sensitive of these measures, but is vulnerable to interobserver reliability.

The right ventricular myocardial performance index (MPI; also known as the Tei index) has been used as a surrogate for increased PVR in BPD, and has been shown to remain increased in infants with BPD compared with preterm infants without BPD.[64] Another study showed that respiratory failure requiring mechanical ventilation from multiple causes, including BPD, was associated with significantly increased right ventricular MPI compared with controls,[65] suggesting that MPI may be a surrogate for worse respiratory disease. Further studies are needed to determine whether high right ventricular MPI is associated with BPD and/or PH.

In the past few years, several studies have attempted to determine the incidence of PH among preterm infants using echocardiograms as the screening tool, albeit with slightly different criteria to diagnose PH (**Fig. 2**).[15–17,66] The first of these was a retrospective review at a single center in South Korea identifying 116 preterm infants born at less than 32 weeks' PMA and diagnosed with BPD.[15] Echocardiograms performed

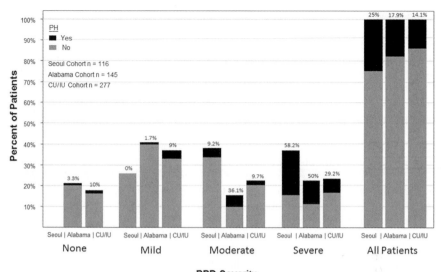

Fig. 2. The incidence of PH according to the degree of BPD severity. Incidence of PH among preterm infants from 3 studies (Seoul,[15] Alabama,[16] and Colorado/Indiana[17]). The percentage of patients listed on the Y axis represents the proportion of patients in each study in whom BPD status was ascertained. Please see text for inclusion criteria of each of the studies. BPD severity was based on National Institutes of Health criteria.[38] Physiologic assessment of oxygenation to determine BPD status[93] was applied in the Alabama and Colorado University/Indiana University (CU/IU) cohorts. The Seoul cohort did not include preterm infants without BPD. Numbers above the bars indicate the percentage of patients with PH.

after 2 months of age at the discretion of the primary caregivers were used to determine PH, but the number and timing of echocardiograms performed were not reported. PH criteria were based on clinical interpretation of echocardiograms and included a TRJV greater than or equal to 3 m/s in the absence of pulmonary stenosis, and/or a flat or left-deviated interventricular septal configuration with right ventricular hypertrophy and chamber dilation. These investigators identified 29 (25%) infants with BPD with PH at a median postnatal age of 65 days, and the diagnosis of PH was significantly correlated with severity of BPD (see **Fig. 2**). All patients diagnosed with PH were reported to have some degree of tricuspid regurgitation (trivial in 27.6%, mild in 44.8%, and moderate in 27.6%), but the proportion meeting the PH threshold was not reported.

The second study was a prospective analysis of preterm infants at the University of Alabama at Birmingham (United States) with birth weight less than 1000 g who survived to 28 days.[16] All patients underwent echocardiogram between 4 and 6 weeks of age and subsequent echocardiograms were performed if severe lung disease or clinical signs suggestive of right-sided heart failure were present. PH was diagnosed if at least 1 of the following findings was present: (1) right ventricular hypertrophy, (2) flattening of interventricular septum, (3) presence of tricuspid regurgitation in the absence of pulmonary stenosis, and (4) increased right ventricular pressures as estimated by Doppler studies of tricuspid regurgitation jet (although the threshold for increased pressure was not provided). Of 145 eligible patients, 9 (6.2%) were identified by the initial echocardiogram. Another 17 (11.7%) infants were diagnosed by subsequent echocardiograms; median age of diagnosis was 112 days. Of the patients

diagnosed with PH, tricuspid regurgitation was identified in 58%, an increased estimated systolic pulmonary pressure in 69%, right ventricular hypertrophy in 42%,
and a flattened interventricular septum in 54%. Fifty-eight percent of infants had
persistent signs of PH at neonatal intensive care unit (NICU) discharge, and 3 patients
died of complications of PH.

The third study was a prospective evaluation at hospitals affiliated with 2 academic
centers in the United States. Two-hundred seventy-seven preterm infants with gestational age at birth less than 34 weeks and birth weights between 500 and 1250 g were
screened with echocardiograms at 7 days of age and 36 weeks PMA.[17] All echocardiograms were interpreted by a single cardiologist, but this study used 3 different a
priori criteria for PH to determine which was most closely associated with outcome.
The most liberal of the criteria were met if subjects had any of the following findings:
an estimated RVSP greater than 40 mm Hg, RVSP/systemic systolic blood pressure
greater than 0.5, any cardiac shunt with bidirectional or right-to-left flow, or any degree of ventricular septal wall flattening were most similar to the 2 studies described
earlier. According to these criteria, the incidence of PH was 14% at 36 weeks' PMA,
with the highest incidence of PH (29%) occurring in infants with severe BPD, but
consistent rate of PH (about 10%) in infants with none, mild, and moderate BPD.
PH diagnosed by these criteria was associated with greater mortality and increased
duration of respiratory support after adjustment for gestational age at birth, BPD status, and other clinical factors. Applying alternate, more strict, criteria for PH dramatically reduced the incidence of PH (3.3% for criteria only using a TRJV-based
threshold or reversal of cardiac shunt, and 4.7% for criteria that included TRJV,
reversal of shunt, or moderate to severe septal flattening).

A fourth prospectively conducted study at the Women & Infants Hospital of Rhode
Island (United States) enrolled 120 infants born at less than 28 weeks' PMA who
underwent echocardiogram screening at 10 to 14 days of age and 36 weeks'
PMA.[66] The study used stricter criteria for PH (estimated systolic pulmonary artery
pressure/systemic systolic artery pressure ratio >0.5 or moderate or severe interventricular septal flattening). Using these criteria, the investigators found an incidence of
PH of 8% at 36 weeks' PMA, which is comparable with the incidence of 4.7% found
by Mourani and colleagues[17] using similar criteria.

Aligning similar criteria for PH, these studies reveal comparable rates of PH in
patients diagnosed with BPD, with most patients with PH having severe BPD. Note
that PH can be identified as a late finding, with 65% of infants with BPD with PH being
diagnosed after having a normal echocardiogram between 4 and 6 weeks of age.[16]
With the exception of the study by Mirza and colleagues,[66] these studies used liberal
criteria for PH, only requiring any evidence of septal flattening, and 1 only requiring the
presence of a tricuspid regurgitant jet without applying a threshold for pressure estimates.[16] However, using liberal criteria for PH, these studies and others have reported
higher death rates and increased morbidities in preterm infants with BPD and PH
compared with those without PH.[15–17,61,63,67] These data suggest that routine
screening of preterm infants near term, especially those with more severe BPD, will
result in identification of a substantial number of infants with PH who are at risk
for increased morbidity and mortality. These data may further provide useful prog-
nostic information for parents and caregivers and may allow the opportunity for early
intervention.

Despite its usefulness for diagnostic screening, echocardiograms still have
limitations that may preclude diagnosis of PH, fail to accurately diagnose the severity
of PH[14] in patients identified by echocardiogram, or fail to identify additional cardiovascular abnormalities that contribute to PH. Thus, we recommend cardiac

catheterization (**Box 1**) for preterm infants (1) with persistent signs of severe cardio-respiratory disease or clinical deterioration not directly explained by other diagnostic evaluations; (2) suspected of having significant PH despite optimal management of their lung disease and associated morbidities; (3) in whom chronic vasodilator therapy is being considered; (4) with unexplained, recurrent pulmonary edema. The goals of cardiac catheterization are to assess the severity of PH, exclude or document the severity of associated anatomic cardiac and vascular lesions that may be amenable to intervention during catheterization, and to assess pulmonary vascular reactivity in patients who fail to respond to oxygen therapy alone.

RISK FACTORS FOR PERIPHERAL VASCULAR DISEASE AND PULMONARY HYPERTENSION IN PRETERM INFANTS

Past clinical studies have suggested that sustained increases of pulmonary artery pressure as assessed by serial echocardiograms may be associated with increased

---

Box 1
Approach to PH in BPD

Screening echocardiograms for:

Severe BPD at 36 weeks

Infants with prolonged ventilator and/or oxygen requirements

Cyanotic episodes

Marked hypercarbia

Persistent pulmonary edema, diuretic dependence

Poor growth, IUGR, oligohydramnios

General evaluation and treatment of factors contributing to persistent respiratory disease and PH

Ensure adequate oxygenation (awake, asleep, feeds)

Assess the adequacy of ventilation

Chronic aspiration (barium swallow, swallowing study, pH probe, impedance study)

Structural airway disease: malacia, subglottic stenosis

Optimal treatment of reactive airways disease

Neurologic abnormalities: hydrocephalus

Ensure optimal nutrition

Consider cardiac catheterization when work-up fails to reveal a clear cause for poor clinical status or when optimal management of these factors fails to achieve clinical improvement

Assess severity of PH

Anatomic heart disease/shunt lesions

Structural vascular abnormalities (eg, arterial stenosis, pulmonary venous obstruction, systemic-to-pulmonary collateral vessels, others)

Catheter-based interventions

Assess cardiac function (LV diastolic dysfunction)

Acute vasoreactivity/hypoxia testing for selection of chronic therapy

Abbreviations: IUGR, intrauterine growth restriction; LV, left ventricular.

risk for BPD,[64,68] supporting the hypothesis that PH in premature newborns may be an early clinical marker for predicting BPD. Early echocardiographic signs of PVD in preterm infants have now been associated with increased risk for both BPD and late PH as well as with prolonged oxygen treatment.[17,66] Sustained evidence of increased right ventricular pressure through the first week after birth may reflect early pulmonary vascular injury that increases risk for BPD. Whether these changes are secondary to delayed transition to extrauterine life, injury caused by excessive hemodynamic stress from patent ductus arteriosus (PDA), or other shunts as has been previously reported,[69–71] or other forms of vascular injury remains to be determined. Understanding the drivers behind these early vascular changes will be crucial to developing novel intervention strategies to prevent both BPD and PH in these infants.

In addition to early hemodynamic indicators of PVD, clinical factors associated with late PH in most studies include lower gestational age, birth weight, and longer periods of respiratory support. PDA,[15] infection,[15] oligohydramnios,[63] small for gestational age,[16,47] and low-birth-weight z score[17] have also been identified as risk factors for PH in infants born preterm. Further examination of clinical factors associated with PH, including prenatal risks, along with translational investigations and rigorous screening of infants will help elucidate how these clinical factors impair normal pulmonary vascular development and lead to BPD and PVD.

OTHER PULMONARY VASCULAR AND CARDIAC ABNORMALITIES ASSOCIATED WITH BRONCHOPULMONARY DYSPLASIA

Although PH is an extreme form of PVD in preterm infants, other cardiac and pulmonary vascular abnormalities may contribute to increased PVR and exacerbate PH in these infants (**Table 1**). Several of these abnormalities may be detected by echocardiogram and others may require alternate imaging such computed tomography (CT), MRI, and/or cardiac catheterization to detect. Echocardiographic assessment of anatomic cardiac disease, especially shunt lesions, is an important aspect of cardiovascular evaluation of infants with BPD. Excessive left-to-right flow through cardiac-level shunts can lead to pulmonary artery remodeling and increased PVR. However, the degree of shunt flow cannot always be accurately estimated by echocardiogram and may require cardiac catheterization to quantify the degree of shunt. Other pulmonary vascular abnormalities, such as systemic-to-pulmonary collaterals or pulmonary venous stenosis, can occasionally be detected with echocardiogram, but often require cardiac catheterization to identify. However, these abnormalities may be amenable to treatment intervention during the catheterization, such as coiling or balloon dilation, respectively.[72] Impaired cardiac function may result from PH (right-sided dysfunction) or may contribute to it (left-sided dysfunction). Preterm birth has

Table 1
Factors contributing to increased PVR in PH

PVD	Cardiac Disease	Lung Disease
High tone and reactivity	RV dysfunction	Hypoxemia
Hypertensive vascular remodeling	Impaired LV contractility	Hyperinflation
Decreased vascular growth	LV diastolic dysfunction	Atelectasis
Systemic-to-pulmonary collateral vessels	Left-to right shunt lesions	Hypercarbia
Pulmonary vein stenosis	—	—

Abbreviations: LV, left ventricular; RV, right ventricular.

been associated with alterations in right ventricular structure and reduced function in young adults, suggesting that the heart in addition to the vasculature may be susceptible to perinatal events.[73] Decreased shortening fraction, left ventricular ejection fraction, or signs of left ventricular hypertrophy may be signs of left ventricular dysfunction, which may require catheterization for confirmation.[14,74,75] Diastolic function may also lead to increased PVR, but is difficult to ascertain by echocardiogram, and often requires catheterization for diagnosis as well.[74] In one study, the combined modality of CT scans (21 patients) and catheterizations (14 patients) identified cardiovascular anomalies in 19 of 29 infants with BPD with PH, including systemic-to-pulmonary collaterals (n = 9), pulmonary vein stenosis (n = 7), atrial septal defects (n = 5), and PDA (n = 9).[76] MRI of the chest may provide an additional modality for evaluating pulmonary vascular function and hemodynamics. Phase-contrast flow measurements via MRI could estimate pulmonary artery velocities and pulmonary arterial pressure. These techniques have been applied in other forms of PH, detecting changes of PVD before symptoms.[77–81]

BPD lung disease can also increase PVR, exacerbating PVD and contributing to PH. Air trapping and hyperinflation from airways disease can overstretch small pulmonary arteries, increasing PVR. In contrast, atelectasis constrains pulmonary vessels, also increasing PVR. Acute episodes of hypoxia and hypercarbia can induce pulmonary artery vasoconstriction, especially within remodeled/dysmorphic vessels.

TREATMENT OF PULMONARY HYPERTENSION IN BRONCHOPULMONARY DYSPLASIA

Despite recent evidence that PH is more common in preterm infants than previously thought and is associated with increased morbidity and mortality, proven strategies to improve outcomes are lacking. Several studies have shown improvement in the severity of PH with various strategies,[13,15,82] but controlled trials of PH treatment in BPD have not been performed. As pointed out earlier, animal and clinical data suggest that contributions from impaired pulmonary vascular development, cardiac abnormalities and dysfunction, and parenchymal lung disease all contribute to increased PVR and PH in preterm infants with BPD and may contribute to evolving PVD over time. Therefore, targeted strategies to optimize these areas form the approach to PH therapy in infants with BPD (see **Box 1**; **Fig. 3**).

Because a higher rate of PH has been found in patients with more severe lung disease, it seems reasonable to aggressively target factors contributing to lung disease, including episodes of hypoxia, ventilatory insufficiency, bronchoconstriction, chronic reflux and aspiration, and upper and lower airway obstruction.[40] Immunoprophylaxis against respiratory infections, including respiratory syncytial virus, is also an important strategy.

The goal to wean infants with severe BPD from respiratory support in preparation for discharge from the NICU should be carefully weighed against the risks for intermittent hypoxia and hypercarbia, which can trigger vasoconstriction and further vascular remodeling. Assessments of oxygenation during feeding and sleep should be performed before weaning infants completely from supplemental oxygen. Targeting oxygen saturations to 92% to 95% should be sufficient to prevent the adverse effects of hypoxia in most infants without increasing the risk of additional lung injury or other systemic effects of hyperoxia. Chronic mechanical ventilation support should be considered for infants who are failing to wean from noninvasive positive pressure support or for infants with frequent episodes of hypoxia and/or impaired ventilation or with inadequate growth velocity despite supplemental oxygen.

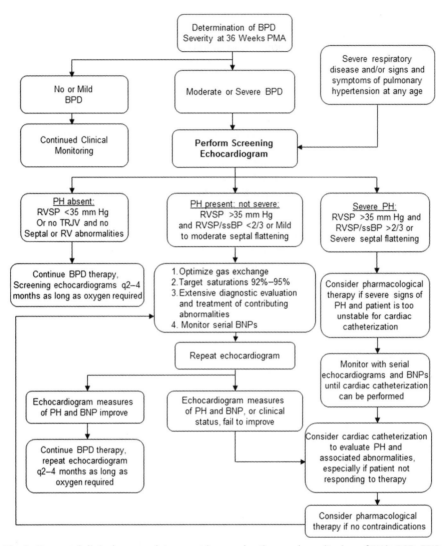

Fig. 3. Proposed clinical approach to screening, evaluation, and monitoring of PH in BPD. BNP, brain natriuretic protein; q, every; RV, right ventricle; ssBP, systemic systolic blood pressure. (*Adapted from* Mourani PM, Abman SH. Pulmonary vascular disease in bronchopulmonary dysplasia: physiology, diagnosis, and treatment. In: Abman SH, editor. Bronchopulmonary dysplasia. New York: Informa Healthcare; 2010. p. 347–63; with permission.)

As noted earlier, identifying or ruling out anatomic cardiovascular abnormalities (see **Table 1**) that contribute to increased PVR and PH and could benefit from specific targeted interventions is important before considering chronic vasodilator therapy because vasodilators could result in adverse clinical effects in the presence of these lesions. Although the use of vasodilators targeted at pulmonary arterial structural remodeling and vasoreactivity is a rational approach, none of the medications approved for adult use are approved for children in the United States. Given the complex maturational influences related to lung vascular development in preterm infants,[83,84] special consideration should be given to the use of these medications in infants and children relative to adults (see **Fig. 3**). In addition, the use of systemic vasodilators (delivered via the bloodstream) may worsen ventilation/perfusion mismatch and oxygenation in infants with BPD.

Inhaled nitric oxide (iNO) is approved for treatment of persistent PH of the newborn and is the drug with the most safety data available in preterm infants, having been used in several clinical trials for the prevention of BPD.[85–87] Although the studies performed to date do not justify routine use of iNO for BPD, prolonged iNO therapy for PH may be considered for hospitalized infants who are ventilated or are receiving nasal cannula therapy.[88,89] In such patients, dose-response studies performed during cardiac catheterization may help to optimize the level of iNO therapy. The acute hemodynamic response to iNO in patients with BPD and PH has been shown to be greater than the response to calcium channel blockers,[90] with doses as low as 2 ppm showing improvements in pulmonary pressure. iNO is easiest to deliver via mechanical ventilation and available data suggest that it can be safely administered for prolonged periods. If PH improves in response to iNO, it can gradually be weaned off over days to weeks with careful monitoring before discontinuation of mechanical ventilation. For infants in whom iNO fails to improve PH sufficiently as the sole agent, or for those whose clinical setting and needs (on extubation from mechanical ventilation) may benefit from alternate vasodilator therapy because of limitations with iNO administration, a second-line agent such as sildenafil may be added.

Sildenafil, a selective type 5 phosphodiesterase inhibitor, is approved by the US Food and Drug Administration (FDA) for the treatment of PH in adults, but has had a large appeal for use in infants and children because of the ease of administration compared with other PH medications. It has been used extensively off label for the treatment of PH in BPD based on several case reports and a couple of retrospective studies suggesting safety with potential efficacy.[13,82] A recent pilot trial of sildenafil did not improve short-term respiratory outcomes (development of BPD) of extremely preterm infants, but further studies are warranted to determine whether treatment could mitigate development of severe PVD. In 2012, the FDA issued a recommendation against the use of sildenafil in children aged 1 to 17 years (http://www.fda.gov/Safety/MedWatch/SafetyInformation/SafetyAlertsforHumanMedicalProducts/ucm317743.htm). The decision was based on reports of increasing mortality with increasing sildenafil doses in a long-term clinical trial in pediatric patients with PH secondary to idiopathic pulmonary arterial hypertension and congenital heart disease.[91] In 2014, the FDA issued a clarification of the statement (http://www.fda.gov/Safety/MedWatch/SafetyInformation/SafetyAlertsforHumanMedicalProducts/ucm391152.htm) stating there may be situations in which the benefit-risk profile of sildenafil may be acceptable in individual children in whom treatment options are limited and close monitoring can be provided. Thus, careful consideration and extreme caution should be exercised when contemplating sildenafil treatment of infants and children. Other vasodilators, including prostacyclin analogues, endothelin receptor antagonists, and soluble guanylate cyclase modulators, could be considered for use in infants with BPD with PH, but there are limited data available for the effectiveness and safety of these medications for this population.

At present, there is limited evidence on how long to continue these therapies if initiated. Often, many infants are discharged from the NICU on these medications and followed up by pediatric pulmonologists, cardiologists, or centers focusing on PH. If PH gradually resolves with lung growth as expected, the medications may either be gradually tapered off, or the infant allowed to outgrow the dose before discontinuation of the drugs one by one (usually the most invasive or least effective medication is weaned off first).

Infants with BPD treated with PH medication require close monitoring of pulmonary and hemodynamic status. Objective assessments of oxygenation should be performed when weaning infants from oxygen therapy or when infants develop respiratory infection. Serial echocardiograms, which should be obtained at least every 2 to 4 weeks with the acute initiation of therapy and at 4-month to 6-month intervals with stable disease, are recommended. Brain natriuretic peptide may augment monitoring,[92] but evidence does not support its use in the absence of echocardiography and other monitoring modalities. Acute worsening of PH or failure to respond to therapy may reflect several factors, including late pulmonary vascular anatomic abnormalities. Repeat diagnostic procedures, including cardiac catheterization, may be indicated for these patients (see **Fig. 3**). We recommend weaning medications with serial normal or near-normal echocardiogram findings over weeks with careful monitoring of pulmonary function and growth velocities.

SUMMARY

PVD in preterm infants with BPD is characterized by altered lung vascular development, growth, structure, or function, which precedes the onset of measureable PH. PVD caused by disruption of normal pulmonary vascular development in association with preterm birth is an important determinant of the pathobiology of BPD and contributes significantly to morbidity and mortality. Exposure to adverse stimuli during the antenatal and/or early postnatal periods impairs normal pulmonary vascular development and creates and imbalance between risk and resiliency factors. Recent studies have revealed the magnitude of PH in preterm infants, but many aspects of PVD remain understudied, and ongoing investigations continue to explore risk factors, mechanisms of disease, and long-term outcomes. Prospective studies are needed to definitively establish standardized clinical criteria for PVD and PH in BPD, and to determine the best methods for early diagnosis, risk stratification, and disease monitoring. Larger collaborative studies and improved clinical infrastructure to conduct these important investigations will provide answers to these critical questions.

REFERENCES

1. Northway WH Jr, Rosan RC, Porter DY. Pulmonary disease following respirator therapy of hyaline-membrane disease. Bronchopulmonary dysplasia. N Engl J Med 1967;276(7):357–68.
2. Furman L, Baley J, Borawski-Clark E, et al. Hospitalization as a measure of morbidity among very low birth weight infants with chronic lung disease. J Pediatr 1996; 128(4):447–52.
3. Smith VC, Zupancic JA, McCormick MC, et al. Rehospitalization in the first year of life among infants with bronchopulmonary dysplasia. J Pediatr 2004;144(6): 799–803.
4. Baraldi E, Filippone M. Chronic lung disease after premature birth. N Engl J Med 2007;357(19):1946–55.
5. Smith VC, Zupancic JA, McCormick MC, et al. Trends in severe bronchopulmonary dysplasia rates between 1994 and 2002. J Pediatr 2005;146(4):469–73.
6. Stoll BJ, Hansen NI, Bell EF, et al. Neonatal outcomes of extremely preterm infants from the NICHD Neonatal Research Network. Pediatrics 2010;126(3):443–56.
7. Bancalari E, Gonzalez A. Clinical course and lung function abnormalities during development of neonatal chronic lung disease. In: Bland R, Coalson J, editors.

Chronic lung disease in early infancy. New York: Marcel Dekker; 2000. p. 41–64.

8. Charafeddine L, D'Angio CT, Phelps DL. Atypical chronic lung disease patterns in neonates. Pediatrics 1999;103(4 Pt 1):759–65.

9. Hislop AA, Haworth SG. Pulmonary vascular damage and the development of cor pulmonale following hyaline membrane disease. Pediatr Pulmonol 1990;9(3): 152–61.

10. Abman SH. Bronchopulmonary dysplasia: "a vascular hypothesis". Am J Respir Crit Care Med 2001;164(10 Pt 1):1755–6.

11. Abman SH. The dysmorphic pulmonary circulation in bronchopulmonary dysplasia: a growing story. Am J Respir Crit Care Med 2008;178(2):114–5.

12. Jobe AH. An unknown: lung growth and development after very preterm birth. Am J Respir Crit Care Med 2002;166(12):1529–30.

13. Mourani PM, Sontag MK, Ivy DD, et al. Effects of long-term sildenafil treatment for pulmonary hypertension in infants with chronic lung disease. J Pediatr 2009; 154(3):379–84, 384.e1–2.

14. Mourani PM, Sontag MK, Younoszai A, et al. Clinical utility of echocardiography for the diagnosis and management of pulmonary vascular disease in young children with chronic lung disease. Pediatrics 2008;121(2):317–25.

15. An HS, Bae EJ, Kim GB, et al. Pulmonary hypertension in preterm infants with bronchopulmonary dysplasia. Korean Circ J 2010;40(3):131–6.

16. Bhat R, Salas AA, Foster C, et al. Prospective analysis of pulmonary hypertension in extremely low birth weight infants. Pediatrics 2012;129(3):e682–9.

17. Mourani PM, Sontag MK, Younoszai A, et al. Early pulmonary vascular disease in preterm infants at risk for bronchopulmonary dysplasia. Am J Respir Crit Care Med 2015;191(1):87–95.

18. Khemani E, McElhinney DB, Rhein L, et al. Pulmonary artery hypertension in formerly premature infants with bronchopulmonary dysplasia: clinical features and outcomes in the surfactant era. Pediatrics 2007;120(6):1260–9.

19. Lassus P, Turanlahti M, Heikkila P, et al. Pulmonary vascular endothelial growth factor and Flt-1 in fetuses, in acute and chronic lung disease, and in persistent pulmonary hypertension of the newborn. Am J Respir Crit Care Med 2001; 164(10 Pt 1):1981–7.

20. D'Angio CT, Maniscalco WM. The role of vascular growth factors in hyperoxia-induced injury to the developing lung. Front Biosci 2002;7:d1609–23.

21. Kumar VH, Ryan RM. Growth factors in the fetal and neonatal lung. Front Biosci 2004;9:464–80.

22. Thebaud B, Abman SH. Bronchopulmonary dysplasia: where have all the vessels gone? Roles of angiogenic growth factors in chronic lung disease. Am J Respir Crit Care Med 2007;175(10):978–85.

23. Maniscalco WM, Watkins RH, Pryhuber GS, et al. Angiogenic factors and alveolar vasculature: development and alterations by injury in very premature baboons. Am J Physiol Lung Cell Mol Physiol 2002;282(4):L811–23.

24. Bhandari V, Bizzarro MJ, Shetty A, et al. Familial and genetic susceptibility to major neonatal morbidities in preterm twins. Pediatrics 2006;117(6):1901–6.

25. Bhandari V, Gruen JR. The genetics of bronchopulmonary dysplasia. Semin Perinatol 2006;30(4):185–91.

26. Abman SH. Impaired vascular endothelial growth factor signaling in the pathogenesis of neonatal pulmonary vascular disease. Adv Exp Med Biol 2010;661:323–35.

27. Cornfield DN. Developmental regulation of oxygen sensing and ion channels in the pulmonary vasculature. Adv Exp Med Biol 2010;661:201–20.

28. Jakkula M, Le Cras TD, Gebb S, et al. Inhibition of angiogenesis decreases alveolarization in the developing rat lung. Am J Physiol Lung Cell Mol Physiol 2000; 279(3):L600–7.

29. Thebaud B, Ladha F, Michelakis ED, et al. Vascular endothelial growth factor gene therapy increases survival, promotes lung angiogenesis, and prevents alveolar damage in hyperoxia-induced lung injury: evidence that angiogenesis participates in alveolarization. Circulation 2005;112(16):2477–86.

30. Galambos C, Ng YS, Ali A, et al. Defective pulmonary development in the absence of heparin-binding vascular endothelial growth factor isoforms. Am J Respir Cell Mol Biol 2002;27(2):194–203.

31. De Paepe ME, Mao Q, Powell J, et al. Growth of pulmonary microvasculature in ventilated preterm infants. Am J Respir Crit Care Med 2006;173(2):204–11.

32. Janer J, Andersson S, Kajantie E, et al. Endostatin concentration in cord plasma predicts the development of bronchopulmonary dysplasia in very low birth weight infants. Pediatrics 2009;123(4):1142–6.

33. Mitchell SH, Teague WG. Reduced gas transfer at rest and during exercise in school-age survivors of bronchopulmonary dysplasia. Am J Respir Crit Care Med 1998;157(5 Pt 1):1406–12.

34. Hakulinen AL, Jarvenpaa AL, Turpeinen M, et al. Diffusing capacity of the lung in school-aged children born very preterm, with and without bronchopulmonary dysplasia. Pediatr Pulmonol 1996;21(6):353–60.

35. Allen J, Zwerdling R, Ehrenkranz R, et al. Statement on the care of the child with chronic lung disease of infancy and childhood. Am J Respir Crit Care Med 2003; 168(3):356–96.

36. Coalson J. Pathology of new bronchopulmonary dysplasia. Semin Neonatol 2003; 8(1):73–81.

37. Husain AN, Siddiqui NH, Stocker JT. Pathology of arrested acinar development in postsurfactant bronchopulmonary dysplasia. Hum Pathol 1998;29(7):710–7.

38. Jobe AH, Bancalari E. Bronchopulmonary dysplasia. Am J Respir Crit Care Med 2001;163(7):1723–9.

39. Galambos C, Sims-Lucas S, Abman SH. Histologic evidence of intrapulmonary anastomoses by three-dimensional reconstruction in severe bronchopulmonary dysplasia. Ann Am Thorac Soc 2013;10(5):474–81.

40. Mourani PM, Abman SH. Pulmonary vascular disease in bronchopulmonary dysplasia: physiology, diagnosis, and treatment. In: Abman SH, editor. Bronchopulmonary dysplasia. New York: Informa Healthcare; 2010. p. 347–63.

41. Hansen AR, Barnes CM, Folkman J, et al. Maternal preeclampsia predicts the development of bronchopulmonary dysplasia. J Pediatr 2010;156(4):532–6.

42. Foidart JM, Schaaps JP, Chantraine F, et al. Dysregulation of anti-angiogenic agents (sFlt-1, PLGF, and sEndoglin) in preeclampsia–a step forward but not the definitive answer. J Reprod Immunol 2009;82(2):106–11.

43. Lapaire O, Shennan A, Stepan H. The preeclampsia biomarkers soluble fms-like tyrosine kinase-1 and placental growth factor: current knowledge, clinical implications and future application. Eur J Obstet Gynecol Reprod Biol 2010;151(2):122–9.

44. Tang JR, Karumanchi SA, Seedorf G, et al. Excess soluble vascular endothelial growth factor receptor-1 in amniotic fluid impairs lung growth in rats: linking preeclampsia with bronchopulmonary dysplasia. Am J Physiol Lung Cell Mol Physiol 2012;302(1):L36–46.

45. Li F, Hagaman JR, Kim HS, et al. eNOS deficiency acts through endothelin to aggravate sFlt-1-induced pre-eclampsia-like phenotype. J Am Soc Nephrol 2012;23(4):652–60.

46. Rozance PJ, Seedorf GJ, Brown A, et al. Intrauterine growth restriction decreases pulmonary alveolar and vessel growth and causes pulmonary artery endothelial cell dysfunction in vitro in fetal sheep. Am J Physiol Lung Cell Mol Physiol 2011;301(6):L860–71.

47. Check J, Gotteiner N, Liu X, et al. Fetal growth restriction and pulmonary hypertension in premature infants with bronchopulmonary dysplasia. J Perinatol 2013; 33(7):553–7.

48. Roberts RJ, Weesner KM, Bucher JR. Oxygen-induced alterations in lung vascular development in the newborn rat. Pediatr Res 1983;17(5):368–75.

49. Nozik-Grayck E, Stenmark KR. Role of reactive oxygen species in chronic hypoxia-induced pulmonary hypertension and vascular remodeling. Adv Exp Med Biol 2007;618:101–12.

50. Jones R, Zapol WM, Reid L. Pulmonary artery remodeling and pulmonary hypertension after exposure to hyperoxia for 7 days. A morphometric and hemodynamic study. Am J Pathol 1984;117(2):273–85.

51. Bhatt AJ, Pryhuber GS, Huyck H, et al. Disrupted pulmonary vasculature and decreased vascular endothelial growth factor, Flt-1, and TIE-2 in human infants dying with bronchopulmonary dysplasia. Am J Respir Crit Care Med 2001; 164(10 Pt 1):1971–80.

52. De Paepe ME, Greco D, Mao Q. Angiogenesis-related gene expression profiling in ventilated preterm human lungs. Exp Lung Res 2010;36(7):399–410.

53. Yee M, White RJ, Awad HA, et al. Neonatal hyperoxia causes pulmonary vascular disease and shortens life span in aging mice. Am J Pathol 2011;178(6):2601–10.

54. Wong PM, Lees AN, Louw J, et al. Emphysema in young adult survivors of moderate-to-severe bronchopulmonary dysplasia. Eur Respir J 2008;32(2):321–8.

55. Walther FJ, Benders MJ, Leighton JO. Persistent pulmonary hypertension in premature neonates with severe respiratory distress syndrome. Pediatrics 1992; 90(6):899–904.

56. Fouron JC, Le Guennec JC, Villemant D, et al. Value of echocardiography in assessing the outcome of bronchopulmonary dysplasia of the newborn. Pediatrics 1980;65(3):529–35.

57. Yock PG, Popp RL. Noninvasive estimation of right ventricular systolic pressure by Doppler ultrasound in patients with tricuspid regurgitation. Circulation 1984; 70(4):657–62.

58. Berger M, Haimowitz A, Van Tosh A, et al. Quantitative assessment of pulmonary hypertension in patients with tricuspid regurgitation using continuous wave Doppler ultrasound. J Am Coll Cardiol 1985;6(2):359–65.

59. Currie PJ, Seward JB, Chan KL, et al. Continuous wave Doppler determination of right ventricular pressure: a simultaneous Doppler-catheterization study in 127 patients. J Am Coll Cardiol 1985;6(4):750–6.

60. Skjaerpe T, Hatle L. Noninvasive estimation of systolic pressure in the right ventricle in patients with tricuspid regurgitation. Eur Heart J 1986;7(8):704–10.

61. Slaughter JL, Pakrashi T, Jones DE, et al. Echocardiographic detection of pulmonary hypertension in extremely low birth weight infants with bronchopulmonary dysplasia requiring prolonged positive pressure ventilation. J Perinatol 2011;31(10):635–40.

62. Benatar A, Clarke J, Silverman M. Pulmonary hypertension in infants with chronic lung disease: non-invasive evaluation and short term effect of oxygen treatment. Arch Dis Child Fetal Neonatal Ed 1995;72(1):F14–9.

63. Kim DH, Kim HS, Choi CW, et al. Risk factors for pulmonary artery hypertension in preterm infants with moderate or severe bronchopulmonary dysplasia. Neonatology 2012;101(1):40–6.

64. Czernik C, Rhode S, Metze B, et al. Persistently elevated right ventricular index of myocardial performance in preterm infants with incipient bronchopulmonary dysplasia. PLoS One 2012;7(6):e38352.
65. Kobr J, Fremuth J, Pizingerova K, et al. Repeated bedside echocardiography in children with respiratory failure. Cardiovasc Ultrasound 2011;9:14.
66. Mirza H, Ziegler J, Ford S, et al. Pulmonary hypertension in preterm infants: prevalence and association with bronchopulmonary dysplasia. J Pediatr 2014;165(5): 909–14.e1.
67. Stuart BD, Sekar P, Coulson JD, et al. Health-care utilization and respiratory morbidities in preterm infants with pulmonary hypertension. J Perinatol 2013;33(7): 543–7.
68. Skinner JR, Boys RJ, Hunter S, et al. Pulmonary and systemic arterial pressure in hyaline membrane disease. Arch Dis Child 1992;67(4 Spec No):366–73.
69. Brown ER, Stark A, Sosenko I, et al. Bronchopulmonary dysplasia: possible relationship to pulmonary edema. J Pediatr 1978;92(6):982–4.
70. Rojas MA, Gonzalez A, Bancalari E, et al. Changing trends in the epidemiology and pathogenesis of neonatal chronic lung disease. J Pediatr 1995;126(4): 605–10.
71. Gonzalez A, Sosenko IR, Chandar J, et al. Influence of infection on patent ductus arteriosus and chronic lung disease in premature infants weighing 1000 grams or less. J Pediatr 1996;128(4):470–8.
72. Drossner DM, Kim DW, Maher KO, et al. Pulmonary vein stenosis: prematurity and associated conditions. Pediatrics 2008;122(3):e656–661.
73. Lewandowski AJ, Bradlow WM, Augustine D, et al. Right ventricular systolic dysfunction in young adults born preterm. Circulation 2013;128(7):713–20.
74. Mourani PM, Ivy DD, Rosenberg AA, et al. Left ventricular diastolic dysfunction in bronchopulmonary dysplasia. J Pediatr 2008;152(2):291–3.
75. Yates AR, Welty SE, Gest AL, et al. Myocardial tissue Doppler changes in patients with bronchopulmonary dysplasia. J Pediatr 2008;152(6):766–70, 770.e1.
76. Del Cerro MJ, Sabate Rotes A, Carton A, et al. Pulmonary hypertension in bronchopulmonary dysplasia: clinical findings, cardiovascular anomalies and outcomes. Pediatr Pulmonol 2014;49(1):49–59.
77. Vonk-Noordegraaf A, van Wolferen SA, Marcus JT, et al. Noninvasive assessment and monitoring of the pulmonary circulation. Eur Respir J 2005;25(4):758–66.
78. Ley S, Mereles D, Risse F, et al. Quantitative 3D pulmonary MR-perfusion in patients with pulmonary arterial hypertension: correlation with invasive pressure measurements. Eur J Radiol 2007;61(2):251–5.
79. Okajima Y, Ohno Y, Washko GR, et al. Assessment of pulmonary hypertension what CT and MRI can provide. Acad Radiol 2011;18(4):437–53.
80. Skrok J, Shehata ML, Mathai S, et al. Pulmonary arterial hypertension: MR imaging-derived first-pass bolus kinetic parameters are biomarkers for pulmonary hemodynamics, cardiac function, and ventricular remodeling. Radiology 2012; 263(3):678–87.
81. Ley S, Mereles D, Puderbach M, et al. Value of MR phase-contrast flow measurements for functional assessment of pulmonary arterial hypertension. Eur Radiol 2007;17(7):1892–7.
82. Nyp M, Sandritter T, Poppinga N, et al. Sildenafil citrate, bronchopulmonary dysplasia and disordered pulmonary gas exchange: any benefits? J Perinatol 2012;32(1):64–9.
83. Robbins IM, Moore TM, Blaisdell CJ, et al. Improving outcomes for pulmonary vascular disease. Am J Respir Crit Care Med 2012;185(9):1015–20.

84. Abman SH, Kinsella JP, Rosenzweig EB, et al. Implications of the FDA warning against the use of sildenafil for the treatment of pediatric pulmonary hypertension. Am J Respir Crit Care Med 2012;187(6):572–5.
85. Ballard RA, Truog WE, Cnaan A, et al. Inhaled nitric oxide in preterm infants undergoing mechanical ventilation. N Engl J Med 2006;355(4):343–53.
86. Schreiber MD, Gin-Mestan K, Marks JD, et al. Inhaled nitric oxide in premature infants with the respiratory distress syndrome. N Engl J Med 2003;349(22): 2099–107.
87. Kinsella JP, Cutter GR, Walsh WF, et al. Early inhaled nitric oxide therapy in premature newborns with respiratory failure. N Engl J Med 2006;355(4):354–64.
88. Channick RN, Newhart JW, Johnson FW, et al. Pulsed delivery of inhaled nitric oxide to patients with primary pulmonary hypertension: an ambulatory delivery system and initial clinical tests. Chest 1996;109(6):1545–9.
89. Ivy DD, Parker D, Doran A, et al. Acute hemodynamic effects and home therapy using a novel pulsed nasal nitric oxide delivery system in children and young adults with pulmonary hypertension. Am J Cardiol 2003;92(7):886–90.
90. Mourani PM, Ivy DD, Gao D, et al. Pulmonary vascular effects of inhaled nitric oxide and oxygen tension in bronchopulmonary dysplasia. Am J Respir Crit Care Med 2004;170(9):1006–13.
91. Barst RJ, Ivy DD, Gaitan G, et al. A randomized, double-blind, placebo-controlled, dose-ranging study of oral sildenafil citrate in treatment-naive children with pulmonary arterial hypertension. Circulation 2012;125(2):324–34.
92. Ambalavanan N, Mourani P. Pulmonary hypertension in bronchopulmonary dysplasia. Birth Defects Res A Clin Mol Teratol 2014;100(3):240–6.
93. Walsh MC, Wilson-Costello D, Zadell A, et al. Safety, reliability, and validity of a physiologic definition of bronchopulmonary dysplasia. J Perinatol 2003;23(6): 451–6.

Airway Disease and Management in Bronchopulmonary Dysplasia

Raouf S. Amin, MD[a,b],*, Michael J. Rutter, MBChB, FRACS[c,d]

KEYWORDS

- Subglottic stenosis • Tracheomalacia • Bronchomalacia • Tracheotomy
- Failure to extubate • Bronchopulmonary dysplasia

KEY POINTS

- Early use of continuous positive airway pressure significantly reduces the incidence of extubation failure.
- Early use of continuous positive airway pressure significantly shortens the duration of mechanical ventilation.
- Prolonged intubation in neonates may be tolerated for months, but, if there is no realistic prospect of extubation, tracheotomy should be considered once the infant weighs more than 1500 g.
- The ideal size of an endotracheal tube is the smallest tube that permits adequate ventilation of an infant.
- In an infant who is difficult to intubate, tracheotomy should be considered early if the reason for intubation difficulty is not correctable.

INTRODUCTION

Over the previous 2 decades, increased survival rates of preterm infants have paralleled improvements in prenatal, obstetric, and neonatal care. However, significant morbidity and mortality among extremely preterm infants (ie, gestational age between

Financial disclosures: Dr M.J. Rutter holds a patent for an airway balloon dilator that may eventually be marketed. At present, he has received no income from this device. A suprastomal stent designed by him and bearing his name is also on the market; however, he has declined royalties for this product.

[a] Division of Pulmonary Medicine, Cincinnati Children's Hospital Medical Center, 3333 Burnet Avenue, Cincinnati, OH 45229, USA; [b] Department of Pediatrics, University of Cincinnati College of Medicine, 231 Albert Sabin Way, Cincinnati, OH 45267, USA; [c] Division of Pediatric Otolaryngology–Head and Neck Surgery, Cincinnati Children's Hospital Medical Center, 3333 Burnet Avenue, Cincinnati, OH 45229-3039, USA; [d] Department of Otolaryngology–Head and Neck Surgery, University of Cincinnati College of Medicine, 231 Albert Sabin Way, Cincinnati, OH 45267, USA
* Corresponding author. Division of Pulmonary Medicine, Cincinnati Children's Hospital Medical Center, 3333 Burnet Avenue, Cincinnati, OH 45229.
E-mail address: Raouf.Amin@cchmc.org

22 and 28 weeks) remain high and have reached a plateau. Bronchopulmonary dysplasia (BPD) is the most common cause of pulmonary morbidity in this patient population. Moderate to severe BPD occurs in 41% of all extremely preterm infants, with an incidence ranging from 85% to 23% in those born at 22 and 28 weeks' gestation respectively. Almost all (93%) of these infants develop respiratory distress and 62% require either conventional or high-frequency ventilation.[1] The strategies for the discontinuation of mechanical ventilation include nasal continuous positive airway pressure (NCPAP) and high-flow nasal cannula (HFNC).

The incidence of extubation failure in preterm infants remains significant, because it ranges from 25% to 30%.[2,3] This problem is more evident among the most premature infants, those with lower gestational age, and those with residual lung disease who require supplemental oxygen at the time of extubation.

Although prolonged intubation has permitted the survival of increasingly premature infants with increasingly premature lungs, it has also brought about a concurrent marked increase in the incidence of tracheotomy-dependent children with acquired subglottic stenosis (SGS), which in turn has precipitated the development of surgical techniques to manage this disease.[4,5]

Airway disease in premature infants may therefore present as an inability to extubate or an inability to wean off noninvasive positive pressure support. Although management generally consists of tracheotomy placement and potentially positive pressure support, in selected cases, airway reconstructive surgery may prevent the need for tracheotomy. If tracheotomy is required, the intent is that eventually the infant will be weaned off positive pressure support and ultimately be decannulated; however, in some case, airway reconstructive surgery is required to achieve decannulation.

This article presents an overview of the neonatal pulmonary and airway problems that are frequently encountered when managing infants with BPD and briefly describes the management of these problems.

RESPIRATORY SUPPORT OF CHILDREN WITH BRONCHOPULMONARY DYSPLASIA

NCPAP has become an effective option for noninvasive respiratory support and is widely used to facilitate weaning from mechanical ventilation and preventing the recurrence of respiratory failure in preterm infants.[6,7]

A randomized controlled trial of 2 NCPAP levels after extubation in preterm infants found that extubation failure with residual lung disease was less common in infants with an NCPAP range of 7 to 9 cm H_2O compared with 4 to 6 cm H_2O.[8] The mechanism by which a larger distending airway pressure decreases the rate of extubation failure is yet to be determined. Alternative settings, such as unsynchronized nasal intermittent positive pressure ventilation (NIPPV), were superior to NCPAP in achieving successful extubation.[9,10]

WEANING FROM NASAL CONTINUOUS POSITIVE AIRWAY PRESSURE

Methods of weaning from NCPAP vary among centers and providers. A randomized controlled trial tested the outcomes of 3 different approaches to weaning. The study compared (1) the discontinuation of CPAP with the view to staying off, (2) cycled on and off CPAP with incremental time off, and (3) cycled on and off CPAP but during off periods infants were supported with 2-mm nasal cannula at a flow of 0.5 L/min. The first approach significantly shortened CPAP weaning time, CPAP duration, oxygen duration, and admission time. Bi-level CPAP was compared with NCPAP as an approach to achieve faster weaning from positive pressure ventilation and oxygen supplementation. It was associated with better respiratory outcomes compared with NCPAP, and allowed earlier discharge.[11]

HEATED HUMIDIFIED HIGH-FLOW NASAL CANNULA THERAPY IN CHILDREN

The concept of providing positive distending pressure through a nasal cannula was developed to decrease the risk of nasal trauma caused by NCPAP. The first-generation nasal cannulae were limited to flow rates up to 2 L/min. However, heated humidification allowed better tolerance of higher nasal flow.[12] In the last 5 years, HFNC has been widely used in neonatal intensive care units,[13] well before evidence to support its use. The concerns about the early introduction of this therapy to clinical care without thorough evaluation of its efficacy have frequently been expressed in the medical community. Specifically, the question is whether the positive pressure delivered by the HFNC is equivalent to that delivered by NCPAP. This subject was addressed by a study that examined the nasal cannula flow required to generate positive distending pressure that is equivalent to an NCPAP of 6 cm H_2O.[14] The study showed that a nasal cannula at flows of 1 to 2.5 L/min could deliver positive distending pressure similar to that of NCPAP. Progress has been made in comparative effectiveness between HFNC and NCPAP both as a primary respiratory support and after extubation. Nevertheless, concern remains regarding whether a leak from the mouth that is large enough could reduce the efficiency of HFNC. Among infants with a postmenstrual age of between 29 and 44 weeks and a birth weight of 835 to 3735 g, no pressure was generated when the infants' mouths were open, regardless of whether flow rates of up to 5 L/min were used.[15] Differences among HFNC devices have also been observed.[16] Although at a low flow rate some devices generate similar positive pharyngeal pressure, differences among devices increase with increasing flow rate.

High-flow Nasal Cannula for Primary Respiratory Support

Few studies have assessed the efficacy of HFNC as first-line management of respiratory distress in premature infants. A retrospective study reported by Shoemaker and colleagues[17] comparing a cohort of infants who received either NCPAP or HFNC as an early mode of respiratory support found no differences in deaths, ventilator days, BPD, blood infections, or other outcomes. More infants were intubated for failing early NCPAP compared with early HFNC.

In a randomized controlled unblinded noncrossover trial in 432 infants ranging from 28 to 42 weeks' gestation by Yoder and colleagues,[18] there was no difference in treatment failure in the first 72 hours between HFNC and NCPAP. Treatment failure for the infants having NCPAP was defined as the need for intubation, and that for infants having HFNC was the transition to NCPAP. Infants having HFNC remained on support significantly longer than infants having NCPAP; however, there were no differences between study groups for days on supplemental oxygen, BPD, or discharge from the hospital on oxygen. The main shortcoming of the study was the more advanced gestational age of the study population, with only 35% of infants younger than 32 weeks' gestation. To date, although data on the use of HFNC are emerging, there is insufficient evidence to support the use of HFNC in preterm infants soon after birth for treatment or prophylaxis of respiratory distress syndrome.

High-flow Nasal Cannula in Extremely Preterm Infants After Extubation

Few studies have examined whether HFNC is as effective as NCPAP in weaning infants from positive pressure and oxygen after extubation. Campbell and colleagues[19] compared the use of HFNC with NCPAP for prevention of reintubation among preterm infants with a birth weight of less than 1250 g. Sixty percent of infants randomized to HFNC were reintubated compared with 15% using NCPAP. The high-flow cannula group had increased oxygen use and more apneas and bradycardias.

A randomized noninferiority trial was conducted to compare HFNC (5–6 L/min) with NCPAP (7 cm H_2O) after extubation.[20] Noninferiority was determined by calculating the absolute difference in the risk of the primary outcome; the margin of noninferiority was 20 percentage points. Treatment failure occurred in 34.2% of infants treated with HFNC compared with 25.8% of infants treated with NCPAP. Fifty percent of infants who failed treatment with HFNC were successfully treated with NCPAP and avoided reintubation. Although the study showed the noninferiority of HFNC to NCPAP, the findings suggest that, for unidentified reasons, some infants are likely to receive more benefit from NCPAP.

Another study by Collins and colleagues[21] enrolled 132 infants younger than 32 weeks' gestation and randomly assigned them to either HFNC or CPAP. Although this study showed a greater treatment failure rate for infants on NCPAP compared with those on HFNC, this difference was not statistically significant.

Careful consideration is needed when interpreting these conflicting results. Although the 2 randomized trials suggest that statistically there is no difference in the performance between HFNC and NCPAP in extremely premature infants, the clinical significance of these conclusions warrants further investigations.

POSITIVE PRESSURE VENTILATION FOR TREATMENT OF APNEA OF PREMATURITY

Apnea of prematurity (AOP) occurs in most premature infants and is frequently a cause of failure of extubation. The response to treatment with NCPAP and NIPPV was investigated in 2 studies.[22,23] According to these studies, the benefit of NIPPV compared with NCPAP is either marginal or nonexistent. Treatment of AOP with HFNC has not been investigated and represents a major gap in knowledge about the safety and efficacy of this intervention in extremely premature infants.

OUTCOMES OF CHILDREN WITH SEVERE BRONCHOPULMONARY DYSPLASIA WHO ARE VENTILATOR DEPENDENT AT HOME

A small percentage of infants with severe BPD cannot wean from mechanical ventilation when they reach medical stability and are eligible to be discharged home. Although these children represent a small percentage of all children requiring long-term mechanical ventilation, the growth has been exponential. A recent single-center study of the outcome of ventilator-dependent children with severe BPD showed that the incidence of chronic respiratory failure requiring long-term mechanical ventilation has almost quadrupled in the last 2 decades.[24] The overall survival of ventilator-dependent children is 80%. For children with severe BPD, the 5-year survival is also 80%.[25] Among survivors, approximately 85% are permanently liberated from mechanical ventilation; of these children, 87%% are decannulated. The median ages of liberation from mechanical ventilation and decannulation are 24 months (interquartile range, 19–33 months) and 37.5 months (interquartile range, 31.5–45 months) respectively.[24]

According to a recent report, 49% of deaths among all ventilator-dependent children occur unexpectedly.[25] Although many of these deaths are secondary to underlying disease, a significant percentage of these mortalities are caused by tracheostomy-related or ventilator-related problems and therefore are avoidable. The management of ventilator-dependent children from the time of initiation of home mechanical ventilation to the time of decannulation requires a high level of vigilance from a dedicated multidisciplinary team that partners with caregivers to ensure safe, high-quality care.

The fundamental principles that govern successful outcomes of ventilator-dependent children have been outlined in several reviews.[25,26] This article briefly describes the essential elements of care before and after discharge.

Predischarge Planning Includes the Following

- Assessment of the family unit and readiness for assuming care.
- Enrolling more than 1 caregiver in a structured training and education program.
- Educating care providers on the underlying medical conditions that contribute to chronic respiratory failure and ventilator dependence.
- Specific training on the mode of ventilation pertaining to each patient.
- Special training on noninvasive pressure ventilation or tracheostomy care as it pertains to each patient.
- Educating care providers on the anticipated clinical course and frequency of visits with the medical team.
- Developing a partnership between medical and care providers that is based on mutual trust.
- Addressing financial challenges that ensure uninterrupted medical services.
- Advocating on behalf of caregivers to receive adequate home nursing support.
- Defining the roles and responsibilities of the company providing durable medical equipment to ensure adequate supply and ventilator function.

Postdischarge Management

The weaning from ventilatory support in children with severe BPD but without large airway abnormalities usually occurs within the first 2 to 3 years of life. Medical management during this period requires a strong partnership between caregivers and the medical team. After discharge of a technology-dependent child to home, the family and home nurses become the eyes and ears of the medical team. An easily accessible and experienced care manager, a social worker, a nutritionist, and a physician are essential to provide safe postdischarge care. Although there is no literature to support the concept of a multidisciplinary team in the care of ventilator-dependent children, all large programs that serve this population follow this structure. To ensure that adequate ventilation is delivered from the time of initiation of home mechanical ventilation until liberation from the ventilator, it is crucial to prevent acute or gradual respiratory decompensation. The General guidelines for postdischarge medical care are presented here.

Prevention of Acute Superimposed on Chronic Respiratory Failure

- Education on modes of transmission of infectious organisms and ways to mitigate the spread of infection in the household.
- Education on hygienic tracheostomy tube care.
- Timely administration of childhood vaccination and Synagis (passive respiratory syncytial virus prophylaxis).
- Yearly administration of influenza vaccine.
- Prevention of atelectasis secondary to inadequate ventilation.

Prevention of Gradual Respiratory Decompensation

One of the main goals of long-term mechanical ventilation in children is to meet the ventilator demands, so as to leave much of their energy available for other activities.

In the absence of parenchymal lung disease, ventilators are adjusted to maintain an oxygen saturation greater than 95% and a CO_2 tension within the range of 35 to 40 mm Hg during wakefulness and sleep. In the presence of parenchymal lung disease, oxygen supplementation might be needed to maintain normal oxygen saturation. Normal CO_2 tension in the presence of parenchymal lung disease might not be achievable with safe ventilator settings that could be used at home. Positive pressure ventilation via a tracheostomy is complicated because, during sleep, children could develop a larger degree of leakage from around the tracheostomy tube than during wakefulness. The leak from around the tracheostomy tube can reach a significant degree during rapid eye movement sleep because of the generalized muscle atonia that develops during that stage of sleep. This leakage can be qualitatively and quantitatively measured using polysomnography. Qualitative assessment of ventilation and degree of leakage from around the tracheostomy tube can be performed by examining the changes in inspiratory and expiratory flows obtained from a pneumotachograph, end-tidal CO_2 measured by a capnograph, and changes in tidal volume measured by respiratory inductive plethysmography. General guidelines for outpatient management of ventilator-dependent children with severe BPD are presented here.

Regular outpatient visits to:

- Evaluate the adequacy of the ventilator settings and the degree of air leakage from around the tracheostomy tube.
- Measure end-tidal CO_2 and oxygenation.
- Assess the child's readiness for weaning from ventilator support.
- Assess growth and development.
- Assess nutrition and feeding.
- Determine the need for airway evaluation by bronchoscopy to identify stoma-related complications.

The approach to weaning from ventilator support varies among providers and institutions. Although some centers rely on regular evaluation of ventilation and readiness for weaning from the ventilator in the sleep laboratory, many rely solely on clinical assessment. The American Thoracic Society consensus statement published in 1996 recommends obtaining a polysomnogram periodically to determine the adequacy of ventilation and oxygenation provided by artificial ventilatory support, including diaphragmatic pacing. The frequency of follow-up study varies depending on the clinical stability of the child, but such studies should occur at least annually.[27] A retrospective study of ventilator-dependent children showed that changes in continuous positive pressure and/or ventilator settings are frequently made after a polysomnogram.[28]

AIRWAY MANAGEMENT OF CHILDREN WITH BRONCHOPULMONARY DYSPLASIA

Failure to extubate encompasses both the inability to extubate and unsuccessful attempts at extubation. The inability to extubate may be caused by continued need for positive pressure ventilation or oxygen requirements, or other nonpulmonary factors such as abnormal central control of breathing. In infants with an inability to extubate and in whom that status is unlikely to change in the near to intermediate future, tracheotomy is an option. In infants in whom ventilator requirements permit extubation but reintubation is required, the reason for reintubation should be sought. If there is a potentially correctable cause such as oversedation, extubation should be attempted again. However, if the infant was extubated for a period of hours or days and/or was reintubated because of airway problems such as stridor and retractions, further evaluation is warranted. In an infant who is extubated but in respiratory distress, awake transnasal flexible laryngoscopy is a valuable method of evaluating supraglottic structures (eg, cysts and laryngomalacia) and glottic function (eg, vocal cord immobility), vocal process granulomas, and edema.[29] However, transnasal flexible laryngoscopy usually does not permit an adequate evaluation of the subglottis, trachea, or bronchi. A more comprehensive evaluation may be performed with rigid and/or flexible laryngoscopy and bronchoscopy, usually in an operative setting. Rigid bronchoscopy allows an excellent evaluation of the posterior glottis and subglottis and is also a good method of evaluating tracheal disorder. Flexible bronchoscopy allows excellent evaluation of airway dynamics, particularly hypopharyngeal collapse, laryngomalacia, tracheomalacia, bronchomalacia, and vascular compression. Flexible bronchoscopy is also of value in obtaining bronchial sampling for culture or for hemosiderin and lipid-laden macrophages. In some infants, these 2 bronchoscopic techniques may be used interchangeably and, in others, one technique has clear advantages compared with the other; there are also infants in whom the two techniques are complementary.

If evaluation confirms a correctable diagnosis such as glottic granulation or a subglottic cyst, then following intervention another attempt at extubation may be warranted. Similarly, bronchoscopy may suggest a diagnosis that requires more comprehensive investigation. For example, in a child with vascular compression of the trachea, bronchoscopic evaluation may confirm the anatomic level of airway compromise and its severity; however, vascular imaging is needed to confirm the diagnosis and evaluate whether surgical intervention could improve the airway.

SUBGLOTTIC STENOSIS

Compared with acquired SGS, congenital SGS is a rare diagnosis. The most common disease entity associated with congenital SGS is Down syndrome (DS), and typically an infant with DS who requires intubation requires an endotracheal tube 0.5 to 1.0 mm smaller than would otherwise be expected in an infant of similar age.[30]

Given that the narrowest point in an infant's airway is the subglottis, intubation is most likely to carry an adverse consequence in this anatomic area. In infants, acquired SGS is often a consequence of intubation, and the primary risk factors include the duration of intubation, reintubation and traumatic intubation, tube composition, nasal versus oral intubation, and cofactors such as gastroesophageal reflux disease (GERD). However, the single most important factor is endotracheal tube size. The lowest risk is intubation with an endotracheal tube that is appropriately sized for the patient (as opposed to the age of the patient). Ideally, a tube that leaks at less than 20 cm H_2O subglottic pressure is ideal, but, with more severe BPD, higher pressures may have to be tolerated, even though they carry a higher risk of SGS. Because the leak pressure is a direct consequence of how tight the endotracheal tube is in the subglottis, an alternative is the use of a smaller diameter, low-pressure, cuffed endotracheal tube. This type of tube is more forgiving to the subglottic mucosa, because the leak pressure depends on the seal of the cuff in the trachea. Although this may be less damaging to the subglottis, care must be taken not to overfill the tracheal cuff, because this in turn could cause damage to the trachea. Again, a leak pressure of less than 20 cm H_2O is desirable if the ventilator needs of the patient permit. SGS is generally an easier problem to manage than distal tracheal stenosis.

Although the diagnosis of SGS may be made from radiographs, with airway films showing subglottic steepling, or on close-cut computed tomography scans, which delineate the stenosis, the diagnostic gold standard is endoscopy. Laryngoscopy and bronchoscopy allow inspection of the stenotic area, with evaluation of the severity, extent, and presence of any other coexistent airway lesions. The degree of SGS is typically graded using the Myer-Cotton grading scale. The size of the sub-glottis is evaluated by using endotracheal tubes (the largest tube that still leaks at <20 cm H_2O pressure).[31] A grade 1 stenosis is less than 50% stenotic, a grade 2 is 51% to 70% stenotic, a grade 3 is 71% to 99% stenotic, and a grade 4 is 100% stenotic.

Although assessment of the severity of the stenosis is important, evaluation should also encompass factors that may influence the outcome of a subsequent intervention. More specifically, management is influenced by inflammation, granulation, and edema, and intervention and optimization improve the outcome of surgery, whether endoscopic or open. In neonates, the relative risk of eosinophilic esophagitis (a negative factor in older children) is low.[32] However, GERD has the potential to exacerbate laryngeal edema and, ideally, should be controlled before surgical intervention. Assessment may therefore include an esophagogastroduodenoscopy or impedance probe testing for evaluation of GERD, and a flexible bronchoscopy for evaluation of dynamic airway collapse and pulmonary secretion management.

Treatment options comprise initial nonoperative measures, endoscopic surgery, open surgery, and tracheotomy. Nonoperative measures include trying to resolve edema and inflammation to either avoid other intervention or to permit surgical intervention with less risk of failure. For example, a smaller endotracheal tube that permits a leak combined with topical steroid and antibiotic drops being delivered down the endotracheal tube may improve subglottic granulation and edema.

Endoscopic surgery may include removal of granulation tissue, marsupialization of subglottic cysts (a disease exclusively of intubated premature infants), and balloon dilation. Balloon dilation is rapid, straightforward, and fairly safe, with infants usually requiring a 5-mm or 6-mm balloon. Although effective at dilation of subglottic scar tissue, balloon dilation is not effective at treating SGS resulting from a congenital elliptical cricoid. Balloon dilation frequently is required on 3 to 4 occasions at 1-week to 2-week intervals until the subglottic scar stabilizes.[33]

Open airway reconstruction in neonates, namely the anterior cricoid split, was originally described by Cotton and Seid[34] as an alternative to tracheotomy in premature infants failing extubation because of SGS. This operation involved a small horizontal neck incision over the cricoid and a vertical incision in the anterior airway, from the lower third of the thyroid cartilage, through the anterior cricoid and the upper 2 tracheal rings. The incision is loosely closed over a Penrose drain to prevent air from accumulating beneath the skin, and the patient is left intubated for 10 days as the airway heals by secondary intention. With appropriate selection criteria, this procedure carried a high success rate and was widely adopted. However, the success rate has steadily decreased, primarily because the infants who most benefited from the operation are now unlikely to be intubated and hence do not develop SGS. Modifications to the surgery include placement of an anterior thyroid alar graft to close the airway and permit earlier extubation,[35] and, in more severe stenosis, an anterior thyroid alar graft is combined with a posterior cricoid split.[36] Again, in selected patients, the outcomes are excellent. In cases in which a cartilage graft is used, the operation is termed a laryngotracheal reconstruction.

In infants with SGS who have a larynx that is extremely inflamed, or in cases in which endoscopic or open surgery has failed, tracheotomy is the best alternative. Typically, further attempts at airway surgery to achieve decannulation are delayed for months or even years until the larynx is quiescent and the infant is otherwise healthy. Although, in the past, guidelines for later airway reconstruction have depended on the weight of the child, laryngeal inflammation and the overall health status of the child are increasingly seen as better indicators for when to attempt further surgery.

TRACHEOMALACIA AND TRACHEOBRONCHOMALACIA

In premature infants who require prolonged intubation and positive pressure ventilation, there is a risk that the continued positive pressure will result in distention of the airway, with resultant tracheobronchomalacia. This condition is not always easy to diagnose, and bronchoscopy in a deeply anesthetized child masks dynamic collapse. The gold standard for diagnosis is flexible bronchoscopy, with the infant lightly anesthetized and with spontaneous ventilation. Mild tracheobronchomalacia may be tolerable, with the expectation of resolution with time and growth, although the symptoms frequently get worse before they get better. Moderate tracheobronchomalacia may present with extubation difficulty; respiratory distress, including both inspiratory stridor and expiratory wheeze; and a honking cough. Children with severe tracheobronchomalacia may have dying spells, even while intubated and even with positive pressure ventilation. In extubated infants, chronic CO_2 retention and inability to wean off noninvasive positive pressure support may be present.

Other frequently encountered causes of tracheobronchomalacia include coexistent disorders such as a tracheoesophageal fistula or a laryngeal cleft, or malacia associated with vascular compression. Vascular compression of the trachea, especially the double aortic arch and the more severe cases of innominate artery compression, primarily affect the trachea, and appropriate corrective vascular surgery may greatly improve both the endoscopic appearance and the symptoms. However, severe vascular compression still leaves the affected cartilage weakened, and tracheomalacia may persist for months in the affected segment of trachea.[37]

In more severe cases of tracheomalacia or tracheobronchomalacia, the ongoing need for positive pressure ventilation for months or even years requires consideration of tracheotomy tube placement and pressure support with CPAP, biphasic positive airway pressure (BiPAP), or a ventilator. However, for patients with isolated tracheomalacia, an aortopexy may be a viable alternative to tracheotomy, with forward suspension of the innominate artery or ascending aorta to the sternum. The key to this operation is creating space to allow the artery to be suspended to the back of the sternum, which is usually achieved by removal of the thymus gland. It follows that children without a thymus (DiGeorge syndrome) gain much less benefit from an aortopexy.

INDICATIONS FOR TRACHEOTOMY PLACEMENT

The indications for tracheotomy placement in an infant are diverse and encompass problems of access, problems of impaired ventilation, and inability to extubate (**Box 1**). Problems of access include nasal or oropharyngeal tumors, macroglossia, retrognathia, or any other condition that might make intubation challenging. In an infant who is difficult to intubate and if the problem is not readily correctable, consideration should be given to performing an early tracheotomy to minimize the risks associated with inadvertent extubation.

Problems of impaired ventilation include an inability to wean from noninvasive forms of positive pressure support, whether HFNC, CPAP, or BiPAP. This inability is often associated with chronic compensated nonacidotic CO_2 retention.

Inability to extubate may be caused by anatomic factors (SGS, vocal cord paralysis, tracheobronchomalacia), ventilation failure (neurologic or neuromuscular), or by other congenital anomalies that preclude extubation. In some cases, the problem can be corrected and tracheotomy avoided; however, the disorder is often not readily resolved,

---

Box 1
Indications for tracheotomy in infants

Pulmonary/chest conditions (conditions needing prolonged mechanical ventilation)

BPD

Poor lung compliance

Pulmonary hypoplasia

Neuromuscular weakness of diaphragm and chest wall muscles

Upper/lower airway obstruction

SGS

Vocal cord paralysis

Tracheobronchomalacia

Vascular compression of trachea/bronchi

Oropharyngeal tumors

Congenital tracheal stenosis

Macroglossia

Retrognathia

---

such as an extremely inflamed larynx. The contraindications to tracheotomy are all relative, with the most relevant being extremely low weight. The smallest tracheotomy tube available has a 2.5-mm inner diameter and may be too large to easily be placed in the trachea of some children weighing less than 1 kg. Ideally, tracheotomy placement should therefore wait until an infant has reached a weight of 1.5 kg, unless the risk of waiting outweighs the risk of early tracheotomy; this may occur in infants who are difficult to intubate. Another contraindication is congenital tracheal stenosis, especially complete tracheal rings, because even the smallest tracheotomy tube may not fit through a segment of complete tracheal rings without rupturing the trachea. In this circumstance, it is better to repair the rings and try to avoid a tracheotomy.[38] Other patients in whom a tracheotomy should be performed with caution include infants with laryngeal clefts and infants with proximal tracheoesophageal fistulae or fistulae pouches.

TRACHEOTOMY TECHNIQUES AND GUIDELINES IN NEONATES

Numerous techniques have been described for performing tracheotomy and no universal standard currently exists. Nevertheless, the following overview outlines the procedure that we recommend and perform at our institution. Ideally, the patient is intubated under general anesthesia. A transverse neck incision is made over the second tracheal ring and the pad of subcutaneous fat dissected out and removed. The strap muscles are split in the midline and retracted laterally to expose the anterior trachea. The thyroid isthmus is identified and divided. The cricoid cartilage is noted and the second to fourth tracheal rings are identified. Nonabsorbable stay sutures are then placed to either side of the midline between the second and fourth tracheal rings, and the trachea incised in the midline between the stay sutures. The stoma is then matured by sewing the skin down to the tracheal incision to minimize the risk of a false passage, especially if the tracheotomy tube should displace. The endotracheal tube is then pulled back until just proximal to the tracheal incision and a tracheotomy tube is inserted. The anesthetic circuit is connected to the tracheotomy tube and ventilation is confirmed before the endotracheal tube is removed. The tracheotomy tube is then secured with twill or Velcro ties, and a small flexible endoscope is passed down it to ensure that the tube is in the trachea, not too long, and lying in a bronchus. We routinely change the tracheotomy ties on the third day and change the tracheotomy itself on the fifth day, after which the family should learn to perform this task. The choice of tracheotomy tube depends on the needs of the child, although typically a single-lumen 3.0-mm or 3.5-mm neonatal tracheotomy tube is placed. In infants expected to be on a ventilator for a period postoperatively, a cuffed tracheotomy may be used. The risk of skin breakdown around a tracheotomy tube is high in neonates, especially because of the weight of attached ventilator tubing. This risk is significantly decreased if an extended collar design of tracheotomy tube is used (Flextend).[39]

Typically, a neonatal tracheotomy tube is exchanged for a longer pediatric tracheotomy tube at around 9 months of age. Once off a ventilator, even an infant may benefit from the use of a speaking valve, although we recommend that an in-line pressure manometer has confirmed subglottic pressures of less than 10 cm H_2O during quiet breathing.

In children who are no longer reliant on a tracheotomy and in whom there is no anatomic reason (such as SGS) to prevent decannulation, we recommend performing a bronchoscopy to confirm anatomic suitability for decannulation and suggest that the tracheotomy tube be replaced by a very small tracheotomy tube, which is then plugged. The child is observed for 48 hours and sent home for several weeks with a pulse oximeter available at night. If no problems arise, the child is then decannulated and observed for a further 48 hours. If the tracheocutaneous fistula does not close spontaneously within 3 months, it may require a minor operation for closure.

TRACHEOTOMY IN THE SETTING OF CHRONIC VENTILATOR DEPENDENCY

An infant requiring a tracheotomy for SGS is not expected to require positive pressure support, and hence an uncuffed tracheotomy tube is adequate to bypass the stenosis and permit spontaneous ventilation. However, in the setting of neuromuscular compromise, positive pressure ventilation may be required for months or even years in an infant with poor respiratory effort. The most challenging infants are those in whom higher ventilator pressures are required to stent open the distal airways; this includes those with severe tracheobronchomalacia, vascular compression, stenosis, or noncompliant lungs. In infants requiring very high ventilator settings, it may be preferable to delay tracheotomy, because there are significant risks associated with high-pressure ventilation, such as an air leak causing subcutaneous emphysema at the tracheotomy site.

Strategies for managing tracheotomies in ventilated infants include having a larger diameter tracheotomy tube that more closely accommodates the walls of the trachea to help minimize the air leak, or a cuffed tube. Cuffed tracheotomy tubes include water filled tight to the shaft designs, high volume low-pressure air cuffs, and occasionally foam-filled cuffs, though these are rare in infants. Low-volume high-pressure cuffs are not recommended. Cuff pressures should be tailored to allow an air leak at a designated acceptable pressure that still permits ventilation of the infant. There is also the option of extended collar designs, to which it is easier to attach a ventilator circuit.

The intent is that, if possible, the ventilation pressures will be steadily weaned as the child grows and gains strength. The child may transition to requiring positive pressure only when sleeping, to BiPAP, to CPAP, and eventually to decannulation. This transition is often driven by sleep study parameters, especially CO_2 retention. However, in severely neurologically damaged children or children with progressive neuromuscular problems, weaning off positive pressure may be unachievable.

TIMING OF TRACHEOTOMY AND OUTCOMES IN PRETERM INFANTS

Among preterm infants with less than 30 weeks' gestation, roughly 3% to 7% ultimately require tracheotomy for the indication of BPD. There are no prospective studies or randomized trials to indicate the optimum timing for tracheotomy in ventilator-dependent infants with BPD. In a recent large multicenter retrospective study from the National Institute of Child Health and Human Development Neonatal Research Network including infants born at less than 30 weeks' gestation from 2001 to 2011, 304 of 8683 (3.5%) infants required tracheotomy.[40] In this large study, 132 infants with a tracheotomy performed at less than 120 days of life had better neurodevelopmental outcomes than 172 infants in whom a tracheotomy was performed at greater than 120 days. The investigators speculated that improved attention to neurodevelopment afforded by a tracheotomy rather than an endotracheal tube might have contributed to the improved outcomes. However, the adjusted odds ratio for severe neurodevelopmental delay was 5 in tracheotomized infants versus those without tracheotomy. Although the investigators corrected for a multitude of confounding factors, poor neurodevelopmental outcomes in the group requiring tracheotomy placement were likely caused by the infants with BPD requiring tracheotomy being the sickest. Lower mortality after early (<45 weeks' postmenstrual age [PMA]) rather than later (>45 weeks' PMA) tracheotomy was reported by Rane and colleagues[41] in a single-center study. However, the patient populations in early versus late tracheotomy were different in this study, making comparisons difficult. In other single-center studies, preterm infants with BPD and high ventilator requirements with a mean airway pressure of around 14 cm H_2O tolerated tracheotomy well and had decreases in respiratory severity scores 1 month posttracheotomy.[42] Infants with BPD who have a tracheotomy require a long hospital stay. Overman and colleagues[43] reported that infants weighing less than 1000 g with a tracheotomy needed an average of 505 days of positive pressure ventilation and 479 days to decannulation, whereas infants weighing greater than 1000 g at birth needed an average of 372 days of positive pressure ventilation and 437 days to decannulation. Thus, the infants needing tracheotomy require long-term care and are at an increased risk for neurodevelopmental delays. However, in most of these reports, the survival rate exceeds 80%. Although firm guidelines for deciding the timing for tracheotomy cannot be made, a reasonable approach in preterm infants who are ventilator dependent largely for BPD is to consider performing a tracheotomy at less than 4 months of age if the pulmonary status has plateaued over the previous few weeks. Parents should be made aware that these infants are at an increased risk for neurodevelopmental delays.

REFERENCES

1. Stoll BJ, Hansen NI, Bell EF, et al. Neonatal outcomes of extremely preterm infants from the NICHD Neonatal Research Network. Pediatrics 2010;126:443–56.
2. Kavvadia V, Greenough A, Dimitriou G. Prediction of extubation failure in preterm neonates. Eur J Pediatr 2000;159:227–31.
3. Mikhno A, Ennett CM. Prediction of extubation failure for neonates with respiratory distress syndrome using the MIMIC-II clinical database. Conf Proc IEEE Eng Med Biol Soc 2012;2012:5094–7.
4. Cotton RT, Evans JN. Laryngotracheal reconstruction in children. Five-year follow-up. Ann Otol Rhinol Laryngol 1981;90:516–20.
5. Cotton RT, Gray SD, Miller RP. Update of the Cincinnati experience in pediatric laryngotracheal reconstruction. Laryngoscope 1989;99:1111–6.

6. Andreasson B, Lindroth M, Svenningsen NW, et al. Effects on respiration of CPAP immediately after extubation in the very preterm infant. Pediatr Pulmonol 1988;4: 213–8.

7. Engelke SC, Roloff DW, Kuhns LR. Postextubation nasal continuous positive airway pressure. A prospective controlled study. Am J Dis Child 1982;136:359–61.

8. Buzzella B, Claure N, D'Ugard C, et al. A randomized controlled trial of two nasal continuous positive airway pressure levels after extubation in preterm infants. J Pediatr 2014;164:46–51.

9. Kahramaner Z, Erdemir A, Turkoglu E, et al. Unsynchronized nasal intermittent positive pressure versus nasal continuous positive airway pressure in preterm infants after extubation. J Matern Fetal Neonatal Med 2014;27:926–9.

10. Todd DA, Wright A, Broom M, et al. Methods of weaning preterm babies <30 weeks gestation off CPAP: a multicentre randomised controlled trial. Arch Dis Child Fetal Neonatal Ed 2012;97:F236–40.

11. Lista G, Castoldi F, Fontana P, et al. Nasal continuous positive airway pressure (CPAP) versus bi-level nasal CPAP in preterm babies with respiratory distress syndrome: a randomised control trial. Arch Dis Child Fetal Neonatal Ed 2010;95:F85–9.

12. Woodhead DD, Lambert DK, Clark JM, et al. Comparing two methods of delivering high-flow gas therapy by nasal cannula following endotracheal extubation: a prospective, randomized, masked, crossover trial. J Perinatol 2006;26:481–5.

13. Hough JL, Shearman AD, Jardine LA, et al. Humidified high flow nasal cannulae: current practice in Australasian nurseries, a survey. J Paediatr Child Health 2012; 48:106–13.

14. Sreenan C, Lemke RP, Hudson-Mason A, et al. High-flow nasal cannulae in the management of apnea of prematurity: a comparison with conventional nasal continuous positive airway pressure. Pediatrics 2001;107:1081–3.

15. Kubicka ZJ, Limauro J, Darnall RA. Heated, humidified high-flow nasal cannula therapy: yet another way to deliver continuous positive airway pressure? Pediatrics 2008;121:82–8.

16. Collins CL, Holberton JR, Konig K. Comparison of the pharyngeal pressure provided by two heated, humidified high-flow nasal cannulae devices in premature infants. J Paediatr Child Health 2013;49:554–6.

17. Shoemaker MT, Pierce MR, Yoder BA, et al. High flow nasal cannula versus nasal CPAP for neonatal respiratory disease: a retrospective study. J Perinatol 2007;27: 85–91.

18. Yoder BA, Stoddard RA, Li M, et al. Heated, humidified high-flow nasal cannula versus nasal CPAP for respiratory support in neonates. Pediatrics 2013;131: e1482–90.

19. Campbell DM, Shah PS, Shah V, et al. Nasal continuous positive airway pressure from high flow cannula versus infant flow for preterm infants. J Perinatol 2006;26:546–9.

20. Manley BJ, Owen LS, Doyle LW, et al. High-flow nasal cannulae in very preterm infants after extubation. N Engl J Med 2013;369:1425–33.

21. Collins CL, Holberton JR, Barfield C, et al. A randomized controlled trial to compare heated humidified high-flow nasal cannulae with nasal continuous positive airway pressure postextubation in premature infants. J Pediatr 2013;162: 949–54.e1.

22. Lin CH, Wang ST, Lin YJ, et al. Efficacy of nasal intermittent positive pressure ventilation in treating apnea of prematurity. Pediatr Pulmonol 1998;26:349–53.

23. Ryan CA, Finer NN, Peters KL. Nasal intermittent positive-pressure ventilation offers no advantages over nasal continuous positive airway pressure in apnea of prematurity. Am J Dis Child 1989;143:1196–8.

24. Cristea AI, Carroll AE, Davis SD, et al. Outcomes of children with severe broncho-pulmonary dysplasia who were ventilator dependent at home. Pediatrics 2013; 132:e727–34.

25. Edwards JD, Kun SS, Keens TG. Outcomes and causes of death in children on home mechanical ventilation via tracheostomy: an institutional and literature review. J Pediatr 2010;157:955–9.e2.

26. Amin RS, Fitton CM. Tracheostomy and home ventilation in children. Semin Neonatol 2003;8:127–35.

27. Standards and indications for cardiopulmonary sleep studies in children. American Thoracic Society. Am J Respir Crit Care Med 1996;153:866–78.

28. Tan E, Nixon GM, Edwards EA. Sleep studies frequently lead to changes in respiratory support in children. J Paediatr Child Health 2007;43:560–3.

29. Albert DM, Mills RP, Fysh J, et al. Endoscopic examination of the neonatal larynx at extubation: a prospective study of variables associated with laryngeal damage. Int J Pediatr Otorhinolaryngol 1990;20:203–12.

30. Shott SR. Down syndrome: analysis of airway size and a guide for appropriate intubation. Laryngoscope 2000;110:585–92.

31. Myer CM 3rd, O'Connor DM, Cotton RT. Proposed grading system for subglottic stenosis based on endotracheal tube sizes. Ann Otol Rhinol Laryngol 1994;103:319–23.

32. Dauer EH, Ponikau JU, Smyrk TC, et al. Airway manifestations of pediatric eosinophilic esophagitis: a clinical and histopathologic report of an emerging association. Ann Otol Rhinol Laryngol 2006;115:507–17.

33. Maresh A, Preciado DA, O'Connell AP, et al. A comparative analysis of open surgery vs endoscopic balloon dilation for pediatric subglottic stenosis. JAMA Otolaryngol Head Neck Surg 2014;140:901–5.

34. Cotton RT, Seid AB. Management of the extubation problem in the premature child. Anterior cricoid split as an alternative to tracheotomy. Ann Otol Rhinol Laryngol 1980;89:508–11.

35. Fraga JC, Schopf L, Forte V. Thyroid alar cartilage laryngotracheal reconstruction for severe pediatric subglottic stenosis. J Pediatr Surg 2001;36:1258–61.

36. White DR, Bravo M, Vijayasekaran S, et al. Laryngotracheoplasty as an alternative to tracheotomy in infants younger than 6 months. Arch Otolaryngol Head Neck Surg 2009;135:445–7.

37. Rutter MJ, deAlarcon A, Manning PB. Tracheal anomalies and reconstruction. In: DaCruz E, Ivy DI, Jaggers J, et al, editors. Pediatric and congenital cardiology, cardiac surgery and intensive care. London: Springer-Verlag; 2013. p. 3129–34.

38. Manning PB, Rutter MJ, Lisec A, et al. One slide fits all: the versatility of slide tracheoplasty with cardiopulmonary bypass support for airway reconstruction in children. J Thorac Cardiovasc Surg 2011;141:155–61.

39. Boesch RP, Myers C, Garrett T, et al. Prevention of tracheostomy-related pressure ulcers in children. Pediatrics 2012;129:e792–7.

40. DeMauro SB, D'Agostino JA, Bann C, et al. Developmental outcomes of very preterm infants with tracheostomies. J Pediatr 2014;164:1303–10.e2.

41. Rane S, Bathula S, Thomas RL, et al. Outcomes of tracheostomy in the neonatal intensive care unit: is there an optimal time? J Matern Fetal Neonatal Med 2014; 27:1257–61.

42. Mandy G, Malkar M, Welty SE, et al. Tracheostomy placement in infants with bronchopulmonary dysplasia: safety and outcomes. Pediatr Pulmonol 2013;48:245–9.

43. Overman AE, Liu M, Kurachek SC, et al. Tracheostomy for infants requiring prolonged mechanical ventilation: 10 years' experience. Pediatrics 2013;131: e1491–6.

Newer Imaging Techniques for Bronchopulmonary Dysplasia

Laura L. Walkup, PhD, Jason C. Woods, PhD*

KEYWORDS

- Bronchopulmonary dysplasia • Prematurity • Lung development • Imaging
- Computerized tomography • MRI

KEY POINTS

- Bronchopulmonary dysplasia (BPD) is a highly complex, multifactorial condition with high variability patient to patient, and clinical imaging has played an important role in the understanding and assessment of BPD.
- Although chest radiograph will continue to be the first line of radiological inquiry, emerging imaging techniques will allow for objective longitudinal assessment of BPD. New, low-dose computerized tomographic techniques lessen radiation burden, and nonionizing, ultrashort echo time and hyperpolarized-gas MRI techniques are poised to reveal structure-function relationships in BPD.
- These methods offer quantitative measurement of the pathologic abnormalities contributing to a patient's condition, and with wider clinical implementation, are likely to contribute to lower mortality and better outcomes for BPD.

INTRODUCTION

Clinical imaging has played an important role in the description of bronchopulmonary dysplasia (BPD) or chronic lung disease of prematurity since its initial recognition. Northway and colleagues[1] first described elements of fibrosis, atelectasis, and hyperinflation in chest films of premature infants who were subjected to mechanical ventilation at high pressure and high oxygen concentration. As postnatal care strategies for premature infants have changed, so too have the definition of and radiological signatures associated with BPD. Advancements such as surfactant therapies, antenatal steroids, and less-aggressive ventilation including lower pressure and oxygen

Disclosures: None.
Division of Pulmonary Medicine, Department of Radiology, Center for Pulmonary Imaging Research, Cincinnati Children's Hospital Medical Center, 3333 Burnet Avenue, MC 5033, Cincinnati, OH 42229, USA
* Corresponding author.
E-mail address: jason.woods@cchmc.org

concentrations have improved survivability, yet the incidence of BPD is increasing as survivors are more premature and lower birth weight than in the past. This so-called new BPD is clinically diagnosed and graded by a physiologically assessed need for supplemental oxygen at 36 weeks postmenstrual age (PMA) following premature birth (≤28 weeks PMA at birth). Gestational age (PMA minus 2 weeks) and birth weight remain the best predictors for BPD,[2] and BPD is recognized as a common pulmonary complication of premature birth. Although very low birth weight infants (<1500 g) represent a small fraction of live births (1.5% in the United States in 2008),[3] 97% of BPD cases occur in infants with birth weight less than 1250 g.[4] These patients often require long durations in the neonatal intensive care unit (NICU), are sometimes discharged on home ventilator or oxygen therapies, and are at higher risk of rehospitalization due to persistent respiratory complications and illness.[3]

Lung growth and development in premature infants are incompletely understood, and although the current ability to predict future outcomes and personalize care for BPD survivors is concomitantly low, newer imaging techniques hold promise to elucidate the connections between structural and functional abnormalities and long-term outcomes.

The purpose in this work is to review how clinical imaging has contributed to the knowledge of BPD epidemiology and pathology and how imaging measures correlate with clinical data, can inform patient care decisions, and be predictive of future outcomes, with particular focus on emerging techniques and the future of imaging BPD.

CHEST RADIOGRAPH

Standard chest radiograph is a clinically accessible and routine imaging modality and is often the first line of radiologic inquiry in the NICU for BPD patients; **Fig. 1** compares chest radiographs for a control and 2 BPD NICU patients. In 1967, Northway and colleagues[1] noted changes in chest radiographs of premature infants that included linear fibrotic opacities and hyperexpanded regions of lung parenchyma and named this condition bronchopulmonary dysplasia to describe radiological changes as a result of prolonged mechanical ventilation. Toce and colleagues[5] adapted clinical and radiographic scoring systems to objectively determine BPD severity; their scoring system (modified from Edwards[6]) incorporates factors describing cardiovascular abnormalities, hyperexpansion, emphysema, fibrosis/interstitial abnormalities, and overall subjective impression. The investigators remark that given the unspecific clinical characteristics of BPD, radiographic findings were considered key to clinical diagnosis; interestingly, the modern clinical diagnosis of BPD does not incorporate a

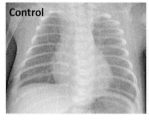 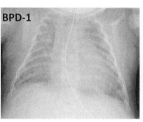 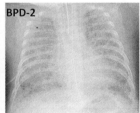

Fig. 1. Comparison of chest radiographs from a control NICU patient (*left*, female patient born 34 weeks PMA, radiograph at 34 weeks PMA) versus 2 BPD patients BPD-1 (male patient, born 23 weeks PMA, radiograph at 38 weeks PMA) and BPD-2 (male patient, born 26 weeks PMA, gestational triplet, radiograph at 39 weeks PMA) with characteristic radiographic findings of BPD including diffused and reticular mixed opacities with some associated increased lung volumes.

radiological component and instead focuses on the clinically assessed need for supplemental oxygen.

These radiographic characteristics are only prevalent in the most severe cases of BPD; however, many patients with significant respiratory symptoms have very minor radiographic abnormalities. A few studies report that these abnormalities are persistent with age even when respiratory function improves. For instance, Breysem and colleagues[7] reported that 1-year-old survivors of BPD had significantly smaller chest depth and width as measured by radiograph compared with other 1-year-old, former NICU patients with respiratory distress syndrome (RDS) but no BPD.

Although chest radiograph has the advantages of accessibility and simplicity, the modality is considered only marginally useful for diagnosis. Although chest films may only provide limited information to guide care, they are clinically routine, because changes in radiograph appearance may be reflective of and are useful for recognizing potential complications with BPD, such as acquired lobar emphysema or overinflation,[8,9] pulmonary edema, atelectasis, and secondary cor pulmonale, which can be diagnosed and further explored by other modalities.

COMPUTERIZED TOMOGRAPHY

Radiograph computerized tomography (CT) provides 3-dimensional spatial resolution compared with conventional radiograph; citing this reason and the fact that radiograph is insensitive to lung abnormalities associated with BPD, Oppenheim and colleagues[10] first described CT findings in older children with BPD (mean age 4 years old) and found regions of hypoattenuation, linear opacities initiating at the pleural surface and radiating inward toward the hilum, and triangular subpleural opacities (small triangles at the pleural surface with interior apexes). Although this cohort would be considered old BPD, recent CT descriptions of BPD (new BPD) include similar abnormalities (**Fig. 2**) and support the notion that BPD is marked by arrested development of the peripheral lung (alveolar simplification) and has limited central airway involvement,[11,12] although bronchial wall thickening and decreased bronchoarterial diameter ratios have been reported in adult survivors of BPD.[13]

Aukland and colleagues[14] conducted a population-based CT study of young children and adults who were born prematurely in the late 1980s and the early 1990s (most of whom were clinically diagnosed with BPD), and for their analysis, developed a 14-parameter scoring system; they reported BPD survivors had higher CT scores for the 4 most common findings in their study (ie, linear and triangular opacities, air trapping, and mosaic attenuation) than other premature survivors without diagnosed BPD; however, the differences were not statically significant. Ochiai and colleagues[15] developed a clinical scoring system to describe the abnormalities found in CT scans of BPD patients and compared their system with the Edwards system for chest radiographs. Their scoring system, similar to Edwards, assigns points based on 4 categories: hyperexpansion (including mosaic attenuation and intercostal bulging), emphysema (bullae and blebs), fibrous/interstitial abnormalities (triangular subpleural opacities and bronchovascular thickening/distortion), and overall subjective impression. They report significant correlations between CT score and BPD clinical scores at 36 weeks PMA (based on the National Institutes of Health workshop guidelines[5]) and duration of oxygen support, whereas only the Edwards radiograph score at 28 days correlated with clinical score and duration of oxygen support, suggesting that CT may provide better predischarge assessment of BPD patients than chest radiograph. Another recent CT scoring system developed by Shin and colleagues[16] counts the number of bronchopulmonary segments with elements of hyperaeration (eg, hypoattenuated

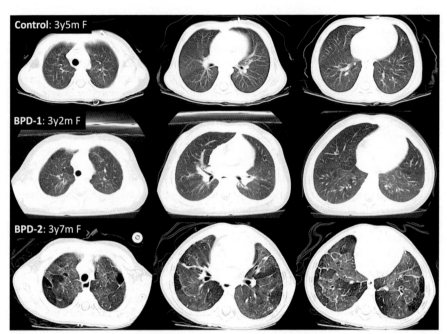

Fig. 2. Comparison of chest CT from ~3.5-year-old female BPD survivors versus a control with normal CT findings. The typical appearance of BPD in CT with abnormalities including bronchiectasis, linear and triangular subpleural opacities, mosaic attenuation, and alveolar simplification is demonstrated in BPD-1 (born 24 weeks PMA, twin), whereas the findings in BPD-2 (PMA not reported, but born prematurely and progressively worsened to a chronic supplemental oxygen need) are atypical of BPD and demonstrate the potential for imaging to identify variants of disease.

regions, mosaic attenuation, bullae, and blebs) and parenchymal lesions (eg, triangular subpleural opacities, subpleural lines, atelectasis, and elements of architectural distortion) in an effort to develop a more objective system, and they showed correlation between their CT scores and physician-assessed clinical severities of BPD.

Aquino and colleagues[12] correlated CT findings in older children and adult BPD survivors with results from pulmonary function tests (PFTs) and reported abnormal CT findings in most of their patients (92%) and that the amount of hypoattenuated lung correlated with PFT findings, consistent with obstructive disease and air trapping (ie, elevated functional residual capacity, decreased forced expiratory volume in 1 second). Persistent structural abnormalities could predispose some adult BPD survivors to respiratory symptoms and morbidities, as supported by the work of Wong and colleagues,[17] who found linear and triangular opacities and emphysema in CT examinations of adult BPD survivors (**Fig. 3**) and correlated these findings with diminished respiratory function (PFT results including decreased forced expiratory volume in 1 second and elevated residual volume).[18] Longitudinal CT studies of BPD survivors are sparse, however, largely due to concerns over serial exposure to ionizing radiation.

There is potential for applying quantitative CT (qCT) techniques in pediatrics; nevertheless, these emerging methods are currently more explored in adult populations.[19] Sarria and colleagues[20] measured trachea and airway diameters and lung volumes and densities from CT examinations of preterm infants diagnosed with chronic lung disease of infancy and full-term controls. They found BPD patients had larger first

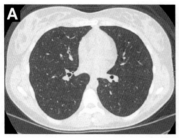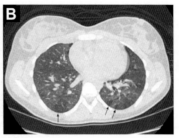

Fig. 3. BPD-associated parenchymal abnormalities can persist into adulthood. Inspiratory (*A*) and expiratory (*B*) CT scans from a 19-year-old, nonsmoking female BPD survivor (born at 25 weeks' gestation, weighing 740 g, on supplementary oxygen for 99 days postnatal) showing multilobular air trapping (*arrows*). (This material has not been reviewed by European Respiratory Society prior to release; therefore the European Respiratory Society may not be responsible for any errors, omissions or inaccuracies, or for any consequences arising there from, in the content. *From* Wong PM, Lees AN, Louw J, et al. Emphysema in young adult survivors of moderate-to-severe bronchopulmonary dysplasia. Eur Respir J 2008;32(2):324; reproduced with permission of the European Respiratory Society.)

and second airway generation diameters than controls and this correlated with duration of mechanical ventilation. However, the effect was only observed in subgroups of shorter subjects. Also, for the BPD group, increased airway cross-section was significantly correlated with days on mechanical ventilation and days on supplemental oxygen. There were no significant differences in total lung volume, air volume, tissue volume, and lung density between the BPD and control groups when corrected for patient size; however, BPD patients had higher heterogeneity (defined as the ratio of mean attenuation divided by the standard deviation) in the lung parenchyma than controls. In a case report from Khan and colleagues,[21] qCT was implemented to quantify air trapping in a BPD patient with acquired lobar emphysema, a rare but serious complication of BPD, as part of an evaluation for lobectomy, and revealed similar volumes on inspiration and expiration of the affected lobe; in this case, qCT measurements helped justify surgery. Multivolume CT analysis is another emerging qCT technique whereby changes in specific gas volume are calculated by segmenting, registering, and warping lungs of expiratory images onto inspiratory lung images, then subtracted pixel-by-pixel to determine regions of emphysema and gas trapping. In patients with emphysema, maps of change-specific gas volume were heterogeneous, identifying regions of trapped gas and emphysema, compared with healthy controls.[22,23] Although multivolume CT is unexplored in BPD survivors, in the future, it could be refined and implemented to quantify alveolar simplification in BPD, and in the rare instances of acquired lobar emphysema, could aid in planning volume reduction surgery.[24] In addition, alveolar simplification and air trapping potentially could be quantified using densitometric histograms in ways similar to emphysema; however, an absolute threshold will likely be inappropriate as lung density decreases as children grow and age.[25] Differences in pediatric CT protocols should also be considered. Virtual bronchoscopic reconstructions of CT data can provide images that simulate traditional endoscopy and allow for visualization of airways,[26] and although the technique has not been reported in BPD patients, there are a few instances of using virtual bronchoscopy in pediatric patients to investigate foreign body aspiration.[27,28]

Despite the increased spatial resolution, CT is not routinely ordered for infants and children unless there is indication from radiograph or elsewhere. The increased (ie, isotropic submillimeter) resolution of CT comes at the price of increased radiation dose as compared with chest radiograph; standard pediatric volumetric or spiral CT protocols have the radiation dose equivalent to ~50 chest radiographs, whereas a low-dose pediatric high-resolution CT protocol (1-mm slices at 10–20-mm spacing) has the radiation dose equivalent to 10 to 15 chest radiographs.[29] Ionizing radiation exposure is the largest drawback to CT; however, there has been much recent work toward optimizing pediatric CT protocols to provide sufficient diagnostic quality yet minimizing the radiation dose.[30–32] Although CT is recognized as the current clinical gold standard for pulmonary imaging, the modality does not have an easy place in routine or longitudinal monitoring of BPD survivors as serial radiation exposure has been linked to increased risk of cancer.[33,34]

NUCLEAR MEDICINE

Both radiograph and CT provide structural information regarding the lung parenchyma and vasculature, and the structural detail provided by both modalities is sometimes used in conjunction with scintigraphy, which provides a spatial distribution of perfusion and ventilation (V/Q) of tracers such as ^{99}Tc, ^{133}Xe, or Technegas.[35,36] **Fig. 4** is an example of a ventilation scan demonstrating uneven radiotracer distribution in the lungs of a 6-month-old BPD survivor. The technique is not routine in neonates and infants due to concerns from radioactive tracers; however, there are limited reports of V/Q scans in BPD patients, many of which focus on BPD patients with acquired lobar emphysema or overinflation.[37,38]

Moylan and Shannon[37] reported ^{133}Xe ventilation scintigraphy in BPD patients with lobar overinflation and showed the overinflated lobe was poorly ventilated, likely due to air trapping. Soler and colleagues[38] demonstrated perfusion scintigraphy in a cohort of BPD survivors and control premature patients without BPD; scintigraphy performed at 6 months corrected age was qualitatively and quantitatively scored and compared with clinical and radiographic scores (ie, Toce radiograph scoring). BPD patients showed abnormal lung perfusion patterns compared with control patients; to quantify the degree of heterogeneity in the perfusion patterns, the investigators developed a lobar-based scoring system and reported BPD patients had higher scores than controls, indicating greater severity of perfusion defects. The investigators suggest that scintigraphy of BPD suffers from low specificity because many diseases can produce similar images, but the modality may be useful for younger patients who cannot perform PFTs.

Murray and colleagues[9] reported V/Q scans in 3 BPD patients with acquired lobar overinflation, and for these few patients, revealed no V/Q mismatch in the overinflated lobes but defects in other collapsed lobes of the lungs; the investigators suggest scintigraphy and bronchoscopy should be implemented to determine if lobectomy is appropriate, because this complication is associated with high mortality and poor outcomes.

In the case study by Khan and colleagues[21] of a BPD patient with acquired lobar emphysema, V/Q scanning revealed a large perfusion defect and correspondingly decreased ventilation in the affected lobe. Hypoperfusion has also been reported in BPD patients with pulmonary hypertension.[39] Recent advancements in single-photon emission computed tomography (SPECT) techniques have allowed for spatial mapping of both ventilation and perfusion in infants and neonates,[35] and Kjellberg and colleagues[36] used SPECT to determine V/Q ratios in infants with BPD and reported a significant negative correlation between the duration of mechanical ventilation and V/Q matching (**Fig. 5**).

MRI

Perhaps the greatest advantage of MRI is that, unlike the imaging modalities previously discussed, it is a nonionizing technique that instead uses radiofrequency energy

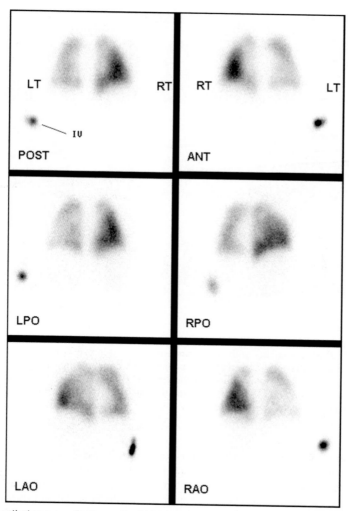

Fig. 4. Ventilation scan of a 6-month-old BPD survivor (female patient, born 26 weeks PMA) showing focal regions of abnormal perfusion in the right upper apex and left lateral basal lung. ANT, anterior; IV, intravenous; LAO, left anterior oblique; LPO, left posterior oblique; POST, posterior; RAO, right anterior oblique; RPO, right posterior oblique; RT, right.

to manipulate nuclear spins to generate images; this is particularly important for imaging children who are more vulnerable to damage from radiation exposure and is significant for cases of chronic illness where longitudinal monitoring is desirable. However, MRI is not without its drawbacks; the equipment is large and expensive, and given the small magnetic moments of the spins producing the signal, a single imaging sequence can take several minutes to acquire, leading to longer examination times than CT.

Conventional ¹H MRI

The technological challenges of conventional ¹H MRI of the lung parenchyma have limited its clinical usefulness until recently. The proton density of the lung parenchyma

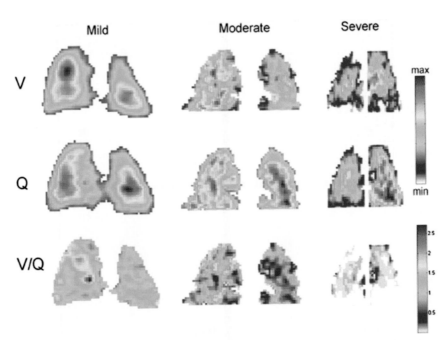

Fig. 5. Representative coronal SPECT slices of lung ventilation (V), perfusion (Q), and V/Q ratio for individual patients with mild, moderate, and severe BPD demonstrating good V/Q matching in the mild and moderate patients but poor V/Q matching in the severe BPD patient. (*Reprinted from* Kjellberg M, Bjorkman K, Rohdin M, et al. Bronchopulmonary dysplasia: clinical grading in relation to ventilation/perfusion mismatch measured by single photon emission computed tomography. Pediatr Pulmonol 2013;48(12):1209; with permission.)

is only about one-fifth that of muscle, and as a result, MRI signal intensity is weakened relative to other soft tissues. Furthermore, the alveoli, which provide the necessary air-tissue surface area for gas exchange, contribute to magnetic inhomogeneity and rapid signal decay (ie, short T_2^*, on the order of 2 milliseconds[40]), and motion artifacts from cardiac and respiratory motion degrade image quality.[41] MRI of neonatal or infant lungs is additionally confounded by the small patient size, rapid respiratory rate, and inability to perform a breath-hold maneuver.

Despite these setbacks, Adams and colleagues[42] at Hammersmith Hospital (London) first reported using a specially designed, small-bore 1.0-T MRI scanner in the NICU to image lung fluid in preterm and full-term neonates and reported that preterm infants had higher, more heterogeneously distributed proton density throughout the parenchyma than term controls; they also demonstrated a gravity-dependent density gradient by imaging patients supine and prone. A second report from the Hammersmith team specific to neonates with BPD found higher relative proton density in BPD patients versus controls and described 2 types of parenchymal abnormalities in BPD infants: focal high-density areas and low-density, cystlike abnormalities.[43]

Colleagues at Cincinnati Children's Hospital Medical Center designed and modified a small-footprint 1.5-T orthopedic MRI scanner for use in the authors' NICU,[44–46] and they recently reported success imaging nonsedate, free-breathing BPD patients using this scanner and standard MRI pulse sequences.[47] Stark and significant differences in parenchymal signal intensity were observed in the BPD patients compared with full-term control NICU patients (**Fig. 6**); focal and diffuse regions of high-signal-intensity parenchyma were observed, and using a modified Ochiai system for CT,[15] BPD patients had higher clinical scores than control NICU patients, indicating more severe parenchymal disease. Although these reports used specially designed MRI scanners, wider implementation of small footprint MRI scanners in NICUs is on the horizon because scanners are becoming increasingly available.

There is still much to be learned about BPD from older children and adult survivors, too, as newer strategies for MRI of the lungs are more widely implemented. As mentioned earlier, the short T_2^* of the lung parenchyma has been a major challenge, meaning that the echo time of the MRI pulse sequence must be short enough to capture the parenchymal signal before it decays; indeed, in most conventional MRIs, the lung parenchyma appears dark and is void of much structural information. Emerging ultrashort and zero echo-time techniques are designed with submillisecond echo times, thereby capturing the parenchymal signal before it decays, and these methods have recently demonstrated their ability to image lung parenchyma and vasculature at resolutions rivaling CT.[48–51] In addition to these structural measures from ^{1}H MRI, sophisticated O_2-enhanced[52,53] and arterial spin-labeling[54,55] techniques use inhaled 100% O_2 or the endogenous contrast of the blood, respectively, rather than a radio-labeled tracer to spatially resolve and quantify ventilation and perfusion.[56] These methods are rapidly emerging, and although applications in BPD remain unexplored as of yet, as clinical implementation widens (many of these techniques are scanner software upgrades and should be disseminated quickly), MRI is poised to make major

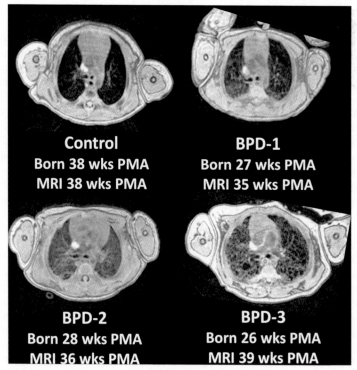

Fig. 6. Differences in parenchymal structure of control and 3 BPD patients using a small-footprint 1.5-T MRI scanner in the NICU. PMA at birth and at MRI are given for each patient.

contributions to pulmonary medicine and, to the knowledge of BPD progression, as well as normal and aberrant lung development.

Hyperpolarized-Gas MRI

Because MRI of the lung parenchyma is challenging, an alternative strategy is to image an inhaled hyperpolarized noble gas (ie, ^{3}He or ^{129}Xe). Since the early 1990s, hyperpolarized gas MRI has been demonstrated in participants, both healthy participants and those with myriad pulmonary conditions, across a wide age range. The magnetic resonance signal from a hyperpolarized gas typically arises from spin-exchange optical pumping—a 2-step process of angular momentum transfer first from circularly polarized laser photons to the electronic spins of an alkali metal vapor, and then onward to the nuclear spins of the noble gas via collisions.[57] Over time, the noble gas polarization builds to exceed the thermal Boltzmann equilibrium by several orders of magnitude; then the gas is dispensed from the polarizer and quickly shuttled to the MRI scanner where it is inhaled for imaging.

Regional functional and microstructural information can be derived from hyperpolarized-gas MRI, the techniques of which can be classified into 3 general categories: ventilation imaging, diffusion imaging, and in the special case of ^{129}Xe, dissolved-phase imaging. Static spin-density images are technologically simple and provide maps of ventilation; healthy, well-ventilated lungs will appear uniformly bright, whereas ventilation defects (ie, poorly ventilated regions of the lung) will appear dark, indicating that the flow of hyperpolarized gas to that region was partially or fully obstructed.[58–60] Imaging hyperpolarized gas with bipolar diffusion-sensing gradients, the apparent diffusion coefficient (ADC)[61–63] of the gas can be used to determine acinar airspace geometry; the walls of the airways and alveoli restrict the Brownian motion of the atoms, and using simple models based on Haefeli-Bleuer and Weibel[64] (ie, cylindrical airways covered with alveoli), acinar duct radii and alveolar lumen radii can be measured noninvasively.[65–67] ADC measurements have been well validated histologically and have been shown to be exquisitely sensitive to airway microstructural changes.[68–71] Finally, because of the slight solubility of ^{129}Xe in tissues and blood, dissolved-phase imaging of hyperpolarized ^{129}Xe can be used to probe gas exchange and perfusion dynamics.[72–76] In general, all of these techniques are possible with a single breath-hold (<20 s, typically much shorter) of hyperpolarized gas. More in-depth reviews of the translational applications of hyperpolarized gas-MRI,[77] as well as applications specific to ^{3}He MRI[78] and ^{129}Xe MRI,[79] can be found elsewhere.

Hyperpolarized-gas MRI has been well tolerated in pediatric patients and healthy volunteers with successful breath-hold maneuvers performed in children as young as 4 years old reported[80] and a recent proof-of-concept demonstrated ^{3}He MRI in a healthy, nonsedated 13-month-old infant (**Fig. 7**).[81] Most of the limited pediatric work with hyperpolarized-gas MRI has focused on asthma and cystic fibrosis[82]; however, Altes and colleagues[83] at University of Virginia performed ^{3}He MRI in BPD survivors (mean age 9.7 years old) and reported that BPD survivors had more heterogeneous ADC maps than age-matched controls (**Fig. 8**). In addition to focal areas of increased ADC, children with BPD had higher mean ADC values than controls, which is consistent with histologic evidence of arrested lung development resulting in simplified alveoli. In addition, Narayanan and colleagues[84] reported that BPD survivors (age range of 10–14 years old) had similar alveolar size and numbers compared with full-term peers as determined with ^{3}He ADC measurements, suggesting catch-up alveolarization in premature infants as they age; although limited to children who had mild to moderate BPD, the study highlights the ability of

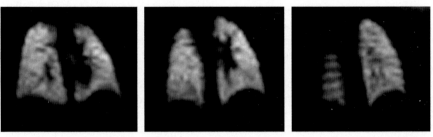

Fig. 7. Hyperpolarized ³He MRI ventilation images in a healthy, nonsedated, nonrestrained 13-month-old infant performed in an adult-sized 1.5-T MRI scanner. (*Reprinted from* Altes TA, Meyer CH, Mata JH, et al. Hyperpolarized helium-3 MR imaging of a non-sedated infant: a proof-of-concept study. Proc Intl Soc Mag Reson Med 2012;20:1355; with permission.)

hyperpolarized-gas ADC measurements to quantify lung microstructure and pediatric lung development.

Beyond these limited reports, there is great opportunity for hyperpolarized-gas MRI to add to the understanding of BPD. Mapping and quantifying trapped gas have been demonstrated using ³He MRI, for example, and correlated well with multivolume CT results in an ex vivo porcine model.[85] These methods can be extended to neonates. The extent of alveolar simplification could be spatially resolved with hyperpolarized-gas ADC mapping, and with longitudinal measurements, lung growth and

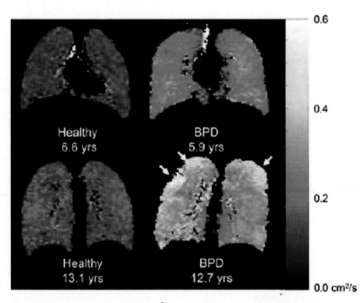

Fig. 8. Coronal slices of hyperpolarized ³He ADC maps in 2 healthy children (*left column*) and 2 BPD survivors (*right column*). The healthy children have homogenously low ADC values, with the older child (*bottom left*) having slightly elevated values. The BPD survivors have higher ADC values, and the older survivor (*bottom right*) has focal regions of marked elevated ADC (*arrows*). (*Reprinted from* Altes TA, Mata J, Froh DK, et al. Abnormalities of lung structure in children with bronchopulmonary dysplasia as assessed by diffusion hyperpolarized helium-3 MRI. Proc Intl Soc Mag Reson Med 2006;14:86; with permission.)

development can be objectively assessed. Although hyperpolarized-gas MRI has been reported for several decades and the safety of ^{3}He and ^{129}Xe demonstrated repeatedly,[86,87] the wider implementation and clinical translation of the technique have been hindered by its limited access and regulation of these noble gases as drugs. If true clinical translation of hyperpolarized-gas MRI is to be realized, compact and simplified "push-button" polarizers must become clinically accessible. Currently, hyperpolarized-gas MRI is limited to several specialized centers with the few commercially available polarizers or the in-house expertise to build their own; however, the recent commercialization efforts from Polarean (Research Triangle Park, NC, USA),[88] as well as so-called open-source polarizers,[89-91] aim to realize wider clinical implementation of hyperpolarized-gas MRI in the near future.

SUMMARY

Clinical imaging has played a pivotal role in recognizing the structural abnormalities associated with BPD since its recognition, and over the past two decades, as standards of postnatal care of premature infants have shifted, the definition and radiological characteristics of BPD have evolved as well. BPD is recognized as a highly complex, multifaceted condition with high variability patient to patient. With emerging imaging techniques, the opportunities to recognize individual phenotypes of BPD, to personalize therapies and assess new ones, and to provide longitudinal monitoring as survivors age are all on the horizon.

Although chest radiograph will continue to be the first line of clinical radiological inquiry, especially for acute morbidity, the future of BPD imaging lies in nonionizing modalities, semiautomated and fully automated quantitative techniques that allow for objective, longitudinal assessment, and the translation of these methods to predict outcomes and personalize patient care. Newer, low-dose CT protocols continue to lessen radiation burden, but for BPD survivors with chronic lung disease, balancing the benefits of longitudinal assessment with the risks of serial radiation exposure must be considered. Many of the major technological hurdles that limited the clinical utility of pulmonary MRI historically are beginning to clear, and furthermore, these technologies are being extended to the youngest, most challenging patients to image, neonates, so there is great opportunity for MRI to add to the knowledge of BPD from its earliest roots and longitudinally as these patients age.

There is exciting opportunity for clinical imaging to expand the definitions and understanding of BPD, to move beyond essentially defining BPD by its treatment. By focusing on the underlying pathologic characteristics contributing to an individual patient's condition, quantitative assessment of disease severity, longitudinal treatment efficacy, and outcomes prediction, clinical imaging is likely to contribute to lower mortality and better outcomes for BPD.

REFERENCES

1. Northway WH Jr, Rosan RC, Porter DY. Pulmonary disease following respirator therapy of hyaline-membrane disease. Bronchopulmonary dysplasia. N Engl J Med 1967;276(7):357–68.
2. Jobe AH. The new bronchopulmonary dysplasia. Curr Opin Pediatr 2011;23(2): 167–72.
3. Johnson TJ, Patel AL, Jegier BJ, et al. Cost of morbidities in very low birth weight infants. J Pediatr 2013;162(2):243–9.e1.
4. Bhandari A, Bhandari V. Biomarkers in bronchopulmonary dysplasia. Paediatr Respir Rev 2013;14(3):173–9.

5. Toce SS, Farrell PM, Leavitt LA, et al. Clinical and roentgenographic scoring systems for assessing bronchopulmonary dysplasia. Am J Dis Child 1984;138(6): 581–5.
6. Edwards DK. Radiology of hyaline membrane disease: transient tachypnea of the newborn, and bronchopulmonary dysplasia, vol. 2. New York: Academic Press Inc; 1982.
7. Breysem L, Smet MH, Van Lierde S, et al. Bronchopulmonary dysplasia: correlation of radiographic and clinical findings. Pediatr Radiol 1997;27(8):642–6.
8. Miller KE, Edwards DK, Hilton S, et al. Acquired lobar emphysema in premature infants with bronchopulmonary dysplasia: an iatrogenic disease? Radiology 1981;138(3):589–92.
9. Murray C, Pilling DW, Shaw NJ. Persistent acquired lobar overinflation complicating bronchopulmonary dysplasia. Eur J Pediatr 2000;159(1–2):14–7.
10. Oppenheim C, Mamou-Mani T, Sayegh N, et al. Bronchopulmonary dysplasia: value of CT in identifying pulmonary sequelae. Am J Roentgenol 1994;163(1): 169–72.
11. Mahut B, De Blic J, Emond S, et al. Chest computed tomography findings in bronchopulmonary dysplasia and correlation with lung function. Arch Dis Child Fetal Neonatal Ed 2007;92(6):F459–64.
12. Aquino SL, Schechter MS, Chiles C, et al. High-resolution inspiratory and expiratory CT in older children and adults with bronchopulmonary dysplasia. AJR Am J Roentgenol 1999;173(4):963–7.
13. Howling SJ, Northway WH Jr, Hansell DM, et al. Pulmonary sequelae of bronchopulmonary dysplasia survivors: high-resolution CT findings. AJR Am J Roentgenol 2000;174(5):1323–6.
14. Aukland SM, Halvorsen T, Fosse KR, et al. High-resolution CT of the chest in children and young adults who were born prematurely: findings in a population-based study. AJR Am J Roentgenol 2006;187(4):1012–8.
15. Ochiai M, Hikino S, Yabuuchi H, et al. A new scoring system for computed tomography of the chest for assessing the clinical status of bronchopulmonary dysplasia. J Pediatr 2008;152(1):90–5, 95.e91–3.
16. Shin SM, Kim WS, Cheon JE, et al. Bronchopulmonary dysplasia: new high resolution computed tomography scoring system and correlation between the high resolution computed tomography score and clinical severity. Korean J Radiol 2013;14(2):350–60.
17. Wong P, Murray C, Louw J, et al. Adult bronchopulmonary dysplasia: computed tomography pulmonary findings. J Med Imaging Radiat Oncol 2011;55(4):373–8.
18. Wong PM, Lees AN, Louw J, et al. Emphysema in young adult survivors of moderate-to-severe bronchopulmonary dysplasia. Eur Respir J 2008;32(2): 321–8.
19. Yoon SH, Goo JM, Goo HW. Quantitative thoracic CT techniques in adults: can they be applied in the pediatric population? Pediatr Radiol 2013;43(3):308–14.
20. Sarria EE, Mattiello R, Rao L, et al. Quantitative assessment of chronic lung disease of infancy using computed tomography. Eur Respir J 2012;39(4):992–9.
21. Khan S, Kurland G, Newman B. Controlled-ventilation volumetric CT scan in the evaluation of acquired pulmonary lobar emphysema: a case report. Pediatr Pulmonol 2007;42(12):1222–8.
22. Aliverti A, Pennati F, Salito C, et al. Regional lung function and heterogeneity of specific gas volume in healthy and emphysematous subjects. Eur Respir J 2013;41(5):1179–88.

23. Pennati F, Salito C, Baroni G, et al. Comparison between multivolume CT-based surrogates of regional ventilation in healthy subjects. Acad Radiol 2014;21(10):1268–75.

24. Salito C, Barazzetti L, Woods JC, et al. Heterogeneity of specific gas volume changes: a new tool to plan lung volume reduction in COPD. Chest 2014; 146(6):1554–65.

25. Long FR, Williams RS, Castile RG. Inspiratory and expiratory CT lung density in infants and young children. Pediatr Radiol 2005;35(7):677–83.

26. Salito C, Barazzetti L, Woods JC, et al. 3D airway tree reconstruction in healthy subjects and emphysema. Lung 2011;189(4):287–93.

27. Adaletli I, Kurugoglu S, Ulus S, et al. Utilization of low-dose multidetector CT and virtual bronchoscopy in children with suspected foreign body aspiration. Pediatr Radiol 2007;37(1):33–40.

28. Bhat KV, Hegde JS, Nagalotimath US, et al. Evaluation of computed tomography virtual bronchoscopy in paediatric tracheobronchial foreign body aspiration. J Laryngol Otol 2010;124(8):875–9.

29. Rossi UG, Owens CM. The radiology of chronic lung disease in children. Arch Dis Child 2005;90(6):601–7.

30. Li X, Samei E, Segars WP, et al. Patient-specific radiation dose and cancer risk for pediatric chest CT. Radiology 2011;259(3):862–74.

31. Macdougall RD, Strauss KJ, Lee EY. Managing radiation dose from thoracic multidetector computed tomography in pediatric patients: background, current issues, and recommendations. Radiol Clin North Am 2013;51(4):743–60.

32. Kim JE, Newman B. Evaluation of a radiation dose reduction strategy for pediatric chest CT. AJR Am J Roentgenol 2010;194(5):1188–93.

33. Brenner DJ, Elliston CD, Hall EJ, et al. Estimated risks of radiation-induced fatal cancer from pediatric CT. Am J Roentgenol 2001;176(2):289–96.

34. Pearce MS, Salotti JA, Little MP, et al. Radiation exposure from CT scans in childhood and subsequent risk of leukaemia and brain tumours: a retrospective cohort study. Lancet 2012;380(9840):499–505.

35. Sanchez-Crespo A, Rohdin M, Carlsson C, et al. A technique for lung ventilation-perfusion SPECT in neonates and infants. Nucl Med Commun 2008;29(2):173–7.

36. Kjellberg M, Bjorkman K, Rohdin M, et al. Bronchopulmonary dysplasia: clinical grading in relation to ventilation/perfusion mismatch measured by single photon emission computed tomography. Pediatr Pulmonol 2013;48(12):1206–13.

37. Moylan FM, Shannon DC. Preferential distribution of lobar emphysema and atelectasis in bronchopulmonary dysplasia. Pediatrics 1979;63(1):130–4.

38. Soler C, Figueras J, Roca I, et al. Pulmonary perfusion scintigraphy in the evaluation of the severity of bronchopulmonary dysplasia. Pediatr Radiol 1997;27(1): 32–5.

39. del Cerro MJ, Sabate Rotes A, Carton A, et al. Pulmonary hypertension in bronchopulmonary dysplasia: clinical findings, cardiovascular anomalies and outcomes. Pediatr Pulmonol 2014;49(1):49–59.

40. Yu J, Xue Y, Song HK. Comparison of lung T2* during free-breathing at 1.5 T and 3.0 T with ultrashort echo time imaging. Magn Reson Med 2011;66(1):248–54.

41. Mulkern R, Haker S, Mamata H, et al. Lung parenchymal signal intensity in MRI: a technical review with educational aspirations regarding reversible versus irreversible transverse relaxation effects in common pulse sequences. Concepts Magn Reson Part A Bridg Educ Res 2014;43A(2):29–53.

42. Adams EW, Counsell SJ, Hajnal JV, et al. Magnetic resonance imaging of lung water content and distribution in term and preterm infants. Am J Respir Crit Care Med 2002;166(3):397–402.

43. Adams EW, Harrison MC, Counsell SJ, et al. Increased lung water and tissue damage in bronchopulmonary dysplasia. J Pediatr 2004;145(4):503–7.
44. Tkach JA, Hillman NH, Jobe AH, et al. An MRI system for imaging neonates in the NICU: initial feasibility study. Pediatr Radiol 2012;42(11):1347–56.
45. Tkach JA, Merhar SL, Kline-Fath BM, et al. MRI in the neonatal ICU: initial experience using a small-footprint 1.5-T system. AJR Am J Roentgenol 2014;202(1): w95–105.
46. Tkach JA, Li Y, Pratt RG, et al. Characterization of acoustic noise in a neonatal intensive care unit MRI system. Pediatr Radiol 2014;44(8):1011–9.
47. Walkup LL, Tkach JA, Higano NS, et al. Quantitative magnetic resonance imaging of bronchopulmonary dysplasia in the NICU environment. Am J Respir Crit Care Med 2015. [Epub ahead of print].
48. Johnson KM, Fain SB, Schiebler ML, et al. Optimized 3D ultrashort echo time pulmonary MRI. Magn Reson Med 2013;70(5):1241–50.
49. Molinari F, Madhuranthakam AJ, Lenkinski R, et al. Ultrashort echo time MRI of pulmonary water content: assessment in a sponge phantom at 1.5 and 3.0 Tesla. Diagn Interv Radiol 2014;20(1):34–41.
50. Lederlin M, Cremillieux Y. Three-dimensional assessment of lung tissue density using a clinical ultrashort echo time at 3 tesla: a feasibility study in healthy subjects. J Magn Reson Imaging 2014;40(4):839–47.
51. Bell LC, Johnson KM, Fain SB, et al. Simultaneous MRI of lung structure and perfusion in a single breathhold. J Magn Reson Imaging 2015;41(1):52–9.
52. Triphan SM, Breuer FA, Gensler D, et al. Oxygen enhanced lung MRI by simultaneous measurement of T and T* during free breathing using ultrashort TE. J Magn Reson Imaging 2015;41(6):1708–14.
53. Kruger SJ, Fain SB, Johnson KM, et al. Oxygen-enhanced 3D radial ultrashort echo time magnetic resonance imaging in the healthy human lung. NMR Biomed 2014;27(12):1535–41.
54. Schraml C, Schwenzer NF, Martirosian P, et al. Non-invasive pulmonary perfusion assessment in young patients with cystic fibrosis using an arterial spin labeling MR technique at 1.5 T. MAGMA 2012;25(2):155–62.
55. Hopkins SR, Prisk GK. Lung perfusion measured using magnetic resonance imaging: new tools for physiological insights into the pulmonary circulation. J Magn Reson Imaging 2010;32(6):1287–301.
56. Miller GW, Mugler JP 3rd, Sa RC, et al. Advances in functional and structural imaging of the human lung using proton MRI. NMR Biomed 2014;27(12):1542–56.
57. Walker TG, Happer W. Spin-exchange optical pumping of noble-gas nuclei. Rev Mod Phys 1997;69(2):629–42.
58. Kauczor HU, Ebert M, Kreitner KF, et al. Imaging of the lungs using 3He MRI: preliminary clinical experience in 18 patients with and without lung disease. J Magn Reson Imaging 1997;7(3):538–43.
59. Spector ZZ, Emami K, Fischer MC, et al. A small animal model of regional alveolar ventilation using HP 3He MRI1. Acad Radiol 2004;11(10):1171–9.
60. Altes TA, Powers PL, Knight-Scott J, et al. Hyperpolarized He-3 MR lung ventilation imaging in asthmatics: preliminary findings. J Magn Reson Imaging 2001; 13(3):378–84.
61. Woods JC, Yablonskiy DA, Choong CK, et al. Long-range diffusion of hyperpolarized He-3 in explanted normal and emphysematous human lungs via magnetization tagging. J Appl Physiol (1985) 2005;99(5):1992–7.
62. Saam BT, Yablonskiy DA, Kodibagkar VD, et al. MR imaging of diffusion of He-3 gas in healthy and diseased lungs. Magn Reson Med 2000;44(2):174–9.

63. Kaushik SS, Cleveland ZI, Cofer GP, et al. Diffusion-weighted hyperpolarized Xe-129 MRI in healthy volunteers and subjects with chronic obstructive pulmonary disease. Magn Reson Med 2011;65(4):1155–65.

64. Haefeli-Bleuer B, Weibel ER. Morphology of the human pulmonary acinus. Anat Rec 1988;220(4):401–14.

65. Mugler JP 3rd, Wang C, Miller GW, et al. Helium-3 diffusion MR imaging of the human lung over multiple time scales. Acad Radiol 2008;15(6):693–701.

66. Yablonskiy DA, Sukstanskii AL, Quirk JD, et al. Probing lung microstructure with hyperpolarized noble gas diffusion MRI: theoretical models and experimental results. Magn Reson Med 2014;71:486.

67. Quirk JD, Chang YV, Yablonskiy DA. In vivo lung morphometry with hyperpolarized (3)He diffusion MRI: reproducibility and the role of diffusion-sensitizing gradient direction. Magn Reson Med 2015;73(3):1252–7.

68. Quirk JD, Lutey BA, Gierada DS, et al. In vivo detection of acinar microstructural changes in early emphysema with (3)He lung morphometry. Radiology 2011; 260(3):866–74.

69. Wang W, Nguyen NM, Guo J, et al. Longitudinal, noninvasive monitoring of compensatory lung growth in mice after pneumonectomy via (3)He and (1) H magnetic resonance imaging. Am J Respir Cell Mol Biol 2013;49(5): 697–703.

70. Cereda M, Emami K, Kadlecek S, et al. Quantitative imaging of alveolar recruitment with hyperpolarized gas MRI during mechanical ventilation. J Appl Physiol (1985) 2011;110(2):499–511.

71. Narayanan M, Owers-Bradley J, Beardsmore CS, et al. Alveolarization continues during childhood and adolescence: new evidence from helium-3 magnetic resonance. Am J Respir Crit Care Med 2012;185(2):186–91.

72. Qing K, Mugler JP 3rd, Altes TA, et al. Assessment of lung function in asthma and COPD using hyperpolarized 129Xe chemical shift saturation recovery spectroscopy and dissolved-phase MRI. NMR Biomed 2014;27(12):1490–501.

73. Kaushik SS, Freeman MS, Cleveland ZI, et al. Probing the regional distribution of pulmonary gas exchange through single-breath gas- and dissolved-phase 129Xe MR imaging. J Appl Physiol (1985) 2013;115(6):850–60.

74. Cleveland ZI, Cofer GP, Metz G, et al. Hyperpolarized Xe MR imaging of alveolar gas uptake in humans. PLoS One 2010;5(8):e12192.

75. Ruppert K, Brookeman JR, Hagspiel KD, et al. Probing lung physiology with xenon polarization transfer contrast (XTC). Magn Reson Med 2000;44(3): 349–57.

76. Patz S, Muradyan I, Hrovat MI, et al. Diffusion of hyperpolarized Xe-129 in the lung: a simplified model of Xe-129 septal uptake and experimental results. New J Phys 2011;13:015009.

77. Walkup LL, Woods JC. Translational applications of hyperpolarized (3) He and (129) Xe. NMR Biomed 2014;27(12):1429–38.

78. Fain S, Schiebler ML, McCormack DG, et al. Imaging of lung function using hyperpolarized helium-3 magnetic resonance imaging: review of current and emerging translational methods and applications. J Magn Reson Imaging 2010;32(6):1398–408.

79. Mugler JP 3rd, Altes TA. Hyperpolarized 129Xe MRI of the human lung. J Magn Reson Imaging 2013;37(2):313–31.

80. Altes TA, Mata J, de Lange EE, et al. Assessment of lung development using hyperpolarized helium-3 diffusion MR imaging. J Magn Reson Imaging 2006;24(6): 1277–83.

81. Altes TA, Meyer CH, Mata JH, et al. Hyperpolarized helium-3 MR imaging of a non-sedated infant: a proof-of-concept study. Proc Intl Soc Mag Reson Med 2012;20:1355.
82. Kirby M, Coxson HO, Parraga G. Pulmonary functional magnetic resonance imaging for paediatric lung disease. Paediatr Respir Rev 2013;14(3):180–9.
83. Altes TA, Mata J, Froh DK, et al. Abnormalities of lung structure in children with bronchopulmonary dysplasia as assessed by diffusion hyperpolarized helium-3 MRI. Proc Intl Soc Mag Reson Med 2006;14:86.
84. Narayanan M, Beardsmore CS, Owers-Bradley J, et al. Catch-up alveolarization in ex-preterm children: evidence from (3)He magnetic resonance. Am J Respir Crit Care Med 2013;187(10):1104–9.
85. Salito C, Aliverti A, Gierada DS, et al. Quantification of trapped gas with CT and 3 He MR imaging in a porcine model of isolated airway obstruction. Radiology 2009;253(2):380–9.
86. Driehuys B, Martinez-Jimenez S, Cleveland ZI, et al. Chronic obstructive pulmonary disease: safety and tolerability of hyperpolarized Xe-129 MR imaging in healthy volunteers and patients. Radiology 2012;262(1):279–89.
87. Lutey BA, Lefrak SS, Woods JC, et al. Hyperpolarized 3He MR imaging: physiologic monitoring observations and safety considerations in 100 consecutive subjects. Radiology 2008;248(2):655–61.
88. Driehuys B, Cates G, Miron E, et al. High-volume production of laser-polarized 129Xe. Appl Phys Lett 1996;69(12):1668–70.
89. Nikolaou P, Coffey AM, Walkup LL, et al. XeNA: an automated 'open-source' (129) Xe hyperpolarizer for clinical use. Magn Reson Imaging 2014;32(5):541–50.
90. Nikolaou P, Coffey AM, Walkup LL, et al. Near-unity nuclear polarization with an open-source 129Xe hyperpolarizer for NMR and MRI. Proc Natl Acad Sci U S A 2013;110(35):14150–5.
91. Nikolaou P, Coffey AM, Walkup LL, et al. A 3D-printed high power nuclear spin polarizer. J Am Chem Soc 2014;136(4):1636–42.

Bronchopulmonary Dysplasia and Chronic Lung Disease: Stem Cell Therapy

Maria Pierro, MD[a,b,]*, Elena Ciarmoli, MD[c],
Bernard Thébaud, MD, PhD[d,e,f]

KEYWORDS

- Bronchopulmonary dysplasia • Prematurity • Stem cells • Newborn
- Clinical translation

KEY POINTS

- In the past few years, increasing insight into stem cell biology has generated excitement about the potential of stem cells to repair, and perhaps to regenerate, damaged organs. Among stem cells, mesenchymal stromal (stem) cells (MSCs) have attracted much attention because of their ease of isolation, multilineage potential, and immunomodulatory properties.
- MSCs ameliorate many critical aspects of bronchopulmonary dysplasia pathogenesis in preclinical models by mitigating lung inflammation, inducing vascular and alveolar growth, and inhibiting lung fibrosis.
- MSCs are preferentially attracted to sites of injury where they exert their therapeutic effects thanks to the interaction with the immune system and to the paracrine secretion of anti-inflammatory, antioxidant, antiapoptotic, trophic, and proangiogenic factors.
- Several details, including timing of administration, route of administration, dose, cell source, and manufacturing processes of the final stem cell product, may influence success or failure of the therapy.

The authors have nothing to disclose.
[a] Department of Clinical Sciences and Community Health, Fondazione IRCCS Cà Granda Ospedale Maggiore Policlinico, University of Milan, Via della Commenda 12, Milan 20122, Italy; [b] Neonatal Intensive Care Unit, IRCCS Istituto Giannina Gaslini, Via Gerolamo Gaslini, 5, Genova 16148, Italy; [c] Neonatal Intensive Care Unit, MBBM Foundation, San Gerardo Hospital, Via Pergolesi 33, Monza 20900, Italy; [d] Division of Neonatology, Department of Pediatrics, Children's Hospital of Eastern Ontario, 401 Smyth Road, Ottawa, ON K1H 8L1, Canada; [e] Regenerative Medicine Program, Sprott Center for Stem Cell Research, Ottawa Hospital Research Institute, The Ottawa Hospital, 501 Smyth Road, Ottawa, Ontario K1H8L6, Canada; [f] Department of Cellular and Molecular Medicine, Sinclair Institute of Regenerative Medicine, University of Ottawa, 501 Smyth Road, Ottawa, ON K1H 8L6, Canada
* Corresponding author. Department of Clinical Sciences and Community Health, Fondazione IRCCS Cà Granda Ospedale Maggiore Policlinico, University of Milan, Via della Commenda 12, Milan 20122, Italy.
E-mail address: maria.pierro@mangiagalli.it

Clin Perinatol 42 (2015) 889–910
http://dx.doi.org/10.1016/j.clp.2015.08.013
0095-5108/15/$ – see front matter © 2015 Elsevier Inc. All rights reserved.

INTRODUCTION

Despite continuous advances of perinatal care, bronchopulmonary dysplasia (BPD) remains a significant burden of extreme prematurity because it lacks a safe and effective treatment.[1,2] In the past few years, increasing insight into stem cell biology has generated excitement about the potential of stem cells to regenerate damaged organs. Stem cells are primitive cells capable of extensive self-renewal with the potential to give rise to multiple differentiated cellular phenotypes. Stem cells play a crucial role in organogenesis and growth during the early stages of development, as well as in organ repair and regeneration throughout life.[3]

MESENCHYMAL STROMAL CELLS

Among stem cells, mesenchymal stromal (stem) cells (MSCs) have attracted much attention because of their ease of isolation, multilineage potential, and immunomodulatory properties.[4] MSCs represent a broad and heterogeneous cell population, defined by 3 minimum criteria: (1) adhesion to plastic when cultured in a tissue culture flask under standard culturing conditions, (2) expression of specific surface markers (CD73, CD90, CD105) and lack of expression of hematopoietic markers, and (3) ability to differentiate into mesodermic (osteogenic, chondrogenic, and adipogenic) lineages on in vitro stimulation.[4]

DISRUPTION OF MESENCHYMAL STROMAL CELL HOMEOSTASIS IN THE EVENTS THAT LEAD TO BRONCHOPULMONARY DYSPLASIA

It is now generally accepted that MSCs reside in all tissues of the human body.[5] Although all MSCs share the 3 minimum criteria, MSCs from different tissues, including lung-resident MSCs, also display distinct functional characteristics to support their specific microenvironment[6] and are considered guardians of tissue repair and maintenance. The role of lung-resident MSCs in the development of BPD remains to be elucidated. Circulating and lung-resident MSCs number and function seems to be perturbed in human and experimental BPD.[7-9] These findings provide a rational for exogenous supplementation of MSCs for the prevention or repair of neonatal lung injury.[9]

PRECLINICAL EVIDENCE OF MESENCHYMAL STROMAL CELL EFFECTS ON ARRESTED LUNG DEVELOPMENT
Bronchopulmonary Dysplasia is an Arrest in Lung Development

BPD is a form of chronic lung disease, peculiar to the extremely premature infants, born at the early stages of pulmonary development, in whom lung growth may be permanently arrested. BPD lungs consist of enlarged and simplified breathing structures (**Fig. 1**A), typical of the canalicular stage, as opposed to the alveolar ducts at term, characterized by smaller, more numerous and more complex alveoli (see **Fig. 1**A), essential to ensure adequate gas exchange.[10] The arrest of lung development, exacerbated by prenatal and postnatal proinflammatory stimuli (see **Fig. 1**), make traditional therapies ineffective in treating this disease.[1]

Animal Models of Arrested Lung Development: the Hyperoxia-Induced Lung Injury

Few models in different animal species have been able to mimic BPD or some of its aspects. Practically, all the studies testing the administration of MSCs in experimental BPD have been carried out in the rodent hyperoxia models.[11,12] Rats and mice are

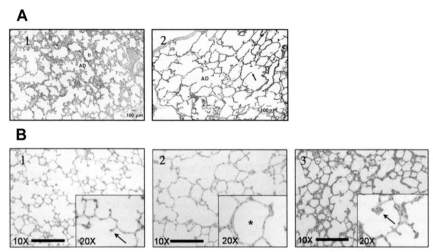

Fig. 1. Arrest of alveolarization in human and experimental BPD and effects of MSCs. (A) Lung histology (newborn). (A1) Autopsy from a term infant who died at 5 months of life. The lung specimen shows numerous secondary crests and alveolar structures within the airspaces and alveolar ducts (AD). (A2) Ex-preterm infant with BPD. Lung specimen from an open lung biopsy at 8 months of age shows enlarged airspaces, ADs with alveolar simplification (arrow). (B) Lung histology (rat). (B1) Normoxic control rat pup at 21 days of life. Lungs show well-organized alveoli with numerous secondary crests (black arrow). (B2) Rat pup exposed to hyperoxia between 4 and 14 days of life. Lungs show enlarged and simplified alveoli (asterisk). (B3) Rat pup exposed to hyperoxia between 4 and 14 days of life and treated endotracheally with MSCs on day 4 of life. Lung architecture with secondary crests (black arrow) is preserved. (Adapted from [A] Coalson JJ. Pathology of new bronchopulmonary dysplasia. Semin Neonatol 2003;8:79, with permission; and [B] Reprinted with permission of the American Thoracic Society. Copyright © 2015 American Thoracic Society. van Haaften T, Byrne R, Bonnet S, et al. Airway delivery of mesenchymal stem cells prevents arrested alveolar growth in neonatal lung injury in rats. Am J Respir Crit Care Med 2009;180:1135. Official Journal of the American Thoracic Society.)

naturally born at the canalicular stage of lung development, equivalent to the developmental stage of extreme preterm infants. Exposure of the developing rat lung to various concentrations of hyperoxic gas during the alveolar stage (day 5 to day 14 of life) impairs normal alveolarization, resulting in fewer and enlarged alveolar air spaces, reminiscent of structural changes seen in human BPD[11,12] (see **Fig. 1B**).

Treatment with Mesenchymal Stromal Cells Ameliorates Hyperoxia-Induced Arrest in Lung Growth

Prophylactic treatment

Prophylactic administration of MSCs (before exposure to hyperoxia) (**Fig. 2**) improves survival in experimental BPD and consistently and remarkably prevents lung injury (see **Fig. 1B**).[9,13–17] Results seem to be most beneficial by endotracheal (ET), compared with intravenous (IV) or intraperitoneal, administration[14] and dose-dependent with no benefit at 5×10^3 (approximately 5×10^2/g body weight) and increased benefit from 5×10^4 (approximately 5×10^3 cells/g) to 5×10^5 cells (approximately 5×10^4 cells/g).[15] Lung compliance and exercise tolerance are also significantly improved by ET administration of MSCs[9,17] (**Table 1**). Effective results have

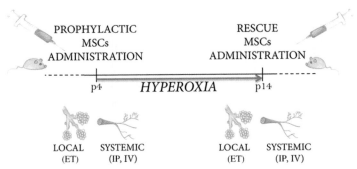

Fig. 2. Experiments testing the therapeutic effect of MSCs in experimental BPD. Rats exposed to hyperoxia during the saccular stage (day 4 to 14 of life). MSCs can be administered prophylactically (before exposure to hyperoxia) or as rescue (after exposure to hyperoxia). In both scenarios, MSCs can be delivered through a systemic route, either intravenously (IV) or intraperitoneally (IP) or through local endotracheal (ET) administration.

been obtained with rodent bone marrow–derived MSCs (BM-MSCs)[9,13] and human cord or cord blood–derived MSCs (hC-MSCs).[13–17]

Rescue treatment

Rescue administration of MSCs (after exposure to hyperoxia) (see **Fig. 2**), have led to less compelling results. Rat BM-MSCs elicited no response at a dose of 1×10^5,[9] whereas hC-MSCs produced only a slight improvement with a dose of 5×10^5, as opposed to early treatment.[16] However, in both rescue studies, the same absolute dose as the prophylactic experiments was used without adjusting for the increase in body weight of the older animals. When the dose was adjusted per body weight, although the prophylactic treatment still elicited a superior response, the rescue administration of hC-MSCs was able to ameliorate lung injury.[17] Taken together, these data suggest a possible beneficial effect of rescue MSC treatment but early timing seems to be more efficient.

PRECLINICAL EVIDENCE OF MESENCHYMAL STROMAL CELL EFFECTS ON DISRUPTED VASCULAR DEVELOPMENT
Hypoplastic Vascular Bed in Human Bronchopulmonary Dysplasia

BPD is also characterized by an abnormal distribution of pulmonary vessels and a reduction in the number of small arteries, which are functionally hyperreactive and hypertonic, culminating in pulmonary arterial hypertension and right ventricular hypertrophy.[18] Early and late pulmonary hypertension, assessed by indirect echocardiographic measurements (**Fig. 3**A), is detected in approximately 20% to 25% of the infants with BPD and worsens outcome.[18,19] Impaired pulmonary vascular growth may contribute to the irreversible arrest of lung development in BPD.[20]

Hyperoxia Induces Pulmonary Vascular Disruption and Pulmonary Hypertension

Exposure of term pups to hyperoxia simulates the typical vascular dysregulation of the dysplastic lung (**Fig. 3**C, D). Lung arterial vessels are reduced in number with thickened medial wall, resulting in right ventricular hypertrophy.[11,12] Echocardiography

Table 1
Studies testing the therapeutic effect of stem or progenitor cells in experimental models of bronchopulmonary dysplasia

Ref	Experiment Number	Dose	Route	Source	Timing	Ctrl Cells	Alveolar Damage	Functional Data	Pulmonary Hypertension	Inflammation	Survival
9	a	$1 \times 10^5 = 1 \times 10^4/g$	IT	Mouse-BM	P4	PASMC	Significant improvement	Improved exercise capacity	Decreased	No reports	Improved
	b	$1 \times 10^5 = 5 \times 10^3/g$	IT	Mouse-BM	P14	PASMC	No effects	Improved exercise capacity	No reports	No reports	No reports
13	—	$5 \times 10^4 = 1 \times 10^4/g$	IV	Mouse-BM	P4	No	Modest improvement	No reports	Decreased	Reduced	No reports
14	a	$5 \times 10^5 = 5 \times 10^4/g$	IT	hC	P5	Fibs	Significant improvement	No reports	No reports	Reduced	No reports
	b	$2 \times 10^6 = 2 \times 10^5/g$	IP	hC	P5	Fibs	No effects	No reports	No reports	Slightly Reduced	No reports
17	a	$3 \times 10^5 = 3 \times 10^4/g$	IT	hC	P4	Fibs	Significant improvement	Improved lung compliance	No reports	No reports	No reports
	b	$6 \times 10^5 = 3 \times 10^4/g$	IT	hC	P14	No	Modest improvement	No reports	No reports	No reports	No reports
15	a	$5 \times 10^3 = 5 \times 10^2/g$	IT	hC	P5	No	No effects	No reports	No reports	No effects	No effects
	b	$5 \times 10^4 = 5 \times 10^3/g$	IT	hC	P5	No	Modest improvement	No reports	No reports	Slightly reduced	Improved
	c	$5 \times 10^5 = 5 \times 10^4/g$	IT	hC	P5	No	Significant improvement	No reports	No reports	Extremely reduced	Improved
16	a	$5 \times 10^5 = 5 \times 10^4/kg$	IT	hC	P3	No	Significant improvement	No reports	No reports	Extremely reduced	Improved
	b	$5 \times 10^5 = 2.5 \times 10^4/g$	IT	hC	P10	No	Modest improvement	No reports	No reports	Slightly reduced	No effects
	c	$5 \times 10^5 = 5 \times 10^4/g+$	IT	hC	P3+P10	No	Significant improvement	No repots	No reports	Extremely reduced	Improved

Abbreviations: BM, bone marrow; Ctrl, control; Fibs, fibroblasts; hC, human cord; IP, intraperitoneal; IT, intratracheal; P, postnatal day; PASMC, pulmonary artery smooth muscle cells.

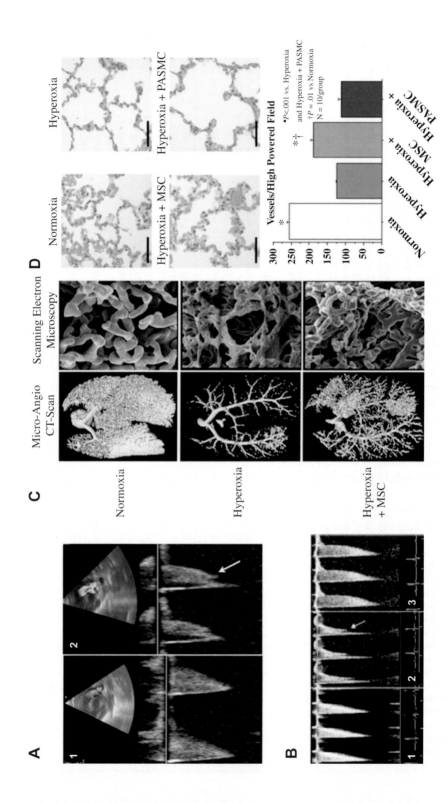

shows surrogate signs of pulmonary hypertension, such as reduced pulmonary arterial acceleration time with a midsystolic notch (**Fig. 3**B).

Mesenchymal Stromal Cells Treatment Mitigates Hyperoxia-Related Pulmonary Hypertension

Prophylactic treatment

Systemic and ET prophylactic administration of murine bone marrow and hC-derived MSCs attenuates pulmonary hypertension, as determined by echocardiographic measurements, right ventricular hypertrophy, medial wall thickness, and vessel count (see **Fig. 3**B–D).[9,13]

Rescue treatment

No studies report on the effects of rescue MSC administration on the vascular component of the lung injury.

PRECLINICAL EVIDENCE OF MESENCHYMAL STROMAL CELL EFFECTS ON INFLAMMATION, OXIDATIVE STRESS, AND FIBROSIS
Mechanisms of Cellular Damage in Bronchopulmonary Dysplasia

Prenatal and postnatal inflammatory stimuli contribute to the development of BPD.[21] Inflammation is documented by higher levels of proinflammatory cytokines and lower levels of anti-inflammatory cytokines in premature infants who will develop BPD.[22] Premature infants have an imbalance of antioxidant defense mechanisms and oxygen reactive species.[23] This dysregulation causes cell apoptosis, contributing to the development of BPD.[24] Moreover, higher number of fibroblasts characterized by increased collagenase activity cause disruption of the extracellular matrix, leading to tissue remodeling and fibrotic areas.[24]

Hyperoxia Induces Lung Inflammation, Fibrosis and Oxidative Stress

Hyperoxia increases the levels of proinflammatory cytokines and the number of polymorphonuclear cells and macrophages.[13–16] Hyperoxia-exposed animals display higher levels of apoptosis, fibrosis, and oxidation than normoxic control.[14–16]

Fig. 3. Lung vascular disease in human and experimental BPD and effects of MSCs. (*A*) Pulmonary artery acceleration time (PAAT) at echocardiography in newborn. (*A1*) Normal PAAT in a term-corrected ex-preterm infant without BPD. (*A2*) Reduced PAAT with midsystolic notch (*white arrow*) characteristic of pulmonary hypertension in a term-corrected patient with BPD. (*B*) Rodent PAAT at echocardiography. (*B1*) Normoxic control rat pup with normal PAAT at 21 days of life. (*B2 and B3*) Rat pups exposed to hyperoxia between 4 to 14 days of life with (*B2*) reduced PAAT and midsystolic notch (*white arrow*) and (*B3*) treated endotracheally with MSCs on day 4 of life, with normal PAAT. (*C*) Microangiography computed tomography (CT) scan and Mercox casts examined by scanning electron microscopy of the lung capillary bed. Endotracheal MSCs preserved lung angiogenesis and a dense capillary network in the lungs of oxygen-exposed rats. (*D*) Hematoxylin and eosin-stained barium angiograms and mean capillary count. Decreased capillary density in oxygen-exposed lungs. Intratracheal MSCs, but not pulmonary artery smooth muscle cells (PASMCs), preserved arterial density. ([A] *Courtesy of* P. Tagliabue, MD, Chief of the Neonatal Intensive Care Unit, MBBM Foundation, San Gerardo Hospital, Monza, Italy; and [C, D] *Reprinted with permission of* the American Thoracic Society. Copyright © 2015 American Thoracic Society. van Haaften T, Byrne R, Bonnet S, et al. Airway delivery of mesenchymal stem cells prevents arrested alveolar growth in neonatal lung injury in rats. Am J Respir Crit Care Med 2009;180:1136–7. Official Journal of the American Thoracic Society.)

Mesenchymal Stromal Cells Reduce Hyperoxia-Induced Inflammation, Fibrosis, and Oxidative Stress

Prophylactic treatment

Early systemic administration of MSCs dramatically decreases the number of both polymorphonuclear cells and macrophages in the bronchoalveolar lavage of hyperoxia-exposed rats.[13] Proinflammatory cytokine are reduced more effectively by local than by systemic administration,[14] in a dose-dependent manner.[15] The degree of lung fibrosis, assessed by alpha-smooth muscle actin and lung collagen, is reduced only by the ET administration of MSCs.[14] The oxidative status in the lung tissue, as documented by the activation of NADPH (nicotinamide adenine dinucleotide phosphate) oxidase, the enzyme responsible for the reactive oxygen species production, is improved by the ET administration of MSCs in a dose-dependent manner.[15]

Rescue treatment

Rescue administration of MSCs shows a milder improvement in terms of inflammation and oxidation compared with early administration. Fibrosis was not attenuated by rescue ET administration of MSCs. However, as previously mentioned, the dose was not increased according to the body weight of older animals.[16]

LONG-TERM CONSIDERATIONS FROM PRECLINICAL STUDIES
Life-Long Consequences of Bronchopulmonary Dysplasia

Ex-preterm infants suffering from BPD continue to show signs of pulmonary damage beyond childhood.[25] Preterm-born children with a history of BPD are significantly more likely to have lung function abnormalities, such as airway obstruction and respiratory symptoms, and receive asthma medication at school age, compared with preterm-born children without BPD.[26,27] Young adults surviving BPD seem to be prone to early-onset emphysema.[28]

Animals Exposed to Hyperoxia in the Neonatal Period Show Long-Term Features of Bronchopulmonary Dysplasia

Hyperoxia-induced lung remodeling persists histologically (**Fig. 4**B) and functionally up to 6 months (equivalent to 25 years in humans),[17] making this model particularly suitable to test long-term therapeutic options for a life-long disease such as BPD. Animals exposed to hyperoxia in the neonatal period also showed functional impairment later in life, as documented by significantly reduced distance running on the treadmill.[17]

Beneficial Effects of Mesenchymal Stromal Cells Persist in Adult Rats

The long-term effects of MSC administration have not yet been extensively investigated. Neonatal prophylactic ET MSC treatment significantly improves exercise capacity and almost normalizes alveolar architecture (see **Fig. 4**B) at 6 months of age in neonatal hyperoxia-exposed animals.[17]

Mesenchymal Stromal Cells Display Long-Term Safety in the Hyperoxia-Induced Lung Injury

Intrapulmonary delivery of MSCs on day 4 of life was safe up to 6 months as assessed by lung structure and exercise capacity.[17] Total body computerized tomography showed no signs of tumor formation (see **Fig. 4**A). These data need to be confirmed by systematic sampling of tissue histology.

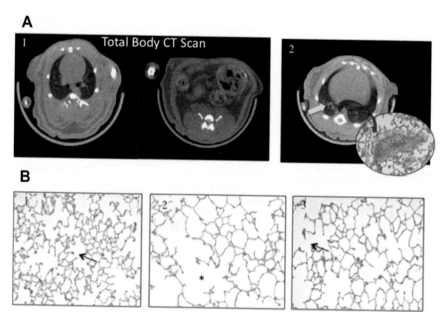

Fig. 4. Long-term safety and efficacy of MSCs in experimental BPD. (*A*) Long-term safety. (*A1*) Representative computed tomography (CT) scan performed at 6 months of age, after neonatal treatment with MSCs. (*A2*) One doubtful image was detected (*yellow arrow*) and the corresponding histology sample ruled out the presence of a possible tumor, indicating a congested blood vessel. (*B*) Long-term efficacy on lung histology (*B1*) Normoxic control rat pup at 6 months of life. Lungs show small and well-organized alveoli with secondary crests (*black arrow*). (*B2*) Rat pup exposed to hyperoxia between 4 to 14 days of life sacrificed at 6 month of life. Lungs show enlarged and simplified alveoli (*asterisk*). (*B3*) A 6-month-old rat exposed to hyperoxia between 4 to 14 days of life and treated endotracheally with MSC on day 4 of life, showing almost normalized alveolar architecture with secondary crests (*black arrow*). (*Adapted from* Pierro M, Ionescu L, Montemurro T, et al. Short-term, long-term and paracrine effect of human umbilical cord derived stem cells in lung injury prevention. Thorax 2013;68:475–84; with permission.)

CONCLUSIONS FROM PRECLINICAL DATA

In summary, evidence from animal models show that MSCs ameliorate many pathologic components leading to BPD. Early, intratracheal administration seems to be most efficient. MSCs also display long-term safety and efficacy in rodents.

MECHANISM OF ACTION OF MESENCHYMAL STROMAL CELLS
Homing to Site of Injury and Regeneration

Chemotactic cytokines and signaling proteins, released by different types of injury, mobilize and recruit resident and remote host MSCs in a process called homing.[29] MSCs express cell adhesion molecules that interact with these cytokines, orchestrating the migration through the local or systemic circulation and the transmigration across the endothelium to reach the target tissue.[30] Homing is a crucial part of the MSC healing process, although the precise mechanisms by which MSCs are recruited into injured organs and the exact site where MSCs are on-call are not yet fully understood. The prevailing hypothesis is that MSCs originate from perivascular precursors, named pericytes.[31] Pericytes surround the blood vessels

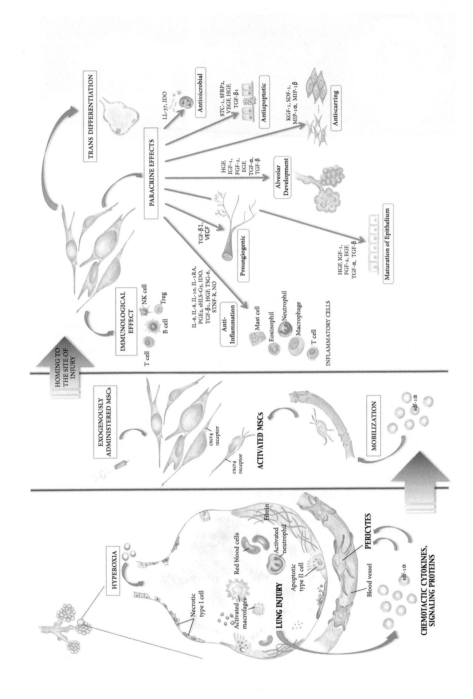

throughout the body,[28] allowing prompt and efficient MSC recruitment and response to injury (see **Fig. 6**).

The homing capacity of systemically and locally exogenously delivered MSCs is a cornerstone of the success of regenerative medicine. Once recruited to the damaged area, MSCs exert their pleiotropic therapeutic benefits. MSCs may be able to differentiate along different lineages, including lung epithelial cells and alveolar type 2 cells.[32,33] However, it has been repeatedly shown that only few exogenously administered cells engraft and differentiate into the damaged tissue,[9,18] suggesting that engraftment and cell replacement plays a minimal, if any, part in the therapeutic benefits of MSCs.

Paracrine Effect

It is now commonly accepted that the therapeutic efficacy of MSCs is greatly depends on their ability to produce paracrine factors that enhance regeneration from endogenous cells.[34,35] In vitro and in vivo studies demonstrated that administration of the cell-free conditioned media, where MSCs have been cultured for 24 hours, protects alveolar epithelial and lung microvascular endothelial cells from oxidative stress, prevents oxygen-induced alveolar growth arrest, and stimulates a subset of host stem or progenitor cells to aid in lung repair.[9,13,17,36] Growth factors and other chemokines that induce cell proliferation and angiogenesis, as well as antiapoptotic, antioxidant, antifibrotic, anti-inflammatory, and antimicrobial factors have been detected in MSC media and are likely responsible for the therapeutic effects of MSCs[37] (**Fig. 5**). Recently, exosomes have been proposed as the paracrine effectors of MSCs.[38] Exosomes are membrane vesicles formed through the fusion of multivesicular endosomes with the plasma membrane.[38] Exosomes, secreted by several cell types, including stem cells, are nanopackages of bioactive molecules and noncoding microRNA (noncoding RNA involved in transcriptional regulation of gene expression) that may mediate cellular function and cell-to-cell interaction and exert therapeutic benefits for lung diseases as demonstrated in hypoxic-induced pulmonary hypertension.[39]

Mitochondrial transfer to resident lung cells via nanotubes seems to be another mechanism of action of MSCs.[40]

Although the option of a cell-free product is appealing, the administration of the entire cocktail containing unidentified products may conjure unforeseen side effects. The near future of regenerative medicine seems to favor cell administration mainly because of the capacity of MSCs to sense their environment, integrate inputs to make decisions, and execute complex response behaviors, an ability that would be

Fig. 5. Mechanism of action of MSCs. Chemokines, cytokines, and growth factors released on injury mobilize perivascular cells (pericytes), which surround the blood vessels throughout the body. Pericytes are believed to be precursors of MSCs. Activated MSCs, derived from pericytes, or exogenously delivered MSCs are recruited to the site of injury through interactions between chemokines, such as stromal cell-derived factor-1α (SDF-1α) and MSC receptors (ie, C × C chemokine receptor type 4, CXCR4, for SDF-1α) in a process called homing. Once homed to the damaged organ, MSCs can exert their therapeutic benefit through multiple mechanisms of action: (1) secretion of anti-inflammatory, antimicrobial, antiapoptotic, and antiscarring molecules; and growth factors and other chemokines, to induce cell proliferation and angiogenesis (paracrine mechanism) and (2) interaction with immune cells, including T cells, natural killer cells, B cells, monocytes, macrophages, and dendritic cells by cell-to-cell contact (immunomodulatory property).

lost with cell-free therapeutic options. Further insight into the mechanism of action of MSCs may eventually lead to new cell-derived therapies for BPD, possibly involving the administration of exosomes, as a combination of bioactive molecules and micro-RNA, that could silence specific genes with deleterious effects during lung injury,[41] mitochondrial transfer, or preconditioned MSC products.[42]

Immunomodulatory Properties

The main mechanism of action of MSCs is the interaction with the immune system. Undifferentiated MSCs express low levels of human leukocyte antigen (HLA) class I and low levels of HLA class II that helps them avoid recognition by the immune system.[43] MSCs also exert immunomodulatory effects by direct cell-to-cell contact, preventing proliferation and function of many inflammatory immune cells, including T cells, natural killer cells, B cells, monocytes, macrophages, and dendritic cells.[44,45] In particular, MSCs derived from the umbilical cord express significantly lower levels of HLA-I, exhibit significantly higher intracellular concentrations of immunosuppressive molecules,[46] and inhibit T-cell proliferation[47] more effectively than bone marrow–derived MSCs, allowing for a theoretic, not yet proven, greater tolerable HLA disparity and decreased frequency of acute or chronic graft versus host disease (GVHD).[48]

On the other hand, immune rejection cannot be ruled out a priori because class I antigen is present at detectable levels and class II antigen expression can be induced,[49] possibly causing MSC recognition by the immune system.[50] Antidonor antibodies, apparently with no clinical consequences, have been detected in 13% of patients receiving allogenic (allo)-MSCs (http://www.prnewswire.com/news-releases-test/positive-results-from-phase-2-trial-of-mesoblasts-adult-stem-cell-therapy-presented-at-the-american-heart-association-annual-meeting-133835958.html). No significant differences have been shown between auto-MSCs and allo-MSCs,[51] or between third-party and haploidentical or HLA-identical MSCs.[52] Although a better understanding of the MSC mechanism of action and results from robust randomized clinical trials are still needed, preliminary data on efficacy of MSCs in preventing and treating GVHD seem to support at least a partial immune privilege of MSCs.[52,53]

CLINICAL TRANSLATION

Although there are still gaps in knowledge about MSCs, the promising animal data have prompted the clinical translation of cell therapies for yet untreatable diseases. The search for currently registered clinical trials, testing MSCs as intervention, retrieves 469 results (https://clinicaltrials.gov/ct2/results?term=&recr=&rslt=&type=Intr&cond=&intr=mesenchymal+stem+cell&titles=&outc=&spons=&lead=&id=&state1=&cntry1=&state2=&cntry2=&state3=&cntry3=&locn=&gndr=&rcv_s=&rcv_e=&lup_s=&lup_e=). Among these, in the United States, a phase I-II, dose-escalation trial is currently recruiting subjects (NCT02381366) and 2 monocentric phase 1 and 2 trials have been registered but are not yet recruiting subjects in Spain and Korea, respectively (https://clinicaltrials.gov/ct2/results?term=mesenchymal+stem+cell+and+BPD&Search=Search).

EFFICACY OF MESENCHYMAL STROMAL CELL TREATMENT

Dosage, timing, and route of administration greatly affect MSC homing, regeneration, and paracrine capacity.[43] In addition to these elements, numerous and more complicated variables, altering the manufacturing of the final MSC product, need to be taken into account when approaching the design and the results of clinical trials assessing MSCs as intervention (**Table 2**).

Factors Affecting Efficacy of Stem Cell Treatment: Considerations

Timing

Rescue administration or treatment of established bronchopulmonary dysplasia Treatment of established BPD requires, by definition, waiting 28 days of life for mild BPD and 36 weeks postmenstrual age (PMA) for moderate and severe BPD. Although this target may be appropriate to prove safety, confirmation of efficacy could be hampered by the delayed timing. Severely injured lungs may be too compromised to be significantly renewed. In addition, the signals, needed to recruit and modulate the effects of MSCs, change with the course of the disease, becoming minimal or absent at a chronic phase of injury.[54]

Prophylactic or early administration Prevention of BPD at birth (prophylactic) and up to 7 days (early administration)[55] is particularly appealing because more than 50% of infants born before 26 weeks' gestation will develop BPD.[56] In addition, based on animal data, prophylactic administration seems the most effective option. Currently, the major limitation to this approach is the risk of overtreatment. Prophylactic or early administration would not be an option until safety of later treatment is well-documented in long-term studies.

Treatment of evolving bronchopulmonary dysplasia Although evolving BPD is not an entirely defined entity, it refers to oxygen-dependent and ventilator-dependent extremely preterm infants, between 7 and 27 days of life,[56] when the respiratory disease represents the leading cause of death.[57] This time-frame may represent the optimal therapeutic window for MSCs. In this population, overtreatment could be easily avoided by selecting the most compromised patients at the highest risk for death and/or severe BPD (https://neonatal.rti.org/index.cfm?fuseaction=tools.main).

Route of administration

Efficacy, bioavailability, and functionality of any pharmacologic drug depend on the route of administration. With regard to lung diseases, the 2 most relevant routes of administration are IV and ET.

Systemic administration Compared with traditional medications, systemic MSC infusion has the advantage of preferential migration and homing into damaged tissues.[54] When considering pulmonary diseases, the localization into the lung is also facilitated by the natural biodistribution of MSCs. After IV transfusion, MSCs initially concentrate into the lung. Afterward, some cells move gradually either to the liver, spleen, kidney, or bone marrow, in noninjurious models; or to the injury sites in various experimental disease models.[58,59] Because several organs may be damaged in severely ill premature infants, MSCs may migrate toward those sites of injury, after the first passage through the lung, eventually improving the overall outcome. The IV route may also be less invasive than the ET route in spontaneously breathing patients.

Endotracheal administration Despite the obvious benefits of the IV route, evidence from animal studies has shown that the ET administration provides superior therapeutic benefit at least in the experimental settings. The ET route allows delivery of MSCs at the alveolar interface and this may alter the interactions and responses of MSCs. In addition, coadministration with surfactant may facilitate the distribution of MSCs. The choice of the most convenient route of administration may be influenced by the timing of intervention because survivors at 36 weeks PMA, are usually supported by

Table 2
Factors affecting efficacy of stem cell treatment

Factor	Subgroup	Pros	Cons
Route	IV	• Less invasive technique • Natural biodistribution of MSCs to the lung • Homing to other damaged organs	May not be as effective as local delivery of MSCs
	ET	Better results in animal studies	• No distribution to other organs • Invasive procedure in case of spontaneous breathing
Timing	Prevention (<7 d)	• Best results in animal studies • Less severely damaged organs	• Overtreatment • Less objective patient selection criteria
	Evolving (7–28 d)	• Minimization of overtreatment • Lungs are likely not completely damaged • Possible benefit for patients dying in the first month of life	—
	Rescue (>28 d)	Avoidance of overtreatment	• Lungs may be too damaged to see an effect • Homing stimuli may not be optimal • Most severe patients may die before this time
Dose	High Low	Better engraftment • Lower volumes • Possibly less side effects	Need for higher volumes Milder results

		Advantages	Disadvantages
Source	Bone marrow	Best studied source of MSCs	• Aging of the cells with donor aging • Painful harvesting procedure • Low number of cells in the bone marrow aspirate
	Adipose tissue	• Higher number of cells • Less invasive harvesting procedure • Optimal availability • No risk or pain for mother and newborn with harvesting	Aging of the cells with donor aging
	Cord-derived (WJ)	• Stronger immunomodulatory potential, improved proliferative capacity, life span and stemness, higher trophic and anti-inflammatory activity	—
Passage	High	Higher number of cells	• Aging of the cells with higher passages • Decreased homing capacity
	Low	Superior cell biological properties	Low number of cells
Type of transplant	Autologous	No rejection	• Hampering of early administration due to lead time. • Need for GMP facilities • Unexplored possible differences between the term and preterm cord MSCs
	Allogeneic	• Facilitates logistics • Off-the-shelf available product	Possible rejection, although rare possibility

Abbreviation: GMP, good manufacturing practice.

noninvasive ventilation, whereas patients with severe evolving BPD are still mechanically ventilated.

Dose

The conversion of the effective preclinical doses, according to the body mass index of the premature infants,[60] results in a theoretic effective dose ranging from 8×10^5/kg up to 8×10^6/kg[15] ET and 1.6×10^6/kg[13] up to 3.2×10^7/kg[14] IV. In a recent phase 1 trial, Chang and colleagues[61] did not report dose-limiting toxicity up to a dose of 2×10^7/kg. The high-dose treatment seemed to be associated with better outcomes, although this study was not designed to show efficacy. These results need to be confirmed in randomized phase 2 trials that are currently ongoing (NCT01828957; NCT01207869). The need for several culture passages and the volumes required to obtain adequate cell concentrations (a crucial variable for the ET route) may influence the quality of the cell product and be limiting factors to the efficacy of higher doses.

Source

The source of MSCs can greatly affect their efficacy. Although MSCs have been isolated from any tissue,[5] some sources are more clinically relevant than others.

Adult sources: bone marrow and adipose tissue Bone marrow is the first described and best known source of MSCs. However, it may not be optimal for patient treatment due to the aging of the cell with the donor aging,[62] the paucity of the MSC among the other cells present in the bone marrow aspirate,[63] and the painful and invasive procedure needed to obtain the cells.

Adipose tissue is an emerging source of MSCs. It offers a greater number of cells and it is more accessible than bone marrow, although aging of the cells with donor aging is still an issue.[64]

Perinatal sources Human extraembryonic tissues (chorion, amniotic membranes, and umbilical cord) as well as human placental fluids (amniotic fluid and umbilical cord blood) **(Fig. 6)** are an appealing source of MSCs. A significant advantage of these perinatal tissues is their availability without invasive and painful harvesting procedures.[48] Even more interestingly, MSCs from these neonatal tissues may be superior to MSCs derived from adult sources. Perinatal MSCs display superior cell biological properties, such as stronger immunomodulatory and immunosuppressive potential,[65] improved proliferative capacity, life span[66] and stemness,[67] and higher trophic[68] and anti-inflammatory[66] activity, compared with adult MSCs.

To date, among the different perinatal sources, the most used and practical is the umbilical cord. In particular, robust and reproducible techniques for harvesting and expansion are available for Wharton Jelly, rather than cord blood or perivascular tissues.

Practical aspects of mesenchymal stromal cell manufacturing

Passage number A passage is the process of removing cells from a culture flask and plating them into more culture flasks. Passaging is necessary to obtain a sufficient number of cells for transplantation. The number of passages is inversely proportional to the efficiency of homing, with freshly isolated cells performing superior results to cultivated cells.[69] Moreover, MSCs tend to show genotypic and phenotypic variation when cultured for extended periods of time,[70] although cord-derived cells seem to be less sensitive to aging in culture.[71] Early-passage cells may have superior homing and therapeutic potential and thus improve the chances of success of the stem cell therapy in clinical trials.

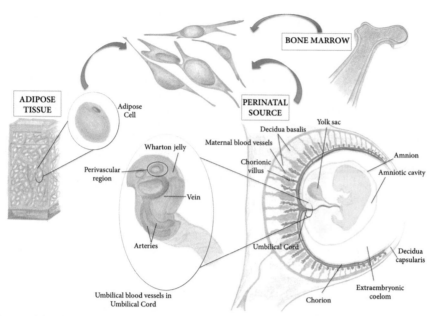

Fig. 6. Clinically relevant sources of MSCs include adult sources (adipose tissue and bone marrow) and perinatal sources (chorion, amniotic membranes, amniotic fluid, and umbilical cord or cord blood).

Culture conditions Several factors, including isolation and characterization techniques, production to scale-up, cryopreservation, and banking, can affect the efficacy of MSC therapy and have been reviewed elsewhere.[72] These details, however, will be important in designing and interpreting the results of clinical trials.

Type of transplantation

Autologous Autologous transplantation of cord MSCs (from the cord of the patient) is particularly appealing in neonates[73] but has some shortcomings: (1) impracticality of the prophylactic or early administration due to lead time, (2) need for on-site good manufacturing practice facilities to handle clinical-grade cell products, and (3) yet to be explored possible differences between the term and preterm cord MSCs.

Allogeneic Considering the low immunogenicity of MSCs, although immune rejection is still possible,[43] allogeneic transplantation (from a donor) may be the most suitable option for preterm infants at risk for BPD[73] by providing a readily available, quality-controlled, off-the-shelf product.

SAFETY OF MESENCHYMAL STROMAL CELL TREATMENT

Safety of MSC administration in the adult[74] and pediatric[75] population has been widely documented. In the neonatal population, Chang and colleagues[61] showed that the ET transplantation of 2 different doses (1×10^7/kg and 2×10^7/kg) of hC-MSCs in preterm infants at high risk for BPD is apparently safe and feasible. The treatment was well tolerated, without dose-limiting toxicity or immediate (up to 6 hours) complications after transplantation. Six severe adverse events were recorded. However, they were typical complications of extreme prematurity and not attributed to the MSC therapy.

This trial was designed to test safety and was not randomized and powered to investigate efficacy measures. The long-term follow-up study is underway (NCT01632475).

SUMMARY

MSCs offer very promising therapeutic options for the prevention of complications of extreme prematurity, including BPD. Although the knowledge of their function and manufacturing process is still incomplete, the documented safety of MSCs in adults and children, and the dramatic benefits observed in experimental models, has prompted the clinical translation of this promising cell therapy. Selection of patients, timing and route of administration, source of cells, and protocols for MSC manufacturing can determine success or failure of this therapy and indelibly influence further research. During the next 5 years, well-designed trials will indicate whether MSC therapy can become a novel breakthrough in neonatal medicine.

REFERENCES

1. Jobe AH, Bancalari E. Bronchopulmonary dysplasia. Am J Respir Crit Care Med 2001;163:1723–9.
2. Farstad T, Bratlid D, Medbo S, et al. Bronchopulmonary dysplasia - prevalence, severity and predictive factors in a national cohort of extremely premature infants. Acta Paediatr 2011;100:53–8.
3. Prockop DJ, Kota DJ, Bazhanov N, et al. Evolving paradigms for repair of tissues by adult stem/progenitor cells (MSCs). J Cell Mol Med 2010;14:2190–9.
4. Dominici M, Le Blanc K, Mueller I, et al. Minimal criteria for defining multipotent mesenchymal stromal cells. The international society for cellular therapy position statement. Cytotherapy 2006;8:315–7.
5. da Silva Meirelles L, Chagastelles PC, Nardi NB. Mesenchymal stem cells reside in virtually all post-natal organs and tissues. J Cell Sci 2006;119:2204–13.
6. Collins JJ, Thébaud B. Progenitor cells of the distal lung and their potential role in neonatal lung disease. Birth Defects Res A Clin Mol Teratol 2014;100(3):217–26.
7. Popova AP, Bozyk PD, Goldsmith AM, et al. Autocrine production of TGF-beta1 promotes myofibroblastic differentiation of neonatal lung mesenchymal stem cells. Am J Physiol Lung Cell Mol Physiol 2010;298:L735–43.
8. Popova AP, Bozyk PD, Bentley JK, et al. Isolation of tracheal aspirate mesenchymal stromal cells predicts bronchopulmonary dysplasia. Pediatrics 2010; 126:e1127–33.
9. van Haaften T, Byrne R, Bonnet S, et al. Airway delivery of mesenchymal stem cells prevents arrested alveolar growth in neonatal lung injury in rats. Am J Respir Crit Care Med 2009;180:1131–42.
10. Coalson JJ. Pathology of new bronchopulmonary dysplasia. Semin Neonatol 2003;8:73–81.
11. Berger J, Bhandari V. Animal models of bronchopulmonary dysplasia. The term mouse models. Am J Physiol Lung Cell Mol Physiol 2014;307:L936–47.
12. O'Reilly M, Thébaud B. Animal models of bronchopulmonary dysplasia. The term rat models. Am J Physiol Lung Cell Mol Physiol 2014;307:L948–58.
13. Aslam M, Baveja R, Liang OD. Bone marrow stromal cells attenuate lung injury in a murine model of neonatal chronic lung disease. Am J Respir Crit Care Med 2009;180:1122–30.
14. Chang YS, Oh W, Choi SJ. Human umbilical cord blood-derived mesenchymal stem cells attenuate hyperoxia-induced lung injury in neonatal rats. Cell Transplant 2009;18:869–86.

15. Chang YS, Choi SJ, Sung DK. Intratracheal transplantation of human umbilical cord blood-derived mesenchymal stem cells dose-dependently attenuates hyperoxia-induced lung injury in neonatal rats. Cell Transplant 2011;20:1843–54.
16. Chang YS, Choi SJ, Ahn SY. Timing of umbilical cord blood derived mesenchymal stem cells transplantation determines therapeutic efficacy in the neonatal hyperoxic lung injury. PLoS One 2013;8:e52419.
17. Pierro M, Ionescu L, Montemurro T, et al. Short-term, long-term and paracrine effect of human umbilical cord-derived stem cells in lung injury prevention and repair in experimental bronchopulmonary dysplasia. Thorax 2013;68:475–84.
18. Rossor T, Greenough A. Advances in paediatric pulmonary vascular disease associated with bronchopulmonary dysplasia. Expert Rev Respir Med 2014;26:1–9.
19. Nagiub M, Lee S, Guglani L. Echocardiographic assessment of pulmonary hypertension in infants with bronchopulmonary dysplasia: systematic review of literature and a proposed algorithm for assessment. Echocardiography 2014;32(5):819–33.
20. Thebaud B, Abman SH. Bronchopulmonary dysplasia: where have all the vessels gone? Roles of angiogenic growth factors in chronic lung disease. Am J Respir Crit Care Med 2007;175:978–85.
21. Speer CP. Role of inflammation in the evolution of bronchopulmonary dysplasia. J Perinatol 2006;(Suppl 1):S57–62.
22. Thompson A, Bhandari V. Pulmonary biomarkers of bronchopulmonary dysplasia. Biomark Insights 2008;3:361–73.
23. Jankov RP, Negus A, Tanswell AK. Antioxidants as therapy in the newborn: some words of caution. Pediatr Res 2001;50:681–7.
24. Saugstad OD. Bronchopulmonary dysplasia-oxidative stress and antioxidants. Semin Neonatol 2003;8:39–49.
25. O'Reilly M, Thébaud B. Using cell-based strategies to break the link between bronchopulmonary dysplasia and the development of chronic lung disease in later life. Pulm Med 2013;2013:874161.
26. Vom Hove M, Prenzel F, Uhlig HH, et al. Pulmonary outcome in former preterm, very low birth weight children with bronchopulmonary dysplasia: a case-control follow-up at school age. J Pediatr 2014;164:40–5.e4.
27. Fawke J, Lum S, Kirkby J, et al. Lung function and respiratory symptoms at 11 years in children born extremely preterm: the EPICure study. Am J Respir Crit Care Med 2010;182:237–45.
28. Wong PM, Lees AN, Louw J, et al. Emphysema in young adult survivors of moderate-to-severe bronchopulmonary dysplasia. Eur Respir J 2008;32:321–8.
29. Ren G, Chen X, Dong F, et al. Concise review: mesenchymal stem cells and translational medicine: emerging issues. Stem Cells Transl Med 2012;1:51–8.
30. Ma S, Xie N, Li W, et al. Immunobiology of mesenchymal stem cells. Cell Death Differ 2014;21:216–25.
31. Crisan M, Yap S, Casteilla L, et al. A perivascular origin for mesenchymal stem cells in multiple human organs. Cell Stem Cell 2008;3:301–13.
32. Krause DS, Theise ND, Collector MI, et al. Multi-organ, multi-lineage engraftment by a single bone marrow-derived stem cell. Cell 2001;105:369–77.
33. Sueblinvong V, Loi R, Eisenhauer PL, et al. Derivation of lung epithelium from human cord blood-derived mesenchymal stem cells. Am J Respir Crit Care Med 2008;177:701–11.
34. Murphy MB, Moncivais K, Caplan AI. Mesenchymal stem cells: environmentally responsive therapeutics for regenerative medicine. Exp Mol Med 2013;45:e54.

35. Fung ME, Thébaud B. Stem cell-based therapy for neonatal lung disease: it is in the juice. Pediatr Res 2014;75:2–7.
36. Tropea KA, Leder E, Aslam M, et al. Bronchoalveolar stem cells increase after mesenchymal stromal cell treatment in a mouse model of bronchopulmonary dysplasia. Am J Physiol Lung Cell Mol Physiol 2012;302:L829–37.
37. Lee JW, Fang X, Krasnodembskaya A, et al. Concise review: mesenchymal stem cells for acute lung injury: role of paracrine soluble factors. Stem Cells 2011;29:913–9.
38. Chaput N, Thery C. Exosomes: immune properties and potential clinical implementations. Semin Immunopathol 2011;33:419–40.
39. Lee C, Mitsialis SA, Aslam M, et al. Exosomes mediate the cytoprotective action of mesenchymal stromal cells on hypoxia-induced pulmonary hypertension. Circulation 2012;126:2601–11.
40. Islam MN, Das SR, Emin MT, et al. Mitochondrial transfer from bone-marrow-derived stromal cells to pulmonary alveoli protects against acute lung injury. Nat Med 2012;18:759–65.
41. Dong J, Carey WA, Abel S, et al. MicroRNA-mRNA interactions in a murine model of hyperoxia-induced bronchopulmonary dysplasia. BMC Genomics 2012;13:204.
42. Waszak P, Alphonse R, Vadivel A, et al. Preconditioning enhances the paracrine effect of mesenchymal stem cells in preventing oxygen-induced neonatal lung injury in rats. Stem Cells Dev 2012;21:2789–97.
43. Le Blanc K, Tammik C, Rosendahl K, et al. HLA expression and immunologic properties of differentiated and undifferentiated mesenchymal stem cells. Exp Hematol 2003;31:890–6.
44. Gebler A, Zabel O, Seliger B. The immunomodulatory capacity of mesenchymal stem cells. Trends Mol Med 2012;18:128–34.
45. Le Blanc C, Davies LC. Mesenchymal stromal cells and the innate immune response. Immunol Lett 2015. [Epub ahead of print].
46. Deuse T, Stubbendorff M, Tang-Quan K, et al. Immunogenicity and immunomodulatory properties of umbilical cord lining mesenchymal stem cells. Cell Transplant 2011;20:655–67.
47. Najar M, Raicevic G, Boufker HI, et al. Mesenchymal stromal cells use PGE2 to modulate activation and proliferation of lymphocyte subsets: Combined comparison of adipose tissue, Wharton's Jelly and bone marrow sources. Cell Immunol 2010;264:171–9.
48. Batsali KA, Kastrinaki MC, Papadaki H, et al. Mesenchymal stem cells derived from Wharton's jelly of the umbilical cord: biological properties and emerging clinical applications. Curr Stem Cell Res Ther 2013;8:144–55.
49. Huang X-P, Sun Z, Miyagi Y, et al. Differentiation of allogeneic mesenchymal stem cells induces immunogenicity and limits their long-term benefits for myocardial repair. Circulation 2010;122:2419–29.
50. Crop MJ, Korevaar SS, de Kuiper R, et al. Human mesenchymal stem cells are susceptible to lysis by CD8fl T-cells and NK cells. Cell Transplant 2011;20:1547–59.
51. Hare JM, Fishman JE, Gerstenblith G, et al. Comparison of allogeneic vs autologous bone marrow–derived mesenchymal stem cells delivered by transendocardial injection in patients with ischemic cardiomyopathy: the POSEIDON randomized trial. J Am Med Assoc 2012;308:2369–79.
52. Le Blanc K, Frassoni F, Ball L, et al. Mesenchymal stem cells for treatment of steroid-resistant, severe, acute graft-versus-host disease: a phase II study. Lancet 2008;371:1579–86.

53. Kuzmina LA, Petinati NA, Parovichnikova EN, et al. Multipotent Mesenchymal Stromal Cells for the Prophylaxis of Acute Graft-versus-Host Disease-A Phase II Study. Stem Cells Int 2012;2012:968213.
54. Yan X, Liu Y, Han Q, et al. Injured microenvironment directly guides the differentiation of engrafted Flk-1(1) mesenchymal stem cell in lung. Exp Hematol 2007; 35:1466–75.
55. Stoll BJ, Hansen NI, Bell EF, et al. Neonatal outcomes of extremely preterm infants from the NICHD neonatal research network. Pediatrics 2010;126:443–56.
56. Walsh MC, Szefler S, Davis J, et al. Summary proceedings from the bronchopulmonary dysplasia group. Pediatrics 2006;117:S52–5.
57. Patel RM, Kandefer S, Walsh MC, et al. Causes and timing of death in extremely premature infants from 2000 through 2011. N Engl J Med 2015;372:331–40.
58. Lee RH, Pulin AA, Seo MJ, et al. Intravenous hMSCs improve myocardial infarction in mice because cells embolized in lung are activated to secrete the anti-inflammatory protein TSG-6. Cell Stem Cell 2009;5:54–63.
59. Schrepfer S, Deuse T, Reichenspurner H, et al. Stem cell transplantation: the lung barrier. Transplant Proc 2007;39:573–6.
60. Reagan-Shaw S, Nihal M, Ahmad N. Dose translation from animal to human studies revisited. FASEB J 2008;22:659–61.
61. Chang YS, Ahn SY, Yoo HS, et al. Mesenchymal stem cells for bronchopulmonary dysplasia: phase 1 dose-escalation clinical trial. J Pediatr 2014;164:966–72.
62. Mueller SM, Glowacki J. Age-related decline in the osteogenic potential of human bone marrow cells cultured in three-dimensional collagen sponges. J Cell Biochem 2001;82:583–90.
63. Castro-Malaspina H, Gay RE, Resnick G, et al. Characterization of human bone marrow fibroblast colony-forming cells (CFU-F) and their progeny. Blood 1980; 56:289–301.
64. Dmitrieva RI, Minullina IR, Bilibina AA, et al. Bone marrow- and subcutaneous adipose tissue-derived mesenchymal stem cells: differences and similarities. Cell Cycle 2012;11:377–83.
65. Li X, Bai J, Ji X, et al. Comprehensive characterization of four different populations of human mesenchymal stem cells as regards their immune properties, proliferation and differentiation. Int J Mol Med 2014;34(3):695–704.
66. Jin HJ, Bae YK, Kim M, et al. Comparative analysis of human mesenchymal stem cells from bone marrow, adipose tissue, and umbilical cord blood as sources of cell therapy. Int J Mol Sci 2013;14:17986–8001.
67. Hsieh JY, Fu YS, Chang SJ, et al. Functional module analysis reveals differential osteogenic and stemness potentials in human mesenchymal stem cells from bone marrow and Wharton's jelly of umbilical cord. Stem Cells Dev 2010;19: 1895–910.
68. Hsieh JY, Wang HW, Chang SJ, et al. Mesenchymal stem cells from human umbilical cord express preferentially secreted factors related to neuroprotection, neurogenesis, and angiogenesis. PLoS One 2013;8:e72604.
69. Rombouts WJC, Ploemacher RE. Primary murine MSC show highly efficient homing to the bone marrow but lose homing ability following culture. Leukemia 2003; 17:160–70.
70. Sethe S, Scutt A, Stolzing A. Aging of mesenchymal stem cells. Ageing Res Rev 2006;5:91–116.
71. Kern S, Eichler H, Stoeve J, et al. Comparative analysis of mesenchymal stem cells from bone marrow, umbilical cord blood, or adipose tissue. Stem Cells 2006;24:1294–301.

72. Thirumala S, Goebel WS, Woods EJ. Manufacturing and banking of mesenchymal stem cells. Expert Opin Biol Ther 2013;13:673–91.
73. Alagesan S, Griffin MD. Autologous and allogeneic mesenchymal stem cells in organ transplantation: what do we know about their safety and efficacy? Curr Opin Organ Transplant 2014;19:65–72.
74. Lalu MM, McIntyre L, Pugliese C, et al, Canadian Critical Care Trials Group. Safety of cell therapy with mesenchymal stromal cells (SafeCell): a systematic review and meta-analysis of clinical trials. PLoS One 2012;7:e47559.
75. Zheng GP, Ge MH, Shu Q, et al. Mesenchymal stem cells in the treatment of pediatric diseases. World J Pediatr 2013;9:197–211.

The Natural History of Bronchopulmonary Dysplasia: The Case for Primary Prevention

Cindy T. McEvoy, MD, MCR[a],*, Judy L. Aschner, MD[b,c]

KEYWORDS

- Bronchopulmonary dysplasia • Prematurity • Pulmonary function • Child
- Adolescent • Adult

KEY POINTS

- Premature birth alters lung growth and development and may predispose to pulmonary functional limitations and early chronic obstructive pulmonary disease (COPD) as an adult.
- Measurements of lung function early in life can improve understanding of the determinants of lung growth and facilitate evaluation of current clinical strategies and new therapeutic interventions.
- Primary prevention of bronchopulmonary dysplasia (BPD) is a critical research priority.

INTRODUCTION

BPD is the most common form of chronic lung disease in infancy.[1] Classic BPD, described in 1967 by Northway and colleagues,[2] occurred in modestly premature infants with surfactant deficiency who were exposed to ventilator-induced volutrauma and high oxygen concentrations. At present, BPD primarily occurs in extremely premature infants (23–28 weeks of gestation) born during the late canalicular/early saccular stage of lung development.[3] In contrast to the inflammation, fibrosis, and scarring that characterized classic BPD, BPD today is conceptualized as a

The authors have no conflicts of interest or affiliations with companies that have direct financial interests in the subject matter of this article.
Funding Sources: NHLBI R01 HL105447 and UL1RR024140 01 to C.T. McEvoy; NHLBI 1U01HL101456 to J.L. Aschner.
[a] Department of Pediatrics, Oregon Health & Science University, 707 SW Gaines Street, CDRC-P, Portland, OR 97239-3098, USA; [b] Department of Pediatrics, Children's Hospital at Montefiore, Albert Einstein College of Medicine, Rosenthal Pavilion, Room 402, 111 East 210th Street, Bronx, NY 10467, USA; [c] Department of Obstetrics & Gynecology and Women's Health, Children's Hospital at Montefiore, Albert Einstein College of Medicine, Rosenthal Pavilion, Room 402, 111 East 210th Street, Bronx, NY 10467, USA
* Corresponding author.
E-mail address: mcevoyc@ohsu.edu

consequence of disrupted and impaired lung development ('new BPD').[4] Importantly, a diagnosis of BPD carries the risk of significant clinical and functional respiratory abnormalities into adolescence and adulthood.[5]

As the epidemiology and pathology of BPD has changed and former premature infants have reached adulthood, the life-course trajectory of BPD continues to be studied. It seems that the natural history of the new BPD may not be significantly different from the natural history of the classic BPD. Both groups of individuals manifest with ongoing respiratory symptoms and reduced lung function, with pulmonary function tests (PFTs) showing expiratory flow limitation at school age, which may improve with bronchodilator treatment,[6] and into adulthood.[7,8] There is concern that BPD will predispose to COPD because infants are beginning life with reduced lung function, and longitudinal cohorts indicate that individuals track along their predetermined PFT percentiles throughout life.[9] This fact emphasizes the important need for increased focus on the primary prevention of BPD.

Pathologic data sets from newborns and infants with BPD are limited, and histologic examination of lung tissue from patients with the new BPD is rare. Therefore, the characterization of the natural history of BPD is mostly clinical, consisting of PFTs, respiratory symptoms, radiographic evaluations, and exercise intolerance. This article summarizes the current knowledge of the life course of BPD by emphasizing recent or key articles noting its natural history from the newborn period through adulthood and building the case for a continued focus on its primary prevention.

NATURAL HISTORY OF PULMONARY FUNCTION TESTING MEASUREMENTS

It is unclear when BPD begins, but it is likely that in many cases it originates in utero.[4] Therefore, detailed assessment of neonatal pulmonary function after a premature delivery is important to understand the evolution of disease and to identify potential windows of vulnerability and intervention. In preterm infants, lung development that would normally occur in utero happens postnatally under altered mechanical and environmental conditions, including active tidal breathing with strain and stretch of immature intrathoracic structures and a state of relative hyperoxia, even with room air.[10] Lung development is also affected by conditions precipitating premature delivery, often including inflammatory and infectious processes.[11] While premature delivery impacts normal alveolarization and pulmonary vascularization, it can also affect respiratory mechanical processes.[12]

Neonatal pulmonary mechanics or PFTs have been useful to reproducibly quantify the newborn's response to a variety of antenatal and postnatal exposures, therapies, or conditions, including preterm birth itself. These PFT results correlate with clinical outcomes. PFTs have given useful insights into normal and aberrant lung development in preterm infants and have strengthened the physiologic basis (or lack thereof) for therapies used for the prevention and treatment of respiratory distress syndrome (RDS) and evolving BPD. Antenatal steroids (ASs) and surfactants, which have been shown in randomized controlled trials (RCTs) to significantly decrease the incidence of death and RDS, have also been shown to significantly improve measurements of neonatal PFTs.[13–17] Therapies unproven in large RCTs, such as inhaled nitric oxide (iNO) for BPD prevention, are not associated with improvements in neonatal PFTs.[18] International guidelines are published regarding specific methodology, acceptance criteria, and standardized equipment for PFT testing in neonates and young infants.[19,20]

Neonatal PFTs are challenging because the patient is often not cooperative, but can be accomplished noninvasively during quiet sleep and do not require sedation.

Published studies examining the mechanical properties of the respiratory system of the newborn have primarily applied passive and dynamic techniques to measure respiratory compliance (passive respiratory system compliance [Crs]) and resistance (passive respiratory system resistance [Rrs]).[12,15] Lung volumes have been measured by gas washout methods, helium dilution, or body plethysmography.[21] **Table 1** summarizes PFTs that have been used to monitor the natural history of BPD from the neonatal period through adulthood.

Neonatal Studies

PFTs have been used to examine the effects of pharmacologic agents on the premature lung including those of ASs,[13–16] surfactants,[17,22] and postnatal steroids.[23] Similar to results in animal models, studies have demonstrated a significant increase in Crs and functional residual capacity (FRC) after a timely single course of AS,[13] thereby supporting accelerated lung maturation with AS treatment (**Fig. 1**). These PFT improvements correlated with improved clinical outcomes with less surfactant and supplemental oxygen need. Neonatal PFTs have been used to quantify the duration of the clinical effect of a single course of AS[14] and to quantify the effects of a single rescue course of AS versus placebo given to women who did not deliver for more than 14 days after their first course of AS.[15] This study demonstrated a significantly increased Crs in the preterm infants (n = 113) whose mothers received the rescue course of AS and provided a physiologic basis for a large randomized trial[24] showing improved clinical respiratory outcomes after a rescue course of AS. Clinical studies examined the effect of surfactant in preterm newborns with RDS and demonstrated an increase in FRC before an increase in Crs.[12,17]

Preterm delivery is the most common cause of abnormal lung development with BPD in the extremely preterm infant at one end of that spectrum. Studies have shown that even healthy preterm infants have a lower Crs and higher Rrs when compared with healthy term infants.[25,26] Preterm infants with BPD have lower FRCs than preterm infants without BPD.[27,28] Infants with BPD studied at 34 to 36 weeks had significantly lower Crs and FRC and higher Rrs when compared with matched healthy late preterm infants studied at comparable postmenstrual ages.[29,30] A longitudinal study demonstrated that Crs was 50% of the predicted value during the acute phase of BPD and was associated with abnormal Rrs values. These values normalized over the first 2 years of life, but significant airway dysfunction persisted in many infants.[31] This observation illustrates the importance of defining the trajectory of the healthy premature lung for an appropriate comparison or control for infants at risk for or diagnosed with BPD.[31] Representative PFT studies in neonates and infants are presented in **Table 2**.

Infants

Infant PFTs are perhaps more challenging than neonatal PFTs both because the patients are not cooperative and the techniques applied to this age group require sedation with normative values established during sleep induced with chloral hydrate, a drug no longer available in the United States. However, the most rapid period of lung growth is during the first 2 years of life and therefore may be the most relevant to the investigations of the natural history of BPD. Infant PFTs have primarily been the measurement of forced expiratory flows (FEFs) and volumes with the raised or tidal volume rapid thoracic compression technique and of FRC with the plethysmograph[19] (see **Table 1**).

Extremely preterm infants are born before the onset of alveolar formation, leading to failed septation and a reduced number of alveoli. To understand the growth of the

Table 1
PFTs that have been used to monitor the natural history of BPD

Measurement	Technique	What It Tells Us	Units of Measure	Is Sedation Needed?
Neonates (up to 44 wk PMA)				
Crs	Single breath or multiple breath occlusion	Respiratory system mechanics (stiffness of lungs) Assess effectiveness of medications, ie, prenatal and postnatal steroids, surfactant, and others Decreased in BPD	mL/cm H_2O; mL/cm H_2O/kg	No
Rrs	Single breath or multiple breath occlusion	Respiratory system mechanics (flow in airways/airspaces) Assess effectiveness of medication as above Increased in BPD	cm H_2O/mL/s	No
Cdyn	Least mean square analysis and others; uses a pneumotachograph	Dynamic respiratory system mechanics (stiffness of lungs) Assess effectiveness of medications as above Decreased in BPD	mL/cm H_2O; mL/cm H_2O/kg	No
FRC	Nitrogen washout; helium dilution; SF_6	Volume in the lungs at the end of a normal expiration. Assess effectiveness of medications as above Decreased in new BPD	mL and mL/kg	No
Zrs	Forced oscillation technique	Describes the resistance, compliance, and inertance of the respiratory system; also resonance frequency	—	No
LCI	Multiple breath washout	Measure of lung homogeneity	—	No
Infants (age 44 wk PMA–2 y)				
As above can measure Crs, Rrs, Cdyn, FRC, Zrs,[a] LCI[a]	As above in neonatal tests	As above	As above	Yes
FEFs (FEF$_{75}$; FEF$_{50}$; FEF $_{25\%-75\%}$; V$_{max}$FRC)	Raised volume RTC technique; tidal breathing RTC (also called V$_{max}$FRC)	Expiratory flow during forced expiration; decreased in BPD	mL/s	Yes

(*continued on next page*)

Table 1
(continued)

Measurement	Technique	What It Tells Us	Units of Measure	Is Sedation Needed?
FVC $FEV_{0.5}$	Raised volume RTC; tidal breathing RTC	Volume change between full inspiration and complete expiration Volume change in first 0.5 s $FEV_{0.5}$ decreased in BPD	mL	Yes
FRCp, functional residual capacity	Plethysmography	Volume in the lungs at the end of a normal expiration; assess effectiveness of medications as above Decreased in new BPD	mL	Yes
D_{LCO} V_A	Single breath-hold	Used to assess lung growth and parenchymal lung disease D_{LCO} decreased in BPD; V_A normal in BPD	mL CO/min/ mm Hg mL	Yes
Children/adolescents/adults				
FEFs ($FEF_{25\%-75\%}$; FEF_{75}; FEF_{50})	Spirometry	Expiratory flow during forced expiration Decreased in BPD	mL/s	No
FVC FEV_1	Spirometry	FVC as above Volume change in first 1 s of expiration FEV_1, volume change in first 1 s of expiration Decreased in BPD	mL or L	No
FRC, RV, TLC, other volumes	Spirometry	FRC as above RV/TLC increased with air trapping	mL or L	No
D_{LCO}	Single breath-hold	D_{LCO} as above	mL CO/min/ mm Hg	No

Other techniques have been used in neonates but may require sedation.

The above list is not comprehensive/inclusive; peak oxygen consumption has also been measured during exercise tolerance in children and adults.

Abbreviations: Cdyn, dynamic compliance; CO, carbon monoxide; Crs, passive respiratory compliance; D_{LCO}, diffusing capacity of the lung for carbon monoxide; FEF, forced expiratory flow; FEF_{75}, forced expiratory flow at 75% of expired volume; FEF_{50}, forced expiratory flow at 50% of expired volume; FEF_{25-75}, forced expiratory flows between 25% and 75% of expired volume; FVC, forced vital capacity; $FEV_{0.5}$, forced expiratory volume in 0.5 s; FEV_1, forced expiratory volume in the first second of inspiration; FRC, functional residual capacity; LCI, lung clearance index/mixing efficiency; PMA, postmenstrual age; RTC, rapid thoracic compression; RV, residual volume; SF6, sulfur hexafluoride; TLC, total lung capacity; Va, alveolar volume; Zrs, impedance of respiratory system.

[a] Studies are underway evaluating the ability to measure Zrs and LCI in infants without sedation.

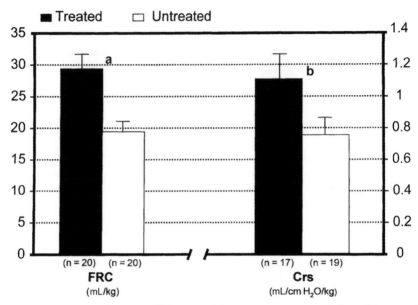

Fig. 1. Measurements of FRC in milliliters per kilogram in 40 preterm infants (20 treated vs 20 untreated infants) and of Crs in milliliters per centimeter water per kilogram in 36 preterm infants (mean ± standard error of mean). FRC and Crs were significantly increased in the betamethasone-treated group compared with the untreated group. [a] $P<.001$ when compared with untreated; [b] $P<.05$ when compared with to untreated. (*From* McEvoy C, Bowling S, Williamson K, et al. Functional residual capacity and passive compliance measurements after antenatal steroid therapy in preterm infants. Pediatr Pulmonol 2001;31(6):428; with permission from the John Wiley & Sons publications.)

preterm lung, a term reference lung is needed. Studies of infants with healthy term lungs show that their lungs grow in concordance with somatic growth and that their lung volume or forced vital capacity (FVC) increases faster than their airway flows.[32,33] Lung growth can occur by 2 possible mechanisms: by increasing the number of alveoli or by increasing the size of existing alveoli. Studies measuring alveolar volumes (V_A) and gas diffusion in healthy term infants between 3 and 23 months of age[34] have shown that the ratio of diffusing capacity of the lung for carbon monoxide (DL_{CO}) to V_A is linear, indicating that lung growth is increasing primarily by the addition of new alveoli rather than by the expansion of existing alveoli and that DL_{CO}/V_A is constant through the first 2 years of life. Infants with BPD have normal V_A but have lower DL_{CO} for the same V_A when compared with term control infants (**Fig. 2**), supporting the premise that in BPD there are fewer (but larger) alveoli.[35] A study using aerosol-derived airway morphometry demonstrated that alveoli number remained constant from 6 years of age and beyond.[36]

In infants with BPD, there are fewer and larger alveoli and less tethering of the airways through the elastic components in alveolar walls,[10] which can affect both gas transfer and elastic recoil. Infants with BPD have lower FEFs when compared with reference values from healthy term controls.[37–40] Infants with BPD who wheeze have lower FEFs than infants with BPD who do not wheeze.[41] Infants with BPD studied at 6 and 12 months of age have decreased FEFs that remain subnormal and may worsen over time.[42] Studies have shown that healthy preterm infants (minimal oxygen

Table 2
Representative PFT in neonates and infants reporting response to therapies and elucidating natural history of BPD

Study/year	Aim	Study Design	Study Groups	Methods	Conclusion/Outcome
Treatment studies (ASs, surfactants, effects of PEEP, postnatal steroids)					
McEvoy et al,[13] 2001	Document changes in Crs and FRC after single course of AS	Case control	20 preterm infants treated with AS vs 20 preterm infants untreated	SBOT; nitrogen washout	A single course of AS within 7 d of delivery significantly increases Crs and FRC
McEvoy et al,[14] 2008	To compare PFTs in infants born at different intervals after AS therapy	Case control	28 preterm infants born within 7 d of AS therapy vs 28 preterm infants born >7 d after AS	SBOT	Infants born >7 d after AS therapy had a significant ↓ in Crs because of the dissipation of the beneficial effects of surfactant induced by AS
McEvoy et al,[15] 2010	To evaluate whether a rescue course of AS improves PFTs in preterm infants	RCT	56 infants randomized to rescue AS vs 57 randomized to placebo	SBOT; nitrogen washout	Preterm infants who received a rescue course of AS had improved Crs and less oxygen need
Hjalmarson & Sandberg,[16] 2011	To evaluate if AS-induced lung changes persist	Case control	22 infants treated with AS but born at term vs 50 term infants untreated with AS	SBOT; nitrogen washout; gas mixing efficiency	No signs of a permanent effect of AS on lung function
Dinger et al,[22] 2002	To understand mechanisms of improved oxygenation after surfactant	Descriptive	90 preterm infants with severe RDS studied before and serially after surfactant	SBOT; SF$_6$ washout	↑ in FRC within 1 h of treatment with ↑ in Crs 3–24 h after treatment depending on the type of surfactant
Dinger et al,[17] 2001	Effect of PEEP levels on lung mechanics	Descriptive	20 infants at 24–32 wk of gestation and 72 h after surfactant	SBOT; SF$_6$ washout	↑ in FRC with ↑ in PEEP but ↓ in Crs with increasing PEEP
Durand et al,[23] 2002	Compare 7 d of low- vs high-dose postnatal steroids on pulmonary function	RCT	24 preterm infants randomized to low-dose and 23 to high-dose dexamethasone	Cdyn	Similar ↑ in Cdyn with both doses by day 7 of treatment, no difference in BPD

(continued on next page)

Table 2
(continued)

Studies in neonates and infants with BPD

Study/year	Aim	Study Design	Study Groups	Methods	Conclusion/Outcome
Kavvadia et al,[27] 1998	Compare FRC in preterm infants with BPD vs preterm infants without BPD	Case control	16 infants with BPD at 28 d and 8 without BPD had FRC done at 14 and 28 d	Helium dilution	Decreased FRC in patients with BPD compared with those without BPD
Kavvadia et al,[28] 2000	Predictive value of FRC, Crs, and Rrs on day 2 of life in 100 VLBW infants	Descriptive	100 consecutive VLBW infants ventilated within 6 h of life and studied on day 2	SBOT; helium dilution	Decreased FRC (<19 mL/kg) best predictor of BPD at 28 d in patients ≤28 wk of gestation
McEvoy & Schilling,[29] 2014	Compare PFTs at 34–36 wk in BPD vs healthy patients born at 34–36 wk	Case control	20 patients with BPD and 20 matched healthy infants	SBOT; nitrogen washout	Infants with BPD have significantly ↓ FRC and ↓ Crs compared with healthy infants studied at same PMA
Hjalmarson & Sandberg,[30] 2005	Compare PFTs of BPD and healthy preterm infants, all studied at term	Case control	50 infants with BPD and 19 healthy preterm controls	SBOT; nitrogen washout; gas mixing efficiency	Infants with severe BPD had lower FRC, less-efficient gas mixing, and ↑ specific conductance than those with mild BPD, moderate BPD, or healthy preterms
Baraldi et al,[31] 1997	Follow PFTs through 2 y in infants with BPD	Longitudinal cohort	24 patients with BPD	SBOT; nitrogen washout; $V_{max}FRC$	Pulmonary mechanics improve over first 2 y but low FEFs persist
Fakhoury et al,[38] 2010	Describe PFTs in BPD infants in the first 3 y of life	Longitudinal cohort	44 patients with BPD	TVRTC	Persistent low partial expiratory flows through 24 mo of age
Filbrun et al,[39] 2011	Assess longitudinal changes in PFTs over first 3 y of life in relation to somatic growth	Longitudinal cohort	18 patients with BPD studied at a mean of 59 and 91 wk of age	RVRTC	Children with BPD have significant and persistent airflow obstruction. Those with above-average somatic growth had greater lung growth

Study	Objective	Design	Population	Technique	Findings
Thunqvist et al,[40] 2014	PFTs at 6 and 18 mo in relation to BPD severity	Longitudinal cohort	55 infants with BPD studied at 6 and 18 mo	SBOT; FRC by plethysmography; TVRTC; RVRTC	Initial low Crs and high Rrs improved over time but FEFs low at 24 mo indicating impaired expiratory flows
Balinnotti et al,[35] 2010	Compare D_{LCO} V_A in patients with BPD compared with term controls	Case control	39 infants with BPD and 61 term infants studied at about 12 mo of age	D_{LCO} with single breath-hold	Infants with BPD had lower D_{LCO} but normal V_A compared with term controls consistent with ↓ alveolarization
Studies in healthy preterm or term neonates and infants (needed as reference group or control group as BPD is studied)					
Hjalmarson & Sandberg,[26] 2002	Compare PFTs in healthy preterm vs term infants	Case control	32 healthy preterm and 53 healthy term infants studied at same PMA	SBOT; nitrogen washout; gas mixing efficiency	Preterm infants show signs of dysfunction of terminal respiratory units
McEvoy et al,[25] 2013	Compare PFTs in healthy LPIs at term vs PFTs in healthy term infants	Case control	31 healthy LPI and 30 healthy term infants studied at 40 wk PMA	SBOT; nitrogen washout	Healthy LPI have ↓ Crs, altered flow volume loops, and ↑ Rrs compared with term infants
Balinotti et al,[34] 2009	To measure the ratio of D_{LCO} to V_A in healthy term infants	Observational	50 healthy infants between 3 and 23 mo of age	D_{LCO} and VA	Lung growth in this age mostly by addition of alveoli rather than by expansion of current alveoli
Jones et al,[33] 2000	Establish reference values for FEFs for term infants	Observational/ normative	155 healthy infants between 3 and 149 wk of age	RVRTC	FEFs increase with increasing length
Friedrich et al,[32] 2007	Compare longitudinal FEFs in healthy preterm vs healthy term infants	Prospective cohort	26 preterm (average GA of 32.7 wk) and 24 term infants studied in year 1 and 2 of life	RVRTC	Healthy preterm infants have persistently lower FEFs than term infants suggesting no catch-up growth in airway function

List of above studies is not inclusive.

↑, increased; ↓, decreased.

Abbreviations: Cdyn, dynamic compliance; D_{LCO}, diffusing capacity of the lung for carbon monoxide; FEF, forced expiratory flows; GA, gestational age; LPI, late preterm infants; PEEP, positive end-expiratory pressure; PMA, postmenstrual age; RVRTC, raised volume rapid thoracic compression technique; SBOT, single breath occlusion technique; TVRTC, tidal volume rapid thoracic compression technique; V_A, alveolar volume; VLBW, very-low-birth-weight infant.

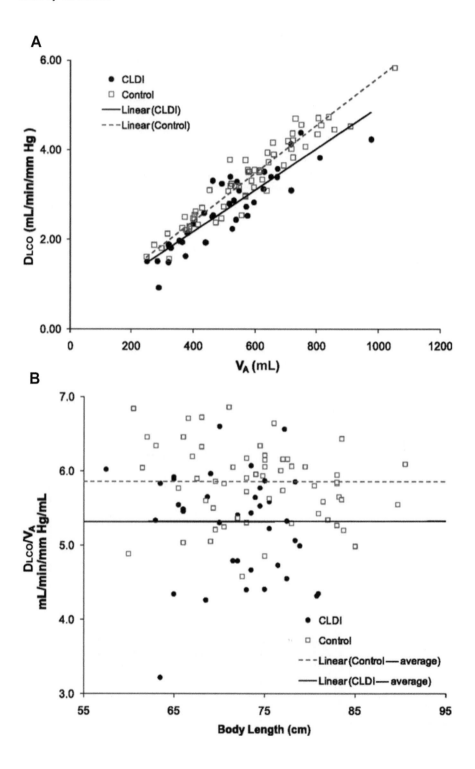

and ventilation need) have decreased FEFs compared with normal term infants and their FEFs do not seem to catch up over time[32] (see **Table 2**).

Children and Adolescents

Studies evaluating the effect of BPD on school-aged children in general document measurements of airflow obstruction with decreased FEFs and forced expiratory volume in the first second of inspiration (FEV$_1$) compared with term controls.[43–45] Measurements of residual volume/total lung capacity suggested air trapping and decrease of diffusing capacity.[45]

Baraldi and colleagues[46] demonstrated that structural abnormalities in the small airways of children with BPD accounts for at least part of their manifested airflow obstruction. These investigators compared children with BPD with children with asthma with a similar degree of airflow obstruction and found that those with BPD had lower levels of exhaled NO and were less responsive to β-agonists, supporting a structural abnormality. Vrijlandt and colleagues[47] applied forced oscillometry in 3- to 5-year-olds with a history of BPD and found higher resonant frequency and lower mean reactance compared with children without BPD, suggesting that those with BPD had decreased peripheral airway patency.

Follow-up of extremely preterm infants from the EPICure (population based studies of survival and later health status in extremely premature infants) study at 11 years of age demonstrated that 56% of the children had significantly decreased FEFs and 27% had a positive bronchodilator response with reductions in lung function being more severe in the infants with a prior BPD diagnosis.[48] A subset of these patients were further tested showing lung function abnormalities in 78% of the extremely preterm children with evidence of airway obstruction, ventilation inhomogeneity, gas trapping, and airway hyperresponsiveness.[49]

Several investigators[50,51] demonstrated that as children, former very-low-birthweight (VLBW) infants with BPD have decreased lung function compared with former VLBW infants without BPD, whereas other investigators reported no differences in lung function or diffusing capacity in VLBW infants with and without BPD.[52] Doyle and colleagues[44] reported a decline in lung function measured at 8 and 18 years of age in BPD survivors. Hospital readmissions in the first 2 years of life and FEV$_1$ and FVC in patients between 8 and 15 years of age have been shown to be significantly associated with initial BPD severity.[53]

Adults

Studies of BPD survivors in adulthood have used case-control or prospective cohort study designs and have consistently reported significantly lower FEFs and FEV$_1$ when

Fig. 2. (A) Pulmonary diffusing capacity, D$_{LCO}$, versus V$_A$. Individual data for subjects with chronic lung disease of infancy (CLDI; *solid circles*) and control subjects (*open squares*) are presented, as well as the linear regressions for each group. D$_{LCO}$ was significantly lower for subjects with CLDI compared with control subjects when adjusted for V$_A$ by analysis of covariance (*P* = .0004). (B) Ratio of pulmonary diffusing capacity to V$_A$, D$_{LCO}$/V$_A$, was not related to body length. Individual data for subjects with CLDI (*solid circles*) and control subjects (*open squares*) are presented, as well as the average data for each group. D$_{LCO}$/V$_A$ was significantly lower for subjects with CLDI compared with control subjects (*P* = .0004). (*Reprinted from* Balinotti JE, Chakr VC, Tiller C, et al. Growth of lung parenchyma in infants and toddlers with chronic lung disease of infancy. Am J Respir Crit Care Med 2010;181(10):1095; with permission from the American Thoracic Society.)

compared with term controls. While several studies have demonstrated significantly decreased FEFs in adult survivors of BPD compared with adults who were preterm without BPD,[7,8] other studies have not demonstrated this difference.[54] A recent regional cohort study[55] reported respiratory outcomes of 26 extremely preterm survivors ($\leq$28 weeks' gestational age or $\leq$1000 g birth weight) at 25 years of age compared with that of matched term-born subjects. Lung function was in the normal range in most extremely preterm survivors and few subjects reported respiratory symptoms, but methacholine responsiveness was more pronounced in the extremely preterm survivors than in the term-born young adults.[55]

NATURAL HISTORY OF RESPIRATORY SYMPTOMS IN PATIENTS WITH BRONCHOPULMONARY DYSPLASIA: CLINICAL PULMONARY OUTCOMES

Several studies using various BPD definitions, study designs, and reference groups have reported the persistent clinical respiratory morbidity of infants, children, adolescents, and adult survivors of BPD.

Infants

An increased incidence of abnormal clinical pulmonary findings are reported in infants with both the old and new BPD when compared with era-matched former premature infants without BPD as well as with contemporaneous term control infants. Greenough[56] reported frequent rehospitalizations through 2 years of age in infants with BPD, which then declined with age with rare hospitalizations by 14 years of age.[57] A single-center birth cohort study followed the outcomes in preterm infants through 12 months of age and showed that 80% had cough, 44% had wheeze, and 25% were rehospitalized with similar respiratory morbidity among preterm infants with and without BPD.[58] Follow-up at 12 months of age of 255 infants with birth weight less than 1250 g who had been randomized to iNO versus placebo after delivery revealed that overall about 53% had wheezing and 22% required respiratory hospitalization.[59]

Children

Hennessy and colleagues[60] reported follow-up of 308 extremely preterm infants ($\leq$25 weeks' gestation with and without BPD) at 30 months and 6 years of age compared with term controls. The investigators reported increased respiratory symptoms and medication use in the premature infants compared with term controls, which was much higher in the premature group with BPD. The EPICure study[48] evaluated 219 of 307 survivors at 11 years of age compared with age-matched term infants. Children delivered extremely preterm were significantly more likely to have a current diagnosis of asthma (25% vs 13%; $P<.01$), recent respiratory symptoms and medication use, and increased asthma-associated sleep disturbance than the term reference group. Those with BPD had significantly more respiratory morbidities. This finding contrasted that of an earlier study of outcomes at 8 years of age, which reported that preterm infants without BPD had a greater incidence of wheezing and asthma compared with preterm infants with BPD.[61]

A recent study[6] of children at 9.5 years of age with a history of moderate to severe BPD demonstrated that patients with BPD had significantly increased rates of persistent respiratory symptoms compared with matched former VLBW infants without BPD (36% vs 7%; $P<.05$). Significantly more patients with BPD received respiratory medications (21% vs 0%; $P<.05$). There was no significant difference in the incidence of doctor-diagnosed asthma, atopy, or allergies between the groups. In this study, one-half of the patients with BPD and 25% of the patients without BPD demonstrated a positive response to bronchodilators. Limitations of this study include its relatively small size (28 infants in each group), absence of a term control group, and differences in the exposure to AS (29% vs 50%, respectively) and surfactant (68% vs 40%, respectively) between the BPD and no BPD groups.

Adolescents and Young Adults

Northway and colleagues[62] compared the clinical findings of 26 BPD survivors (mean age of 18.7 years) with that of 26 age-matched adults born at similar gestational ages but who had not developed BPD and 53 normal term controls. Patients with BPD had more wheezing, episodes of pneumonia, exercise intolerance, and long-term medication use compared with either of the other 2 groups. More contemporary studies of survivors with BPD older than 18 years continue to demonstrate increased respiratory morbidity. Gough and colleagues[7] reported that BPD survivors at 24.1 years of age were twice as likely to report wheeze and three times more likely to use asthma medications than term controls. Vrijlandt and colleagues[63] reported significantly more shortness of breath and wheeze during exercise at 19 years of age in female BPD survivors compared with term controls.

EVOLUTION OF RADIOGRAPHIC/HIGH-RESOLUTION COMPUTED TOMOGRAPHY CHANGES

Aquino and colleagues[64] correlated inspiratory and expiratory high-resolution computed tomographic (CT) findings with pulmonary function in BPD survivors at 10 years of age and found that 92% had abnormal CT findings. There was a significant correlation between abnormal results of PFTs and abnormal CT findings including decreases in density, air trapping on expiratory CT, and architectural distortion. Northway and colleagues[62] evaluated CT scans in young adults with BPD and found that the patients with BPD had extensive bilateral areas of reduced lung attenuation and bronchial wall thickening.

Aukland and colleagues[65] found parenchymal abnormalities in most extremely preterm survivors and that those with BPD had significantly more opacities and hypoattennuated areas than those without BPD. The extent of these abnormalities was positively associated with the duration of oxygen therapy and degree of impaired lung function. In a study of 19 adult survivors of moderate and severe BPD, 84% had emphysema, which was inversely related to low FEV_1 scores.[66]

The process and timing of the postnatal development of alveoli in the human lung remains poorly understood with controversy over the age (2–3 years of age vs 7–8 years of age) at which alveolarization is complete, with studies citing 2 to 3 years of age to as late as 7 to 8 years of age.[67] However, there is recent provocative evidence of ongoing alveolarization into adolescence or early adult life in humans. Narayanan and colleagues[68,69] recently reported the application of a new technique using hyperpolarized helium diffusion during a brief breath-hold and using magnetic resonance to measure alveolar dimensions. Using this technique, they reported measurements consistent with continued alveolarization through adolescence in 109 healthy patients aged 7 to 21 years.[68] The investigators also demonstrated similar alveolar dimensions/size at 11 to 12 years of age in survivors of extreme prematurity and survivors of BPD compared with term and mild preterm survivors.[69] These data suggest that late alveolarization may be able to compensate for early impaired alveolar development. The implication of this finding, if validated, is a longer therapeutic window for interventions that stimulate catch-up alveolar growth than previously thought.

EVOLUTION OF EXERCISE TOLERANCE THROUGH ADULTHOOD

A recent meta-analysis[70] of 20 studies (685 preterm and 680 control subjects) showed that children and adults born preterm with or without BPD have a significantly lower oxygen uptake at maximal exercise than term-born controls, although the effect size was small. Some individual studies have not shown differences in exercise capacity between children born preterm compared with those born full term. In adults with a history of extreme prematurity, Clemm and colleagues[71] found only a minor reduction in exercise capacity that was primarily related to self-reported physical activity.

A recent[72] study performed ventilatory and sensory measurements before and during exercise in 3 groups of adults aged 18 to 31 years: 20 formerly premature without BPD, 15 formerly premature with BPD, and 20 full-term controls. The adults born very premature with and without BPD demonstrated severe dyspnea and leg discomfort, which was associated with critical constraints on tidal volume expansion and reduced exercise tolerance; this occurred despite differences in expiratory flow limitation in the patients with and without BPD, emphasizing the potential limitations of spirometry alone in the assessment of very preterm survivors. In summary, continued research is needed to fully elucidate exercise capacity limitations in patients with BPD as they age.

NEED FOR PRIMARY PREVENTION OF BRONCHOPULMONARY DYSPLASIA

The development of BPD is closely related to gestational age with infants born at the earliest gestational ages at the highest risk. However, there are extremely preterm infants who do not develop BPD, supporting the premise that primary prevention of BPD is attainable. To accomplish this goal, many barriers must be overcome. Also, the refinement of BPD risk and diagnosis by endotypes, inclusion of BPD severity classifications in outcome measures, improvement of the sensitivity and accuracy of a diagnosis of BPD as a modifiable outcome in future trials, and increased understanding of the molecular causal pathways that underlie the pathogenesis of BPD are required to design strategies to prevent BPD.

The recognition and refinement of BPD phenotypes is underway. An increasingly recognized extreme phenotype is BPD associated with pulmonary hypertension (PH). A recent longitudinal study[73] demonstrated that echocardiogram-derived risk factors at 7 days of age were associated with development of both BPD and PH.

The Challenge of Defining a Healthy Lung in the Premature Infant

To define the abnormal trajectory of a premature lung evolving to BPD, normal lung growth, development, and function must be defined in the healthy preterm infant who does not progress to BPD. This task is challenging given that premature infants are born at various junctures of the late canalicular/saccular stage of lung development and are exposed to a wide range of prenatal and postnatal circumstances contributing to lung injury and repair. Also, it necessitates a new paradigm with increased focus and research on the evolution of lung health in the well infant delivered at term, a group largely unstudied particularly in infancy.

BPD-related research has focused on the cause, risk factors, and interventions for this poorly defined and evolving disease. Several studies[74,75] have documented the clinical pulmonary evolution in extremely preterm infants and offer insight into possible postnatal windows for BPD prevention. A study of 1340 extremely preterm infants described 3 patterns of pulmonary disease over the first 2 weeks of life: 20% of infants had consistently low oxygen requirements and 17% of these infants developed BPD, nearly 38% had low initial oxygen needs that increased in week 2 of life and 51%

developed BPD, and 43% of the infants had initial and consistently high oxygen needs and 76% developed BPD.[74] Future studies examining risk factors and exposures in the first 2 weeks of life or earlier (including in utero) and collecting robust functional and molecular biomarkers associated with the different phenotypes of premature infants and their pulmonary dysfunction are crucial to the primary prevention of BPD.

Causal Pathways of Bronchopulmonary Dysplasia

It is critical to understand the causal molecular pathways that underlie BPD development to prevent its occurrence. The current views on several of these pathways are detailed by Mariani TJ and Pryhuber GS.[76,77] Other important areas of focus include genetic, epigenetic, and environmental factors.

Several studies have applied approaches including familial aggregation, twins, candidate genes, and genome-wide association studies to examine genetic factors in the development of BPD. A family-based study[78] found that an SP-B marker locus B-18 within the 5′ untranslated region of SP-B was associated with susceptibility to moderate to severe BPD. Several twin studies have estimated the heritability for moderate to severe BPD to be 50% to 80%.[79,80] The SPOCK2 gene has been shown to have a strong association with BPD.[81] Investigators have evaluated specific alterations in the sequence of candidate genes that might be associated with a change in the risk of developing BPD. Although many genes have been investigated, few studies have been replicated. Progress in this area will require robust prospective multicenter/international population cohort studies.

Although few studies have been done in premature infants, epigenetic changes may alter the expression of genes involved in prenatal and postnatal lung development and may increase BPD susceptibility. For example, in utero smoke exposure has been shown to cause modification of methylation of specific genes and to be associated with changes in indices of global DNA methylation. At birth, DNA methylation of the repetitive element AluYb8 is decreased in the placenta of smokers with a correlation between the degree of AluYb8 methylation and birth weight.[82] Breton and colleagues[83] showed that AluYb8 methylation remains decreased in buccal epithelia of kindergarten-aged children who had prenatal smoke exposure. The degree of Alu methylation has been found to correlate with lung function in adults.[84] Maternal prenatal stress, cortisol, and obesity[85] have been shown to be independently associated with children's wheeze perhaps through programming mechanisms. Studies are needed to understand the relationship between epigenetic factors and lung outcomes in preterm infants at risk for BPD **Box 1**.

FUTURE GOALS AND RESEARCH PRIORITIES FOR BRONCHOPULMONARY DYSPLASIA PREVENTION

BPD is categorized as a rare disease because there are an estimated 10,000 to 15,000 new cases per year in the United States. However, the significance of BPD spans the individual's lifetime, which if estimated to be 65 years places the estimated prevalence of BPD at 1 million.[87]

Although adults with persistent symptoms of wheeze, breathlessness, and reduced exercise tolerance may have bronchial asthma, it is important to consider preterm birth as a potential cause. Future progress will require longitudinal studies in large populations of well-phenotyped individuals born preterm (with and without BPD) and healthy term controls to follow the progression of respiratory disease in the context of lung injury, developmental disruption, environmental exposures, and natural aging. Multifaceted physiologic and quantitative assessments will be needed to

Box 1
Barriers to primary prevention research and clinical trials in BPD

Barriers related to the targeted patient population

- Vulnerable (immature, developing) population of very premature infants
- Need to balance risk/benefit of preventative strategies or interventions—some premature babies that would never get the disease will be exposed to an experimental therapy that could have side effects or cause harm
- Institutional Review Board (IRB) consent and ethical issues of dealing with children and vulnerable populations, including possible harm with no guarantee of benefit in a high-risk population
- BPD is a rare disease necessitating multiinstitutional collaborations:
  - Deregionalization of neonatal care
  - Need to organize academic centers into consortiums with the capacity to collect data and enroll patients in intervention trials for rapid scientific discovery
- Pharmaceutical companies are reluctant to study the neonatal population given limited numbers of patients and inherent risks of studying a critically ill pediatric population with high mortality and long statute of limitations
  - Best Pharmaceutical for Children Act: limitations in studying drug therapies in neonatal population[86]

Barriers related to scientific knowledge gaps

- Limited understanding of normal lung growth and repair mechanisms; few tissue repositories for anatomic studies of lungs of babies who die of BPD or premature babies who recover from BPD and die of other causes
- Poorly understood pathophysiology—multiple pathways to BPD
- Unclear timing for primary prevention—does BPD start in utero or at delivery?
- Need for more information on how various BPD phenotypes evolve/mature over time
  - Limited BPD model systems: rodents may not be an ideal model for studying BPD prevention
  - Long-standing primate model in San Antonio no longer funded
  - History of novel, promising therapies in rodent studies that have not been translated to early phase clinical trials
- Lack of validated early biomarkers that predict later disease onset
- No good surrogates for important long-term respiratory outcomes
  - Relatively poor correlation between a diagnosis of BPD and childhood respiratory disease

Systematic clinical and bureaucratic barriers

- Poor phenotyping/definition of BPD—definition provides no information about pathophysiology, disease progression, or variability in lung pathology.
- Failure to examine severity of disease; some interventions (ie, iNO) may reduce disease severity but not incidence, as currently defined by O_2 use at 36 weeks.
- Failure to identify subpopulations with distinct mechanisms of disease
- Clinical trials of combination therapies are hard to design and interpret but may be what is needed given the various mechanistic pathways and phenotypes
- Double standard for the evidence: high bar for new therapies but not for established approaches, which may cause harm
- Need for redesign of the clinical research machine plagued with inefficiencies and bureaucratic barriers

Adapted from McEvoy CT, Jain L, Schmidt B, et al. Bronchopulmonary dysplasia: NHLBI workshop on the primary prevention of chronic lung diseases. Ann Am Thorac Soc 2014;11(Suppl 3):S146–53; with permission.

define specific phenotypes to facilitate targeted biologic and genetic interventions that may need to begin very early to accomplish primary prevention of BPD.

The holy grail is the prevention of prematurity, which has been proved to be elusive. Aside from prematurity prevention, perinatal interventions represent a unique opportunity in BPD prevention because longitudinal studies show that small improvements in neonatal lung function translates into large improvements in childhood and adult respiratory health.

REFERENCES

1. Baraldi E, Carraro S, Filippone M. Bronchopulmonary dysplasia: definitions and long-term respiratory outcome. Early Hum Dev 2009;85(10 Suppl):S1–3.
2. Northway WH Jr, Rosan RC, Porter DY. Pulmonary disease following respirator therapy of hyaline-membrane disease. Bronchopulmonary dysplasia. N Engl J Med 1967;276(7):357–68.
3. Jobe AH, Bancalari E. Bronchopulmonary dysplasia. Am J Respir Crit Care Med 2001;163(7):1723–9.
4. McEvoy CT, Jain L, Schmidt B, et al. Bronchopulmonary dysplasia: NHLBI workshop on the primary prevention of chronic lung diseases. Ann Am Thorac Soc 2014;11(Suppl 3):S146–53.
5. Stocks J, Hislop A, Sonnappa S. Early lung development: lifelong effect on respiratory health and disease. Lancet Respir Med 2013;1(9):728–42.
6. Vom HM, Prenzel F, Uhlig HH, et al. Pulmonary outcome in former preterm, very low birth weight children with bronchopulmonary dysplasia: a case-control follow-up at school age. J Pediatr 2014;164(1):40–5.
7. Gough A, Linden M, Spence D, et al. Impaired lung function and health status in adult survivors of bronchopulmonary dysplasia. Eur Respir J 2014;43(3): 808–16.
8. Gibson AM, Reddington C, McBride L, et al. Lung function in adult survivors of very low birth weight, with and without bronchopulmonary dysplasia. Pediatr Pulmonol 2014. http://dx.doi.org/10.1002/ppul.23093.
9. Stern DA, Morgan WJ, Wright AL, et al. Poor airway function in early infancy and lung function by age 22 years: a non-selective longitudinal cohort study. Lancet 2007;370(9589):758–64.
10. Colin AA, McEvoy C, Castile RG. Respiratory morbidity and lung function in preterm infants of 32 to 36 weeks' gestational age. Pediatrics 2010;126(1):115–28.
11. Kallapur SG, Kramer BW, Nitsos I, et al. Pulmonary and systemic inflammatory responses to intra-amniotic IL-1alpha in fetal sheep. Am J Physiol Lung Cell Mol Physiol 2011;301(3):L285–95.
12. Gappa M, Pillow JJ, Allen J, et al. Lung function tests in neonates and infants with chronic lung disease: lung and chest-wall mechanics. Pediatr Pulmonol 2006; 41(4):291–317.
13. McEvoy C, Bowling S, Williamson K, et al. Functional residual capacity and passive compliance measurements after antenatal steroid therapy in preterm infants. Pediatr Pulmonol 2001;31(6):425–30.
14. McEvoy C, Schilling D, Spitale P, et al. Decreased respiratory compliance in infants less than or equal to 32 weeks' gestation, delivered more than 7 days after antenatal steroid therapy. Pediatrics 2008;121(5):e1032–8.
15. McEvoy C, Schilling D, Peters D, et al. Respiratory compliance in preterm infants after a single rescue course of antenatal steroids: a randomized controlled trial. Am J Obstet Gynecol 2010;202(6):544–9.

16. Hjalmarson O, Sandberg KL. Effect of antenatal corticosteroid treatment on lung function in full-term newborn infants. Neonatology 2011;100(1):32–6.
17. Dinger J, Topfer A, Schaller P, et al. Effect of positive end expiratory pressure on functional residual capacity and compliance in surfactant-treated preterm infants. J Perinat Med 2001;29(2):137–43.
18. Di Fiore JM, Hibbs AM, Zadell AE, et al. The effect of inhaled nitric oxide on pulmonary function in preterm infants. J Perinatol 2007;27(12):766–71.
19. Beydon N, Davis SD, Lombardi E, et al. An official American Thoracic Society/European Respiratory Society statement: pulmonary function testing in preschool children. Am J Respir Crit Care Med 2007;175(12):1304–45.
20. Rosenfeld M, Allen J, Arets BH, et al. An official American Thoracic Society workshop report: optimal lung function tests for monitoring cystic fibrosis, bronchopulmonary dysplasia, and recurrent wheezing in children less than 6 years of age. Ann Am Thorac Soc 2013;10(2):S1–11.
21. Wanger J, Clausen JL, Coates A, et al. Standardisation of the measurement of lung volumes. Eur Respir J 2005;26(3):511–22.
22. Dinger J, Topfer A, Schaller P, et al. Functional residual capacity and compliance of the respiratory system after surfactant treatment in premature infants with severe respiratory distress syndrome. Eur J Pediatr 2002;161(9):485–90.
23. Durand M, Mendoza ME, Tantivit P, et al. A randomized trial of moderately early low-dose dexamethasone therapy in very low birth weight infants: dynamic pulmonary mechanics, oxygenation, and ventilation. Pediatrics 2002;109(2):262–8.
24. Garite TJ, Kurtzman J, Maurel K, et al. Impact of a 'rescue course' of antenatal corticosteroids: a multicenter randomized placebo-controlled trial. Am J Obstet Gynecol 2009;200(3):248–9.
25. McEvoy C, Venigalla S, Schilling D, et al. Respiratory function in healthy late preterm infants delivered at 33-36 weeks of gestation. J Pediatr 2013;162(3):464–9.
26. Hjalmarson O, Sandberg K. Abnormal lung function in healthy preterm infants. Am J Respir Crit Care Med 2002;165(1):83–7.
27. Kavvadia V, Greenough A, Dimitriou G, et al. Lung volume measurements in infants with and without chronic lung disease. Eur J Pediatr 1998;157(4):336–9.
28. Kavvadia V, Greenough A, Dimitriou G. Early prediction of chronic oxygen dependency by lung function test results. Pediatr Pulmonol 2000;29(1):19–26.
29. McEvoy C, Schilling D. Pulmonary function in extremely low birth weight infants with bronchopulmonary dysplasia before hospital discharge. Abstract publication at the Pediatric Academic Society Meeting. E-PAS2014:3540.6.
30. Hjalmarson O, Sandberg KL. Lung function at term reflects severity of bronchopulmonary dysplasia. J Pediatr 2005;146(1):86–90.
31. Baraldi E, Filippone M, Trevisanuto D, et al. Pulmonary function until two years of life in infants with bronchopulmonary dysplasia. Am J Respir Crit Care Med 1997; 155(1):149–55.
32. Friedrich L, Pitrez PM, Stein RT, et al. Growth rate of lung function in healthy preterm infants. Am J Respir Crit Care Med 2007;176(12):1269–73.
33. Jones M, Castile R, Davis S, et al. Forced expiratory flows and volumes in infants. Normative data and lung growth. Am J Respir Crit Care Med 2000;161(2 Pt 1): 353–9.
34. Balinotti JE, Tiller CJ, Llapur CJ, et al. Growth of the lung parenchyma early in life. Am J Respir Crit Care Med 2009;179(2):134–7.
35. Balinotti JE, Chakr VC, Tiller C, et al. Growth of lung parenchyma in infants and toddlers with chronic lung disease of infancy. Am J Respir Crit Care Med 2010; 181(10):1093–7.

36. Zeman KL, Bennett WD. Growth of the small airways and alveoli from childhood to the adult lung measured by aerosol-derived airway morphometry. J Appl Physiol (1985) 2006;100(3):965–71.

37. Lum S, Hulskamp G, Merkus P, et al. Lung function tests in neonates and infants with chronic lung disease: forced expiratory maneuvers. Pediatr Pulmonol 2006; 41(3):199–214.

38. Fakhoury KF, Sellers C, Smith EO, et al. Serial measurements of lung function in a cohort of young children with bronchopulmonary dysplasia. Pediatrics 2010; 125(6):e1441–7.

39. Filbrun AG, Popova AP, Linn MJ, et al. Longitudinal measures of lung function in infants with bronchopulmonary dysplasia. Pediatr Pulmonol 2011;46(4):369–75.

40. Thunqvist P, Gustafsson P, Norman M, et al. Lung function at 6 and 18 months after preterm birth in relation to severity of bronchopulmonary dysplasia. Pediatr Pulmonol 2014. http://dx.doi.org/10.1002/ppul.23090.

41. Robin B, Kim YJ, Huth J, et al. Pulmonary function in bronchopulmonary dysplasia. Pediatr Pulmonol 2004;37(3):236–42.

42. Hofhuis W, Huysman MW, Van Der Wiel EC, et al. Worsening of V'maxFRC in infants with chronic lung disease in the first year of life: a more favorable outcome after high-frequency oscillation ventilation. Am J Respir Crit Care Med 2002; 166(12 Pt 1):1539–43.

43. Doyle LW. Respiratory function at age 8-9 years in extremely low birthweight/very preterm children born in Victoria in 1991-1992. Pediatr Pulmonol 2006;41(6): 570–6.

44. Doyle LW, Faber B, Callanan C, et al. Bronchopulmonary dysplasia in very low birth weight subjects and lung function in late adolescence. Pediatrics 2006; 118(1):108–13.

45. Korhonen P, Laitinen J, Hyodynmaa E, et al. Respiratory outcome in school-aged, very-low-birth-weight children in the surfactant era. Acta Paediatr 2004;93(3): 316–21.

46. Baraldi E, Bonetto G, Zacchello F, et al. Low exhaled nitric oxide in school-age children with bronchopulmonary dysplasia and airflow limitation. Am J Respir Crit Care Med 2005;171(1):68–72.

47. Vrijlandt EJ, Boezen HM, Gerritsen J, et al. Respiratory health in prematurely born preschool children with and without bronchopulmonary dysplasia. J Pediatr 2007; 150(3):256–61.

48. Fawke J, Lum S, Kirkby J, et al. Lung function and respiratory symptoms at 11 years in children born extremely preterm: the EPICure study. Am J Respir Crit Care Med 2010;182(2):237–45.

49. Lum S, Kirkby J, Welsh L, et al. Nature and severity of lung function abnormalities in extremely pre-term children at 11 years of age. Eur Respir J 2011;37(5): 1199–207.

50. Doyle LW, Ford GW, Olinsky A, et al. Bronchopulmonary dysplasia and very low birthweight: lung function at 11 years of age. J Paediatr Child Health 1996;32(4): 339–43.

51. Ronkainen E, Dunder T, Peltoniemi O, et al. New BPD predicts lung function at school age: follow-up study and meta-analysis. Pediatr Pulmonol 2015. http://dx.doi.org/10.1002/ppul.23153.

52. Cazzato S, Ridolfi L, Bernardi F, et al. Lung function outcome at school age in very low birth weight children. Pediatr Pulmonol 2013;48(8):830–7.

53. Landry JS, Chan T, Lands L, et al. Long-term impact of bronchopulmonary dysplasia on pulmonary function. Can Respir J 2011;18(5):265–70.

54. Vrijlandt EJ, Gerritsen J, Boezen HM, et al. Lung function and exercise capacity in young adults born prematurely. Am J Respir Crit Care Med 2006;173(8):890–6.
55. Vollsaeter M, Clemm HH, Satrell E, et al. Adult respiratory outcomes of extreme preterm birth - a regional cohort study. Ann Am Thorac Soc 2015;12(3):313–22.
56. Greenough A. Long-term respiratory consequences of premature birth at less than 32 weeks of gestation. Early Hum Dev 2013;89(Suppl 2):S25–7.
57. Doyle LW, Cheung MM, Ford GW, et al. Birth weight <1501 g and respiratory health at age 14. Arch Dis Child 2001;84(1):40–4.
58. Pramana IA, Latzin P, Schlapbach LJ, et al. Respiratory symptoms in preterm infants: burden of disease in the first year of life. Eur J Med Res 2011;16(5):223–30.
59. Hibbs AM, Walsh MC, Martin RJ, et al. One-year respiratory outcomes of preterm infants enrolled in the nitric oxide (to prevent) chronic lung disease trial. J Pediatr 2008;153(4):525–9.
60. Hennessy EM, Bracewell MA, Wood N, et al. Respiratory health in pre-school and school age children following extremely preterm birth. Arch Dis Child 2008;93(12):1037–43.
61. Palta M, Sadek-Badawi M, Sheehy M, et al. Respiratory symptoms at age 8 years in a cohort of very low birth weight children. Am J Epidemiol 2001;154(6):521–9.
62. Northway WH Jr, Moss RB, Carlisle KB, et al. Late pulmonary sequelae of bronchopulmonary dysplasia. N Engl J Med 1990;323(26):1793–9.
63. Vrijlandt EJ, Gerritsen J, Boezen HM, et al. Gender differences in respiratory symptoms in 19-year-old adults born preterm. Respir Res 2005;6:117.
64. Aquino SL, Schechter MS, Chiles C, et al. High-resolution inspiratory and expiratory CT in older children and adults with bronchopulmonary dysplasia. AJR Am J Roentgenol 1999;173(4):963–7.
65. Aukland SM, Rosendahl K, Owens CM, et al. Neonatal bronchopulmonary dysplasia predicts abnormal pulmonary HRCT scans in long-term survivors of extreme preterm birth. Thorax 2009;64(5):405–10.
66. Wong PM, Lees AN, Louw J, et al. Emphysema in young adult survivors of moderate-to-severe bronchopulmonary dysplasia. Eur Respir J 2008;32(2):321–8.
67. Schittny JC, Mund SI, Stampanoni M. Evidence and structural mechanism for late lung alveolarization. Am J Physiol Lung Cell Mol Physiol 2008;294(2):L246–54.
68. Narayanan M, Owers-Bradley J, Beardsmore CS, et al. Alveolarization continues during childhood and adolescence: new evidence from helium-3 magnetic resonance. Am J Respir Crit Care Med 2012;185(2):186–91.
69. Narayanan M, Beardsmore CS, Owers-Bradley J, et al. Catch-up alveolarization in ex-preterm children: evidence from (3)He magnetic resonance. Am J Respir Crit Care Med 2013;187(10):1104–9.
70. Edwards MO, Kotecha SJ, Lowe J, et al. Effect of preterm birth on exercise capacity: a systematic review and meta-analysis. Pediatr Pulmonol 2015. http://dx.doi.org/10.1002/ppul.23117.
71. Clemm HH, Vollsaeter M, Roksund OD, et al. Exercise capacity after extremely preterm birth. Development from adolescence to adulthood. Ann Am Thorac Soc 2014;11(4):537–45.
72. Lovering AT, Elliott JE, Laurie SS, et al. Ventilatory and sensory responses in adult survivors of preterm birth and bronchopulmonary dysplasia with reduced exercise capacity. Ann Am Thorac Soc 2014;11(10):1528–37.
73. Mourani PM, Sontag MK, Younoszai A, et al. Early pulmonary vascular disease in preterm infants at risk for bronchopulmonary dysplasia. Am J Respir Crit Care Med 2015;191(1):87–95.

74. Laughon M, Allred EN, Bose C, et al. Patterns of respiratory disease during the first 2 postnatal weeks in extremely premature infants. Pediatrics 2009;123(4): 1124–31.

75. Rojas MA, Gonzalez A, Bancalari E, et al. Changing trends in the epidemiology and pathogenesis of neonatal chronic lung disease. J Pediatr 1995;126(4): 605–10.

76. Mariani TJ. Update on molecular biology of lung development – transcriptomics. Clin Perinatol 2015, in press.

77. Pryhuber GS. Postnatal infections and immunology affecting chronic lung disease of prematurity. Clin Perinatol 2015, in press.

78. Pavlovic J, Papagaroufalis C, Xanthou M, et al. Genetic variants of surfactant proteins A, B, C, and D in bronchopulmonary dysplasia. Dis Markers 2006;22(5–6): 277–91.

79. Parker RA, Lindstrom DP, Cotton RB. Evidence from twin study implies possible genetic susceptibility to bronchopulmonary dysplasia. Semin Perinatol 1996; 20(3):206–9.

80. Bhandari V, Gruen JR. The genetics of bronchopulmonary dysplasia. Semin Perinatol 2006;30(4):185–91.

81. Hadchouel A, Durrmeyer X, Bouzigon E, et al. Identification of SPOCK2 as a susceptibility gene for bronchopulmonary dysplasia. Am J Respir Crit Care Med 2011;184(10):1164–70.

82. Wilhelm-Benartzi CS, Houseman EA, Maccani MA, et al. In utero exposures, infant growth, and DNA methylation of repetitive elements and developmentally related genes in human placenta. Environ Health Perspect 2012;120(2):296–302.

83. Breton CV, Siegmund KD, Joubert BR, et al. Prenatal tobacco smoke exposure is associated with childhood DNA CpG methylation. PLoS One 2014;9(6):e99716.

84. Lange NE, Sordillo J, Tarantini L, et al. Alu and LINE-1 methylation and lung function in the normative ageing study. BMJ Open 2012;2(5):1–7.

85. Wright RJ, Fisher K, Chiu YH, et al. Disrupted prenatal maternal cortisol, maternal obesity, and childhood wheeze. Insights into prenatal programming. Am J Respir Crit Care Med 2013;187(11):1186–93.

86. Davis JM, Connor EM, Wood AJ. The need for rigorous evidence on medication use in preterm infants: is it time for a neonatal rule? JAMA 2012;308:1435–6.

87. Bhandari A, McGrath-Morrow S. Long-term pulmonary outcomes of patients with bronchopulmonary dysplasia. Semin Perinatol 2013;37(2):132–7.

Index

Note: Page numbers of article titles are in **boldface** type.

Clin Perinatol 42 (2015) 933–943
http://dx.doi.org/10.1016/S0095-5108(15)00116-5
0095-5108/15/$ – see front matter © 2015 Elsevier Inc. All rights reserved.

United States Postal Service

Statement of Ownership, Management, and Circulation
(All Periodicals Publications Except Requestor Publications)

1. Publication Title							2. Publication Number								3. Filing Date
Clinics in Perinatology							0	0	1	-	7	4	4	4	9/18/15

4. Issue Frequency	5. Number of Issues Published Annually	6. Annual Subscription Price
Mar, Jun, Sep, Dec	4	$285.00

7. Complete Mailing Address of Known Office of Publication (*Not printer*) (*Street, city, county, state, and ZIP+4®*)

Elsevier Inc.
360 Park Avenue South
New York, NY 10010-1710

Contact Person
Stephen R. Bushing

Telephone (Include area code)
215-239-3688

8. Complete Mailing Address of Headquarters or General Business Office of Publisher (*Not printer*)

Elsevier Inc., 360 Park Avenue South, New York, NY 10010-1710

9. Full Names and Complete Mailing Addresses of Publisher, Editor, and Managing Editor (*Do not leave blank*)

Publisher (*Name and complete mailing address*)

Linda Belfus, Elsevier Inc., 1600 John F. Kennedy Blvd., Ste. 1800, Philadelphia, PA 19103-2899

Editor (*Name and complete mailing address*)

Kerry Holland, Elsevier, Inc., 1600 John F. Kennedy Blvd. Suite 1800, Philadelphia, PA 19103-2899

Managing Editor (*Name and complete mailing address*)

Adrianne Brigido, Elsevier, Inc., 1600 John F. Kennedy Blvd. Suite 1800, Philadelphia, PA 19103-2899

10. Owner (*Do not leave blank. If the publication is owned by a corporation, give the name and address of the corporation immediately followed by the names and addresses of all stockholders owning or holding 1 percent or more of the total amount of stock. If not owned by a corporation, give the names and addresses of the individual owners. If owned by a partnership or other unincorporated firm, give its name and address as well as those of each individual owner. If the publication is published by a nonprofit organization, give its name and address.*)

Full Name	Complete Mailing Address
Wholly owned subsidiary of	1600 John F. Kennedy Blvd. Ste. 1800
Reed/Elsevier, US holdings	Philadelphia, PA 19103-2899

11. Known Bondholders, Mortgagees, and Other Security Holders Owning or Holding 1 Percent or More of Total Amount of Bonds, Mortgages, or Other Securities. If none, check box. ☐ None

Full Name	Complete Mailing Address
N/A	

12. Tax Status (*For completion by nonprofit organizations authorized to mail at nonprofit rates*) (*Check one*)
The purpose, function, and nonprofit status of this organization and the exempt status for federal income tax purposes:
☐ Has Not Changed During Preceding 12 Months
☐ Has Changed During Preceding 12 Months (*Publisher must submit explanation of change with this statement*)

13. Publication Title	14. Issue Date for Circulation Data Below
Clinics in Perinatology	September 2015

15. Extent and Nature of Circulation		Average No. Copies Each Issue During Preceding 12 Months	No. Copies of Single Issue Published Nearest to Filing Date
a. Total Number of Copies (*Net press run*)		1482	1188
b. Legitimate Paid and Or Requested Distribution (By Mail and Outside the Mail)	(1) Mailed Outside-County Paid/Requested Mail Subscriptions stated on PS Form 3541. (*Include paid distribution above nominal rate, advertiser's proof copies and exchange copies*)	860	730
	(2) Mailed In-County Paid/Requested Mail Subscriptions stated on PS Form 3541. (*Include paid distribution above nominal rate, advertiser's proof copies and exchange copies*)		
	(3) Paid Distribution Outside the Mails Including Sales Through Dealers And Carriers, Street Vendors, Counter Sales, and Other Paid Distribution Outside USPS®	248	249
	(4) Paid Distribution by Other Classes of Mail Through the USPS (e.g. First-Class Mail®)		
c. Total Paid and or Requested Circulation (*Sum of 15b (1), (2), (3), and (4)*)	►	1108	979
d. Free or Nominal Rate Distribution (By Mail and Outside the Mail)	(1) Free or Nominal Rate Outside-County Copies included on PS Form 3541	83	74
	(2) Free or Nominal Rate In-County Copies included on PS Form 3541		
	(3) Free or Nominal Rate Copies mailed at Other classes Through the USPS (e.g. First-Class Mail®)		
	(4) Free or Nominal Rate Distribution Outside the Mail (*Carriers or Other means*)		
e. Total Nonrequested Distribution (Sum of 15d (1), (2), (3) and (4))	►	83	74
f. Total Distribution (Sum of 15c and 15e)	►	1191	1053
g. Copies not Distributed (See instructions to publishers #4 (page #3))	►	291	135
h. Total (Sum of 15f and g)	►	1482	1188
i. Percent Paid and/or Requested Circulation (15c divided by 15f times 100)	►	93.03%	92.97%

* If you are claiming electronic copies go to line 16 on page 3. If you are not claiming Electronic copies, skip to line 17 on page 3

16. Electronic Copy Circulation	Average No. Copies Each Issue During Preceding 12 Months	No. Copies of Single Issue Published Nearest to Filing Date
a. Paid Electronic Copies		
b. Total paid Print Copies (Line 15c) + Paid Electronic copies (Line 16a)		
c. Total Print Distribution (Line 15f) + Paid Electronic Copies (Line 16a)		
d. Percent Paid (Both Print & Electronic copies) (16b divided by 16c X 100)		

☐ I certify that 50% of all my distributed copies (electronic and print) are paid above a nominal price

17. Publication of Statement of Ownership

If the publication is a general publication, publication of this statement is required. Will be printed in the **December 2015** issue of this publication.

18. Signature and Title of Editor, Publisher, Business Manager, or Owner

Stephen R. Bushing

Date
September 18, 2015

Stephen R. Bushing – Inventory Distribution Coordinator

I certify that all information furnished on this form is true and complete. I understand that anyone who furnishes false or misleading information on this form or who omits material or information requested on the form may be subject to criminal sanctions (including fines and imprisonment) and/or civil sanctions (including civil penalties).

PS Form 3526, July 2014 [Page 1 of 3 (Instructions Page 3)] PSN 7530-01-000-9931 PRIVACY NOTICE: See our Privacy policy in www.usps.com

PS Form 3526, July 2014 (Page 1 of 3 (Instructions Page 3)) PSN 7530-01-000-9931 PRIVACY NOTICE: See our Privacy policy in www.usps.com (Page 3 of 3)

Moving?

Make sure your subscription moves with you!

To notify us of your new address, find your **Clinics Account Number** (located on your mailing label above your name), and contact customer service at:

Email: journalscustomerservice-usa@elsevier.com

800-654-2452 (subscribers in the U.S. & Canada)
314-447-8871 (subscribers outside of the U.S. & Canada)

Fax number: 314-447-8029

Elsevier Health Sciences Division
Subscription Customer Service
3251 Riverport Lane
Maryland Heights, MO 63043

*To ensure uninterrupted delivery of your subscription, please notify us at least 4 weeks in advance of move.

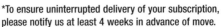
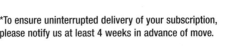